Neurosurgery for Spasticity

Marc Sindou
George Georgoulis
Patrick Mertens

Neurosurgery for Spasticity

A Practical Guide for Treating Children and Adults

Springer

Marc Sindou, M.D., D.Sc.
Department of Neurosurgery
University of Lyon 1
Hôpital Neurologique Pierre Wertheimer, GHE
Lyon
France

George Georgoulis, M.D.
Department of Neurosurgery
University of Lyon 1
Hôpital Neurologique Pierre Wertheimer, GHE
Lyon
France

Patrick Mertens, M.D., Ph.D.
Department of Neurosurgery
University of Lyon 1
Hôpital Neurologique Pierre Wertheimer, GHE
Lyon
France

Additional material to this book can be downloaded from http://extra.springer.com

ISBN 978-3-7091-1958-7 ISBN 978-3-7091-1771-2 (eBook)
DOI 10.1007/978-3-7091-1771-2
Springer Wien Heidelberg New York Dordrecht London

Softcover reprint of the hardcover 1st edition 2014

Printed on acid-free paper

Springer is part of Springer Science+Business Media (www.springer.com)

Preface

Spasticity is a common sequelar condition frequently encountered after a variety of pathologies that affect the upper motor neuron system. Spasticity can be useful by compensating for lost motor strength, but may also become harmful leading to further functional losses and irreducible contractures.

When spasticity fails to be controlled by relaxant medications and physical therapy and special rehabilitation programs, functional neurosurgery can be a recourse. By aiming at diminishing the excess of tone and re-equilibrating the tonic balances, neurosurgical procedures, that often need to be supplemented with orthopedic operations, may help improve function and limit irreversible deformities.

The book is devoted to the neurosurgical management of spasticity. The matter is based on an overall surgical experience of more than a thousand patients, both adults and children. The book reports in a synthetic way the lessons from own clinical observations and main literature data. The authors have attempted to organize the whole in a didactic and practical manner.

Overall, emphasis is placed on the importance of a multidisciplinary approach, including neurologists, pediatricians and rehabilitation specialists. Close collaboration with other surgical disciplines, namely, orthopedic surgery, neuro-urology, among many other specialties, are also outlined.

We hope that the book will be a useful aid for all physicians and professionals directly or indirectly involved in caring these severely affected and disabled patients.

Lyon, France

Marc Sindou
George Georgoulis
Patrick Mertens

Acknowledgements

First of all, we want to express our deep indebtedness to those patients who have to endure their harmful disease, to their family and their caregivers, for their courage to face so often severe handicaps.

We wish then to manifest our gratitude to the neurosurgical team whom we are daily working with, namely doctors Gustavo Polo, Emile Simon, Afif Afif, Andrei Brinzeu, and also the physical therapists, the nurses, the secretaries and all the staff members, so intensively devoted to the task of treating these disabled patients.

Acknowledgements go to our partners who collaborate to the Adult Rehabilitation program, professors Dominique Boisson and Jacques Liauté, and those who are in charge of the Pediatric population: doctors Carole Bérard and Isabelle Poirot, together with their medical network.

We are also indebted to distinguished universitary colleagues for their fruitful cooperation and advices, in particular professors Milan Dimitrijevic, Rick Abbott, Philippe Decq, Takaomi Taira, and eminent others, and also to our many pupils over the world.

Special acknowledgement is to Mrs Silvia Schilgerius for her guidance in the Edition work, as well as for the Editing and Production departments at Springer.

We do hope the book will be useful.

Lyon, France Marc Sindou, M.D., D.Sc.

Contents

1 Introduction

Spasticity – as a component of the upper motor neuron syndrome – is a frequently encountered clinical condition. Spasticity may be either useful – by compensating decrease in motor strength – or harmful – by limiting both passive and active motion and, in the extreme, by leading to irreducible contractures and deformities – or as in most cases and harmful and useful in the same patient. A large population of adults and children in developing countries and in wealthy societies as well is suffering from this locomotor disability. Caring involves a large number and variety of actors.

When spasticity is disabling, an effective therapeutic armamentarium is currently available. If spasticity fails to be controlled by relaxant medications and physical therapy and escapes rehabilitation programs, neurosurgical procedures aiming to diminish the excess of tone and rebalance agonist and antagonist muscle groups can be the remedy. They may help improve function and limit irreversible deformities. Complementary orthopedic surgical corrections are often required though.

Neurosurgery for spasticity is an important field of Functional Neurosurgery. The **concept of Functional Neurosurgery** was developed in the 1950s, and definition given in 1956 by Pierre Wertheimer in his book [1], as follows. "Functional Neurosurgery is that branch of Neurosurgery which aims at correcting the functional disorders that cannot be normalized by direct cure of the causative lesion. Operations are based on neurophysiological information. Procedures consist of removing irritative foci or interrupting excitatory pathways. In the future new procedures will probably be developed to compensate for failing inhibitory systems." This definition is still valid due to the impact of the currently used selective lesioning techniques and visionary in regard to the later developed intrathecal baclofen (ITB) method [2].

Studies on the **underlying mechanisms of spasticity**, whatever the location of the causal lesions, spinal cord or brain, have shown that neurobiological responses of the central nervous system to damages entail the reorganization of synapses, creation of new connectivities, and reestablishment of residual functions in partially impaired structures. Neurorestoration, a newly developed sector of neurology, offers further insight in the adaptive mechanisms after nervous system insults. The

M. Sindou et al., *Neurosurgery for Spasticity*,
DOI 10.1007/978-3-7091-1771-2_1, © Springer-Verlag Wien 2014

concepts of neuroplasticity and neurorestoration should thus be integrated into the contemporary management of spasticity in order to effectively optimize outcome.

Spasticity should not be treated just because it is present. Hypertonia may compensate loss of motor power. **Spasticity should only be treated when excess of tone** leads to further functional losses, impairs locomotion and motricity, or induces deformities.

Because the strategies of evaluation and assessment of the spastic disorders and the decision-making processes with adult patients differ significantly from those with pediatric patients, owing to the rapid locomotor and cognitive development of the child, we present them in separate parts of the book. The book starts with an outline of the history of neurosurgical spasticity treatment and a survey of the anatomical and physiological bases of the disorder. Then the various treatment modalities are described with respect to their impact, whether general or focal, and their effect, whether temporary or permanent. The neurosurgical armamentarium includes: pharmacological therapy with ITB and lesioning techniques with botulinum toxin injections, surgery to the peripheral nerves, the dorsal root entry zone and the dorsal roots. At end, orthopedic surgery and the management of the hyperactive bladder are briefly discussed.

In the following we briefly address the **issues most relevant for the choice of an appropriate treatment of spasticity**.

Spasticity may be hard to differentiate from other types of hypertonia or movement disorders; dystonia is a frequently associated disorder especially in patients with cerebral palsy. Spasticity in the strict sense is defined as the hyperexcitability of the stretch reflex related to the loss of inhibitory influences from descending supraspinal structures.

Differentiation between the harmful component(s) of spasticity and its useful contribution in the antigravity postures and locomotion may not be easy to achieve, the more so as one and the same muscular group may be able to simultaneously produce useful and harmful effects. Meticulous clinical and gait analysis, if necessary with anesthetic blocks, are most helpful in the selection process.

The choice of the most appropriate and optimal technique is far from being obvious in most cases as all of the methods have inherent disadvantages and advantages. First of all, discussing neurological surgery versus orthopedic surgery frequently offers a dilemma, especially for children with cerebral palsy. Regarding neurosurgery, choice must be based on the rationale of each method with respect to the mechanism(s) of the neurological disorders of every particular patient. Surgery should be tailored to each individual case. An essential step is to define the objective(s) of the planned treatment: improvement in function, prevention of deformities, or alleviation of discomfort and pain in the most disabled patients; in other words, what can be gained and what will not be obtained by surgery. These crucial issues must be clearly explained to the patients, relatives, and caregivers. Especially for children, the treatment of spasticity must be considered before fixed musculotendinous contractures and joint deformities appear and as part of a therapeutic program that extends over years.

For **adult patients**, ITB is indicated for paraplegia or tetraplegia with diffuse spasticity, i.e., spasticity from spinal cord origin. ITB can also be used to treat spasticity related to cerebral palsy. Lesioning operations are reserved for severe spasticity in the limbs if treatment with botulinum toxin injections has become insufficient. Peripheral neurotomies are preferred when harmful spasticity affects one (or a few) muscular group(s). An anesthetic block used as a preliminary test may help predict the outcome by mimicking the effect of a planned neurotomy. When harmful spasticity affects the entire limb(s) in paraplegic or hemiplegic patients, surgery directed to the dorsal roots (dorsal rhizotomies in the lumbar or sacral roots) or the dorsal root entry zone (using lumbosacral or cervical microsurgical DREZotomy) may be the solution. Complementary orthopedic operations are frequently needed for patients developing irreducible contractures and/or joint deformities.

For **children** with cerebral palsy it is essential to consider the evolution of their motor abilities and of their cognitive functions; moreover, the capability of the family to participate in the therapeutic program and the quality of the educational environment, which are of paramount importance, have to be taken into account. For diffuse spasticity of the lower limbs, dorsal rhizotomy or ITB administration are available; dorsal rhizotomy is preferred when definitive action is targeted to a number of muscular groups in the lower limbs. For focal spasticity, botulinum toxin injections permit to delay surgery until the child is old enough to undergo a neurotomy. Anesthetic blocks or botulinum toxin injections are administered to particular muscles in order to simulate the effect that would be obtained by the neurotomy. These tests allow the child and her/his environment to estimate the benefits that are expected from the neurotomy. In hemiplegic adolescents harboring severe spasticity and/or dystonia in the upper limb, a (cervical) deep microsurgical DREZotomy may be a remedy. For children with cerebral palsy, orthopedic surgical corrections are frequently needed, either as the first-line treatment or as an adjuvant to neurosurgical treatment.

Timing of surgery is also an object of debate. Its determination is relatively easy for adult patients; but deciding the optimal time is not so obvious for children with cerebral palsy because of their prospective growth and cognitive development.

Whatever the final decision, all steps of the program should be conceived, discussed, and applied within the frame of a **multidisciplinary team**, including specialists in neurology, pediatrics, and rehabilitation, and close collaboration with other specialities, such as orthopedic surgery and neurourology, should be sought.

In this book, we gathered those pieces of **knowledge most relevant to present-day neurosurgical management** of disabling spasticity and synthesized them with the lessons we learned from clinical observations, gained in the treatment of more than a thousand patients. A comprehensive review of personal or published data was not intended. Details of rehabilitation programs and physical therapy are beyond the scope of this book.

An appendix contains scales, schematic drawings, and forms that can be used in dealing with patients.

References

1. Wertheimer P (1956) La neurochirurgie fonctionelle. Masson, Paris
2. Sindou M (2001) Presidential address to the Quadrennial Meeting of the World Society for Stereotactic and Functional Neurosurgery: stereotactic surgery has merged into general neurosurgery; functional neurosurgery is increasingly "applied neurophysiology". Stereotact Funct Neurosurg 76:133–136

Part I

General Information

2 History of Neurosurgical Treatment for Spasticity

Excess of spasticity leads to a disability that is marked by impaired locomotion and, if not controlled, handicapping deformities, discomfort, and pain. Physiologic and clinical studies by Sherrington and Babinski, respectively, helped to improve understanding of mechanisms underlying spasticity and led to the development of effective neurosurgical techniques, first interruptive and then pharmacological. Targets of lesioning procedures are the peripheral nerves (neurotomies), the spinal roots (dorsal rhizotomies), the spinal cord (myelotomies), and the dorsal root entry zone (DREZotomy). Treatment with intrathecal baclofen can be achieved thanks to modern technology, namely, the computerized programmable, implantable, pump. This chapter gives a brief overview of the evolution on this field of functional neurosurgery.

2.1 Pioneering Works

The work of the British physiologist Sherrington (Fig. 2.1) on decerebrate animals led to the demonstration that spasticity was associated with a hyperexcitability of the stretch reflex related to the loss of inhibitory influences from descending supraspinal structures [1, 2].

The loss of inhibitory supraspinal influences on the myotatic reflex does not explain exclusively all aspects of spasticity encountered in clinical situations. Babinski's (Fig. 2.2) observations led to the classification of three clinical types of spastic states [2]. They include (1) the tendon reflex contracture with predominant hyperexcitability of the myotatic reflex; (2) the cutaneous reflex contracture related to dominant hyperactivity of the polysynaptic nociceptive flexion reflex associated with the triple withdrawal phenomenon; (3) the nuclear contracture associated with intramedullary involvement, most certainly caused by modifications of inhibitory medullary interneurons. Spasticity is caused not by one mechanism only but by several more or less linked mechanisms associated with different clinical manifestations, leading to different medical and surgical therapeutic management strategies. The classical definition of spasticity given by Lance in 1980 [3] remains the most widely accepted: "Spasticity is a motor disorder characterized by

M. Sindou et al., *Neurosurgery for Spasticity*,
DOI 10.1007/978-3-7091-1771-2_2, © Springer-Verlag Wien 2014

Fig. 2.1 Sir Charles Scott Sherrington (1857–1952), English neurophysiologist. He received the Nobel Prize in Physiology and Medicine in 1932

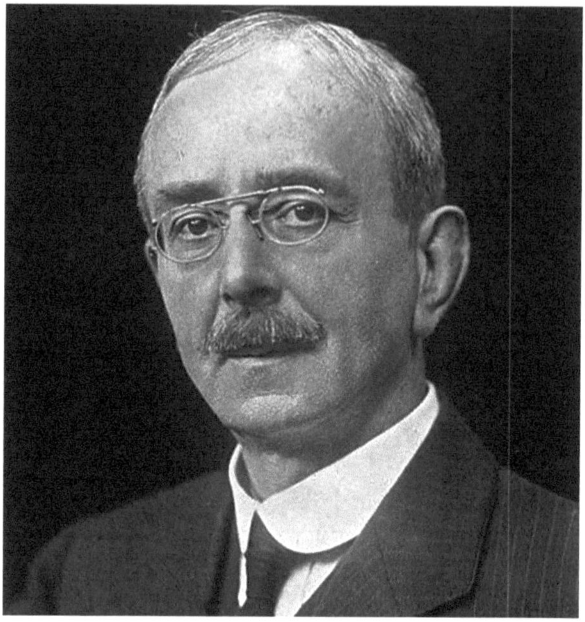

Fig. 2.2 Joseph Jules François Félix Babinski (1857–1932), French neurologist, best known for his 1896 description of the Babinski sign, a pathological plantar reflex indicative of corticospinal tract damage

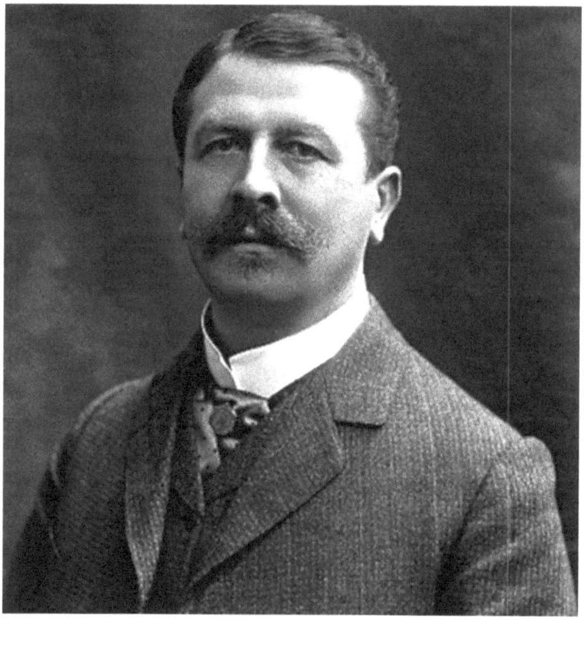

a velocity-dependent increase in tonic stretch reflexes ('muscle tone') with exaggerated tendon jerk, resulting from hyperexcitability of the stretch reflex, as one of the components of the upper motor neuron syndrome."

The first surgical interventions involving the nervous system designed to reduce spasticity were peripheral neurotomies. The first performed one was an obturator

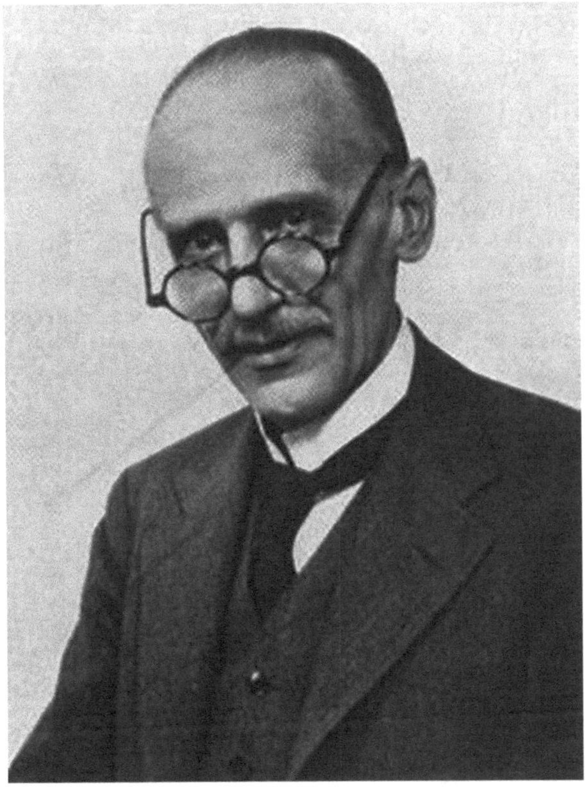

Fig. 2.3 Otfrid Foerster (1873–1941), German neurologist and neurosurgeon who made innovative contributions such as rhizotomy for the treatment of spasticity and anterolateral cordotomy for pain

nerve neurotomy for spasticity of hip adductors performed by Lorenz in 1887 [4]. In 1912, Stoffel performed a tibial nerve neurotomy for spastic foot and a median nerve neurotomy for spastic pronation of the forearm and hand [5]. As early as 1908, Foerster (Fig. 2.3) introduced the principle of dorsal rhizotomy, following Sherrington's observations that posterior rhizotomy reduced spasticity in decerebrate animals [6]. Those two techniques initiated neurosurgical treatment of focalized spasticity. This branch of functional neurosurgery has developed quite extensively, leading to an arsenal of contemporary methods able to improve many disabling situations that previously were without therapeutic solutions.

2.2 Surgery on Peripheral Nerves

The first publications showed the results of obturator neurotomies in association with orthopedic myotomy and tenotomy of adductor muscles for the correction of adduction hip deformities in children with cerebral palsy [7, 8]. To render neurotomies more selective, Gros (Fig. 2.4) and colleagues introduced the use of intraoperative (unipolar) electrical stimulation to identify the functions of the different fascicles composing a nerve [9–11]. At Lyon University we then improved the technique of neurotomy by intraoperative bipolar electrical stimulation combined to fascicular dissections under the operating microscope. In addition, before any surgical decision

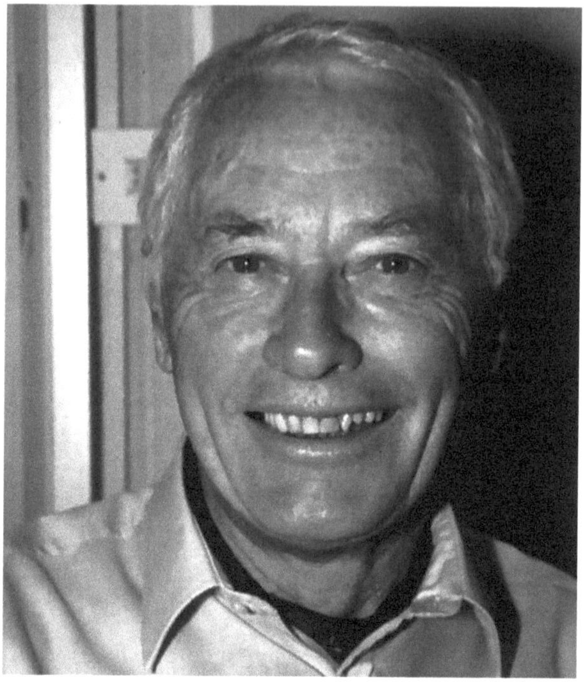

Fig. 2.4 Claude Gros (1915–1998), French neurosurgeon from Montpellier University, who with his pupils favored the concept of selectivity in the destructive procedures for treating spasticity

on the indication of selective neurotomy, we advised to perform nerve block tests with local anesthetic to predict the functional effects of the procedure [12, 13]. Although surgical neurotomies have since then been widely used to treat spasticity of the lower limbs, applications to spasticity of the upper limbs, which is more complex, have evolved more slowly. The pioneering works on upper limbs were performed by orthopedic surgeons who were highly competent in peripheral nerve surgery. Garland and collaborators performed neurotomies of the musculocutaneous nerve for spastic elbow [14]. Brunelli and Brunelli [15, 16] performed microsurgical hyponeurotization of the median nerve, if necessary associated with lengthening of tendons of the wrist and finger flexor muscles, especially of the Scaglietti type. Decq et al. introduced a neurosurgical procedure that involved sectioning branches of the brachial plexus for shoulder spasticity [17]. Kanpolat and collaborators developed percutaneous neurotomies with a thermocoagulation lesion-maker [18], a modern equivalent of percutaneous chemical neurolysis using alcohol or phenol.

There is an increasing tendency to combine peripheral neurotomies with surgical interventions on muscles, tendons, and articulation capsules when severe and irreducible contractures are present.

2.3 Surgery on Spinal Roots

In 1898, using the animal model of mesencephalic transsection, Sherrington showed that decerebrate rigidity could be abolished by cutting dorsal roots. On the basis of these experimental data, Foerster in 1908 performed the first lumbosacral dorsal rhizotomies in four patients for the treatment of lower limb spasticity. The results of his series of 159 patients with cerebral palsy were published in 1913. In his article "On the indications and results of the excision of posterior spinal nerves in men", Foerster made as the conclusion the following recommendations [19]: "For severe spastic paraplegia, I recommend resecting at least five roots. It is necessary to leave the fourth lumbar root, since this root generally guarantees the extensor reflex of the knee so very necessary for standing and walking. Thus the general rule is resection of the second, third and fifth lumbar, and first and second sacral roots. Unfortunately, there exist individual differences. In some cases, the fourth lumbar does not affect knee extension but knee flexion, as the fifth lumbar and first sacral do; the knee extension is affected only by the second and third lumbar roots. To know by which lumbar roots the extension reflex of the knee is effected, we must have recourse to the electrical current during the operation."

Considering these results, Foerster concluded [19], "we must bear in mind that the resection of the posterior roots relieves only the spastic symptoms, but not the paralysis, if such exists besides the spastic state. The disappearance of the spasticity after the root resection is the best proof of the sensory origin of the spastic contracture. But a certain degree of spasm sometimes returns, owing to the fact that the spinal gray matter is gradually recharged by the remaining posterior roots."

In 1945 Munro [20] suggested sectioning ventral roots from the last thoracic roots to the first sacral root to treat irreducible spasticity with severe spasms. This type of procedure was recommended for spasticity associated with spontaneous hyperactivity of motor neurons, as observed after anoxia. In such cases, clinical and experimental data have shown that attempts to sectioning dorsal roots are ineffective, whereas ventral root sectioning abolishes spasms. Side effects on motor function and trophicity are paramount. Ventral rhizotomies are scarcely indicated.

To reduce the sensory secondary effects of Foerster's original technique, Gros and collaborators [21] introduced a slight modification that consisted in preserving one rootlet out of the five (on average) for each root, from L1 to S1. This method significantly decreased spasticity in 75 % of the 25 patients who were followed for a mean period of 3 years and 8 months. The number of preserved rootlets was sufficient to maintain normal sensations in the lower limbs of 70 % of the patients. Apart from the effects on the lower limbs, the authors also observed a decrease in spasticity of the upper limbs. Also, speech and swallowing improved for 18 of 25 cases. This effect is termed an indirect effect.

To further reduce the incidence of secondary effects on the postural tonus of patients who were capable of walking, Gros et al. introduced the topographical selection of rootlets to preserve the innervation of muscles responsible for the so-called useful tonus (quadriceps, abdominal and gluteal muscles in particular). This technique was termed sectorial posterior rhizotomy. The mapping method involves the anatomical identification and stimulation of the roots, which is essential to determine their different functions [11].

In 1977 Fraioli and Guidetti developed a slight variation of the dorsal rhizotomy, the partial dorsal rhizotomy, which consisted in sectioning the dorsal half of each rootlet a few millimeters before their entry into the dorsolateral sulcus [22]. The aim was to avoid significant sensory deficits by leaving a large number of all types of fibers intact.

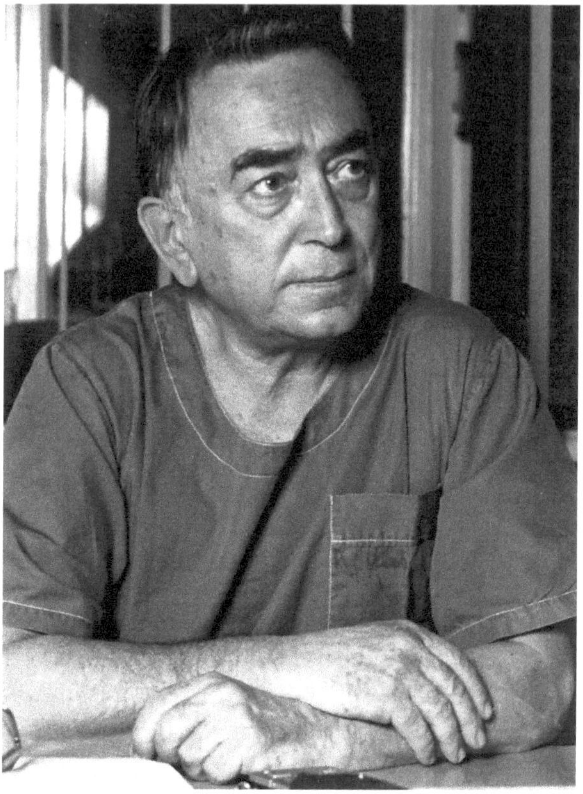

Fig. 2.5 Victor Fasano (1920–1991), Italian neurosurgeon from Torino University, who with his school, developed the concept of functional dorsal rhizotomy to treat spastic diplegic children affected with cerebral palsy. Functional dorsal rhizotomy is based on preferentially cutting those sensory rootlets identified by intraoperative electrostimulation as responsible for hyperactive segmental/intersegmental spinal cord circuitry

In 1976 Fasano (Fig. 2.5) and collaborators introduced the modality termed functional dorsal rhizotomy [23]. This technical variety is based on bipolar intraoperative stimulation of the dorsal rootlets and analysis of the types of muscle responses by electromyographic recordings in which way specially organized circuits responsible for spasticity are detected. Responses characterized by a permanent tonic contraction, an after-discharge pattern, or a large spatial diffusion to distant muscle groups are considered to belong to uninhibited spinal circuits responsible for spasticity.

In 1972 Sindou [24, 25] observed that the technique of microsurgical rhizotomy in the dorsal root entry zone which was developed for treating some forms of neuropathic deafferentation pain and consists in the selective microsurgical destruction of the dorsal root entry zone and dorsal horn led to severe hypotonia in the muscles corresponding to the operated medullary segments. On this basis, he suggested that the technique should be applied to bedridden spastic paraplegic patients and to hemiplegic patients affected with severe spasticity in the upper limb [26–28].

In contrast to the number of dorsal rhizotomies in early attempts to treat lower-limb spasticity, their number remained small for the treatment of the upper limbs. In his article published in 1913, Foerster [19] reported 23 cases of spastic paralysis of the upper limb treated by resection of the dorsal roots from C4 to T2, with the exception of C6. He concluded [19]: "In the majority, the result was not good, satisfactory improvement being obtained in only a few cases; therefore we do not recommend dorsal rhizotomy as a valuable procedure for spasticity of the upper limb."

In the 1970s Kottke [29] and Heimburger and coworkers [30] proposed reducing spasticity in the upper limb by dorsal rhizotomy from C1 to C3, the dorsal root of C4 not being sectioned in order not to affect the diaphragm. The roots of C5 to T1 were not sectioned in order to avoid any impairment of the sensory function of the limb. These superior cervical rhizotomies could (slightly) reduce upper-limb spasticity, possibly because of an indirect effect through the decrease of tonic neck reflexes.

In parallel to open surgical techniques, intrathecal chemical rhizotomies with alcohol, originally introduced by Doglioti for the treatment of pain associated with cancerous lesions [31], were then performed by Guttman in 1953 to treat disabling spasticity in paraplegic patients [32]. Alcohol was replaced by phenol (a hyperbaric solution) as a neurolytic agent, and in 1959 Nathan [33] used phenol to treat spasticity. These chemical rhizotomies are nowadays scarcely indicated, because of the difficulty to selectively direct the agent onto those roots solely involved in the harmful spasticity and because of a lack of specificity to the fibers responsible for tone. These issues explain the frequent appearance of undesirable effects on motricity and sphincterian functions and also why the results were not always maintained for the long term.

Percutaneous radiofrequency rhizotomy with thermocoagulation, also introduced to treat chronic pain [34, 35], was then applied to treat some well-localized spasticities and neurogenic detrusor hyperreflexia of the bladder, particularly on the L2-L3 lumbar roots, for the treatment of flexion-adduction of the spastic hip [36] and on the sacral roots through the sacral foramina for the hyperactive bladder [37].

2.4 Surgery on the Spinal Cord

In 1951 Bischof [38] first described the longitudinal myelotomy procedure. The aim was to interrupt the spinal reflex arc between the ventral and dorsal horns by a vertical coronal incision performed laterally from one side of the spinal cord to the other. For cases with complete paraplegia, the procedure was performed from L1 to S1. Pourpre [39] modified Bischof's technique in order to avoid complete interruption of the corticospinal fibers. Through a laminectomy from T9 to L1, the procedure consisted in making a posterior longitudinal sagittal incision before performing a cruciform myelotomy by transverse incision on either side with a stylet with a right-angled extremity. The purpose of this surgical lesion was to interrupt the spinal reflex arc between the ventral and dorsal horns without sectioning the fibers connecting the pyramidal tract to the motor neurons of the ventral horn. This technique was later popularized by Laitinen and Singounas [40], who designed a special surgical knife to perform less damaging myelotomies [41]. Myelotomies are applied for the treatment of spasticity in bedridden paraplegic patients with triple flexion and severe sphincter disorders.

2.5 Surgery in the Dorsal Root Entry Zone

In 1972 surgery in the dorsal root entry zone of the spinal cord was introduced for the treatment of certain forms of persistent pain [24, 25, 42]. Because the method also induced considerable hypotonia it was used by Sindou and collaborators to treat severe spasticity [26, 43], not only in the lower limbs of paraplegic patients but also in the upper limbs of hemiplegic patients [27, 28]. The purpose of the microsurgical rhizotomy in the dorsal root entry zone is to preferentially interrupt both small- (nociceptive) and large-caliber (myotatic) tonigenic fibers coming from the dorsal root, situated laterally and in the middle of the entry zone, respectively. The surgical lesion must partially, if not totally, preserve the medial large-caliber fibers that reach the dorsal column, as well as their collaterals to the dorsal horn, which also are situated medially in the entry zone. The surgical target includes in addition most of the dorsal horn, where the circuits and neurons that activate the segmental circuitry of the spinal cord are located.

2.6 Stereotactic Lesioning Techniques

Lesioning techniques directed to the basal ganglia (ventrolateral thalamotomies and pulvinarotomies) or to the cerebellum (lesions of the fastigial nucleus, dentatotomies) were attempted. They did not show long-term effects and entailed neurological risks. They lacked a compelling rationale. Consequently they were rapidly abandoned. Those techniques were described and discussed in detail elsewhere [44].

2.7 Intrathecal Infusion of Baclofen

Baclofen, a γ-aminobutyric acid-B (GABA-B) receptor agonist, became part of the therapeutic arsenal in the 1960s [45, 46]. It has a weak capacity to cross the blood–central nervous system barrier. Therefore, oral doses must be increased for cases with severe spasticity, which reduces its potential use in severely affected patients. To counteract this problem, Penn and Kroin [47, 48] developed the method of intrathecal subarachnoid lumbar infusions of the substance. Indeed, the density of GABA-B receptors in the dorsal horn of the spinal cord is high, particularly in layers II and III. Baclofen activates GABA-B presynaptic receptors that inhibit the release of excitatory neurotransmitters (such as aspartate and glutamate) of the dorsal horn. The excitability of monosynaptic and polysynaptic reflexes of the spinal cord is thereby reduced.

The development of implantable and programmable pumps, such as the Synchromed models (Medtronic Co., Minneapolis, MN), has enabled the use of this method in the treatment of handicapped patients, not only adults but also children with cerebral palsy.

This historical synopsis represents only a brief overview of the evolution of concepts related to the neurosurgical treatments of spasticity. More detailed data on these neurosurgical treatments and results can be found elsewhere [49].

References

1. Sherrington CS (1898) Decerebrate rigidity and reflex coordination of movements. J Physiol 22:319–332
2. Babinski J (1912) Contracture tendino-reflèxe et contracture cutanéo-reflèxe. Rev Neurol (Paris) 14:77–80
3. Lance JW (1980) Symposium synopsis. In: Feldman RG, Young RR, Koella WP (eds) Spasticity: disordered motor control. Symposia Specialists, Miami, pp 485–494
4. Lorenz F (1887) Über die chirurgische Behandlung der angeborenen spastischen Gliedstarre. Wien Klin Rdsch 21:25–27
5. Stoffel A (1913) The treatment of spastic contractures. Am J Orthop Surg 2(10):611–644
6. Foerster O (1908) Über eine neue operative Methode der Behandlung spastischer Lähmungen mittels Resektion hinterer Rückenmarkswurzeln. Z Orthop Chir 22:203–223
7. Banks HH, Green WT (1960) Adductor myotomy and obturator neurotomy for the correction of adductive contracture of the hip in cerebral palsy. J Bone Joint Surg Am 42:111–126
8. Keats S (1957) Combined adductor-gracilis tenotomy and selective obturator nerve resection for the correction of adduction deformity of the hips in children with cerebral palsy. J Bone Joint Surg Am 39:1087–1090
9. Gros C, Frerebeau P, Benezech J, Privat JM (1977) Neurotomie ramiculaire selective. In: Simon L (ed) Actualités en rééducation fonctionnelle, ser 2. Masson, Paris, pp 230–235
10. Gros C (1977) Table ronde de la Societé Française de Neurochirurgie sur la chirurgie de la spasticité. Neurochirurgie 23:316–388
11. Gros C (1979) Spasticity: clinical classification and surgical treatment. In: Krayenbühl H, Brihaye J, Loew F, Logue V, Mingrino S, Pertuiset B, Symon L, Troupp H, Yaşargil MG (eds) Advances and technical standards in neurosurgery, vol 6. Springer, Wien/New York, pp 55–97
12. Sindou M, Mertens P (1988) Selective neurotomy of the tibial nerve for the treatment of the spastic foot. Neurosurgery 23:738–744
13. Mertens P, Sindou M (2001) Surgical management of spasticity. In: Barnes MP, Johnson GR (eds) Upper motor neurone syndrome and spasticity: clinical management and neurophysiology. Cambridge University Press, Cambridge, pp 239–265
14. Garland DE, Thompson R, Waters RL (1980) Musculocutaneous neurectomy for spastic elbow flexion in non-functional upper extremities in adults. J Bone Joint Surg Am 62:108–112
15. Brunelli G, Brunelli F (1983) Hyponeurotisation selective microchirurgicale dans les paralysies spastiques. Ann Chir Main 2:277–280
16. Brunelli G, Brunelli F (1988) Hyponeurotization in spastic palsies (selective partial denervation). In: Brunelli G (ed) Textbook of microsurgery. Masson, Milan, pp 861–865
17. Decq P, Filipetti P, Fève A, Djindjian M, Saraoui A, Kéravel Y (1997) Peripheral selective neurotomy of the brachial plexus collateral branches for the treatment of the spastic shoulder: anatomical study and clinical results in five patients. J Neurosurg 86:648–653
18. Kanpolat Y, Cağlar C, Akiş E, Ertürk A, Uluğ H (1987) Percutaneous selective RF neurotomy in spasticity. Acta Neurochir (Wien) Suppl 39:96–98
19. Foerster O (1913) On the indications and results of the excision of posterior spinal nerve roots in men. Surg Gynecol Obstet 16:463–474
20. Munro D (1945) The rehabilitation of patients totally paralyzed below the waist, with special reference to making them ambulatory and capable of earning their living: anterior rhizotomy for spastic paraplegia. N Engl J Med 233:453–461
21. Gros C, Ouaknine G, Vlahovitch B, Frerebeau P (1967) La radicotomie selective postérieure dans le traitement neurochirurgical del'hypertonie pyramidale. Neurochirurgie 13:505–518
22. Fraioli B, Guidetti B (1977) Posterior partial rootlet section in the treatment of spasticity. J Neurosurg 46:618–626
23. Fasano VA, Barolat-Romana G, Ivaldi A, Sguazzi A (1976) La radicotomie postérieure fonctionnelle dans le traitement de la spasticité cérébrale: premieres observations sur la stimulation electrique peropératoire des racines postérieures, et leur utilisation dans le choix des racines à sectionner. Neurochirurgie 22:23–34

24. Sindou M (1972) Etude de la jonction radiculo-medullaire postérieure. La radicellotomie selective postérieure dans la chirurgie de la douleur. Thèse de Médecine, Université de Lyon, Lyon
25. Sindou M, Quoex C, Baleydier C (1974) Fiber organization at the posterior spinal cord–rootlet junction in man. J Comp Neurol 153:15–26
26. Sindou M, Fischer G, Goutelle A, Schott B, Mansuy L (1974) La radicellotomie postérieure selective dans le traitement de spasticité. Rev Neurol (Paris) 30:201–215
27. Sindou M, Jeanmonod D (1989) Microsurgical DREZ-otomy for the treatment of spasticity and pain in the lower limbs. Neurosurgery 24:655–670
28. Sindou M, Mifsud JJ, Boisson D, Goutelle A (1986) Selective posterior rhizotomy in the dorsal root entry zone for treatment of hyperspasticity and pain in the hemiplegic upper limb. Neurosurgery 18:587–595
29. Kottke J (1970) Modification of athetosis by denervation of the tonic neck reflexes. In: annual meeting of the American Academy for Cerebral Palsy, Las Vegas, December 1969, reported by Martin Bax. Dev Med Child Neurol 12:236–237
30. Heimburger RF, Slominski A, Griswold P (1973) Cervical posterior rhizotomy for reducing spasticity in cerebral palsy. J Neurosurg 39:30–34
31. Dogliotti A (1931) Traitement des syndromes douloureux de la périphérie par l'alcoolisation sous-arachnoïdienne des racines postérieures à leur emergence de la moelle epinière. Presse Med 39:1249–1252
32. Guttman L (1953) The treatment and rehabilitation of patients with injuries of the spinal cord. In: Cope VZ (ed) Surgery. Her Majesty's Stationery Office, London, pp 422–516
33. Nathan PW (1959) Intrathecal phenol to relieve spasticity in paraplegia. Lancet 2:1099–1102
34. Lazorthes Y, Verdie JC, Lagarrigue J (1976) Thermocoagulation percutanée des nerfs rachidiens a visée antalgique. Neurochirurgie 22:445–453
35. Uematsu S, Udvarhelyi GB, Benson D, Siebens A (1974) Percutaneous radiofrequency rhizotomy. Surg Neurol 2:319–325
36. Segnarbieux F, Frerebeau P (1991) The different (open surgical, percutaneous thermal, and intrathecal chemical) rhizotomies for the treatment of spasticity. In: Sindou M, Abbott R, Keravel Y (eds) Neurosurgery for spasticity: a multidisciplinary approach. Springer, Wien/New York, pp 133–139
37. Young B, Mulcahy JJ (1980) Percutaneous sacral rhizotomy for neurogenic detrusor hyperreflexia. J Neurosurg 53:85–87
38. Bischof W (1951) Die longitudinale Myelotomie. Zentralbl Neurochir 11:79–88
39. Pourpre H (1960) Traitement neuro-chirurgical des contractures chez les paraplégiques posttraumatiques. Neurochirurgie 6:229–236
40. Laitinen L, Singounas E (1971) Longitudinal myelotomy in the treatment of spasticity of the legs. J Neurosurg 35:536–540
41. Laitinen LV (1973) A myelotome for the treatment of spasticity. In: Proceedings of the 25th Annual Meeting of the Nordisk Neurokirurgisk Förening (Scandinavian Neurosurgical Society), May 31–June 2, 1973, Turku/Abo, compiled by P. Rasmussen. Acta Neurochir (Wien) 29:269
42. Sindou M, Fischer G, Goutelle A, Mansuy L (1974) La radicellotomie postérieure selective. Premières resultats dans la chirurgie de la douleur. Neurochirurgie 20:391–408
43. Sindou M, Millet MF, Mortamais J, Eyssette M (1982) Results of selective posterior rhizotomy in the treatment of painful and spastic paraplegia secondary to multiple sclerosis. Appl Neurophysiol 45:335–340
44. Siegfried J (1991) Destructive stereotactic procedures for spasticity directed to the brain and the cerebellum. In: Sindou M, Abbott R, Keravel Y (eds) Neurosurgery for spasticity: a multidisciplinary approach. Springer, Wien/New York, pp 187–190
45. Birkmayer W, Danielczyk W, Weiler G (1967) Zur objektivierbarkeit des myotonolytischen Effektes eines Aminobuttersäurederivates (CIBA 34647-Ba). Wien Med Wochenschr 117:7–9

46. Jerusalem F (1968) Doppeltblindstudie über den antispastischen Effekt von β-(4-Chlorphenyl)-γ-aminobuttersäure (CIBA) bei Multipler Sklerose. Nervenarzt 39:515–517
47. Penn RD, Kroin JS (1984) Intrathecal baclofen alleviates spinal cord spasticity. Lancet 1:1078
48. Penn RD, Kroin JS (1985) Continuous intrathecal baclofen for severe spasticity. Lancet 2:125–127
49. Sindou M, Abbott R, Keravel Y (eds) (1991) Neurosurgery for spasticity: a multidisciplinary approach. Spinger, Wien/New York

3 Anatomical and Physiological Bases of Motricity Applied to the Study of Spasticity

The spinal motoneuron is under permanent influence of peripheral afferent fibers, interneurons, and descending projections from supraspinal structures. Spasticity corresponds to the exaggeration of the monosynaptic reflex (Fig. 3.1). Various lesions of the central nervous system give rise to spasticity, especially if they affect the supraspinal descending controls, mainly the reticulospinal tracts.

Spasticity has many clinical expressions, with a varied distribution among different muscle groups in a given limb, by different responses to physiological stimuli that may be exteroceptive, proprioceptive, or interoceptive, by variable delays of occurrence after the lesion of the motor pathways, and finally because of the wide range of etiologies and locations of the causal lesions.

Corresponding to this clinical variability, there is a wide variety of experimental models: the model of transection of the brainstem at the intercollicular level by Sherrington, provoking an immediate reaction to decerebration; the model of complete spinal section; the model of resection of the motor cortical areas 4 and 6; finally, the model of spinal ischemia, causing an interneuronal deprivation with motoneuronal hyperactivity.

3.1 Organization of Spinal Cord

3.1.1 Alpha Motoneurons

The alpha motoneurons are located in the ventral horn. Those innervating the same muscle group are associated in a motoneuronal group, itself organized in longitudinal motor columns that can extend over 2–4 metameres. The spinal alpha motoneurons have a somatotopic distribution, as schematically summarized in Fig. 3.2

M. Sindou et al., *Neurosurgery for Spasticity*,
DOI 10.1007/978-3-7091-1771-2_3, © Springer-Verlag Wien 2014

3.1.2 Primary Afferents

All the laminae of Rexed receive primary afferents directly, except lamina VIII, which is an area of intercommissural exchange. The fibers of large diameter project onto laminae III, IV, V, VI, and IX, the fibers of small diameter project onto the superficial laminae I and II and the deeper laminae V and X. Some proprioceptive IA fibers project directly onto the lamina IX motor neurons to trigger the monosynaptic reflex. However, the majority of these proprioceptive afferents ends onto lamina VI, at the base of the dorsal horn, which constitutes a real "proprioceptive layer" where the primary afferent fibers connect with the interneurons that are the origin of the ascending pathways.

a

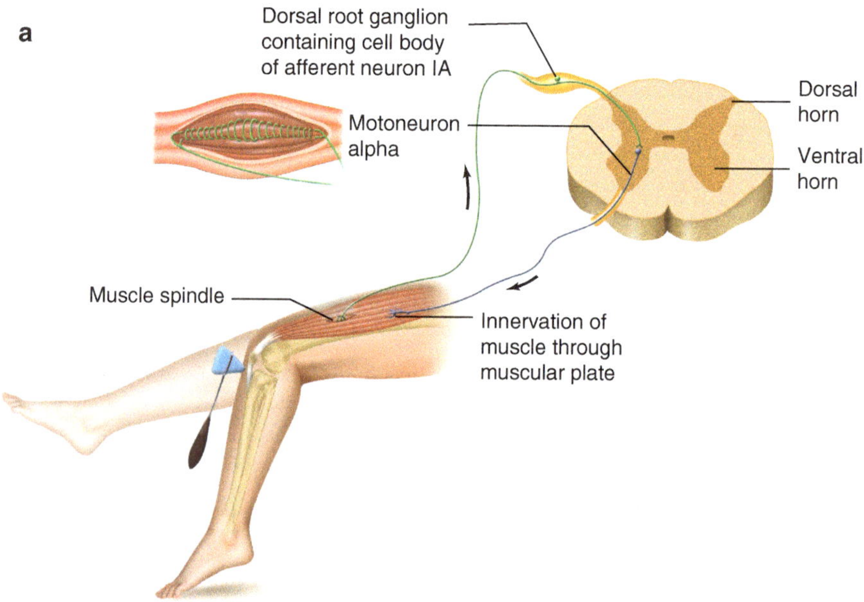

Fig. 3.1 (**a**) Myotatic reflex. The myotatic reflex is a muscle's contraction in response to its stretching (for instance, when the patellar tendon is tapped with a tendon reflex hammer). This reflex provides automatic regulation of the muscle length. When a muscle is lengthened, its spindle, which is its sensory receptor, is stretched, increasing its nerve activity (IA fiber). The afferent volley in IA excites the alpha motoneuron, causing the muscle to contract, thus resisting the stretching. (**b**) H reflex. Method of recording the H reflex, which explores the monosynaptic pathways (IA afferent fiber to alpha motoneuron). Stimulation (*S*) of tibial nerve at popliteal fossa and recording (*R*) of motor response of soleus muscle. Increasing the stimulation intensities results in the occurrence of the H reflex (*I1*, *I2*). When stimulation intensities continue to increase, the H reflex disappears, by collision with the recruitment of motor fibers that is manifested by the increasing amplitude of direct motor response (*M*; *I3*, *I4*)

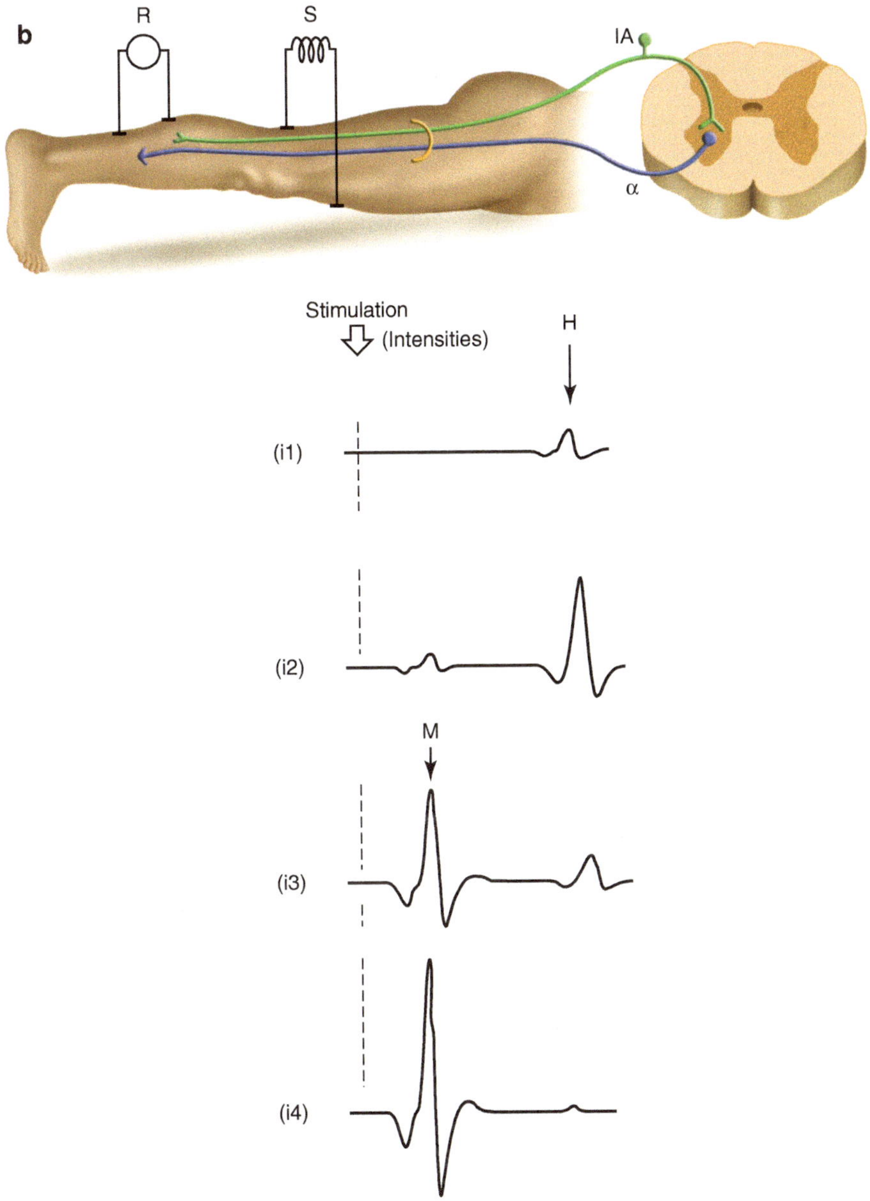

Fig. 3.1 (continued)

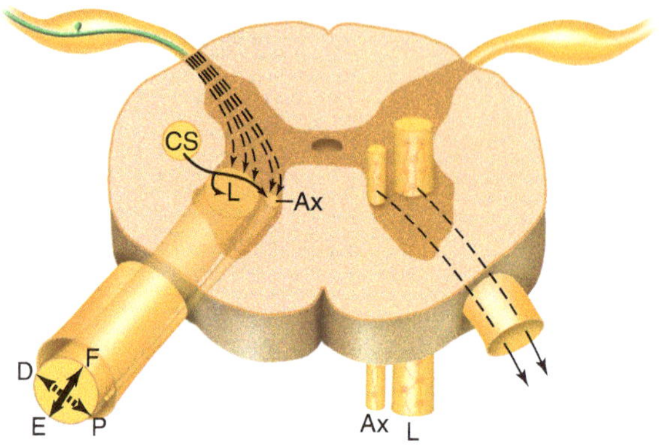

Fig. 3.2 Motoneurons in the ventral horn are organized somatotopically according to their destinations and functional roles into two longitundinal columns: a medial group (medial column), which innervates the axial musculature (neck and trunk), and a lateral group (lateral column), which innervates the extremities musculature (upper limb and lower limb). In this group the motoneurons for extensor muscles are located more ventrally, whereas the motoneurons for flexor muscles are located more dorsally. *Ax* Axial musculature, *L* limbs, *D* for distal muscles of limbs, *P* for proximal muscles of limbs, *F* for flexor muscles, *E* for extensor muscles, *CS* corticospinal tract

For the entry zone of the dorsal rootlets, anatomical and physiological studies in humans revealed the existence of a spatial organization of the primary afferents according to their size and their destination in the spinal cord and therefore to their functions. Thus, the fine fibers (Aδ and C), primarily nociceptive, regroup at the ventrolateral region of the dorsal root entry zone (see Chap. 9); they then cross through the medial part of the tract of Lissauer to reach the uppermost layers of the dorsal horn. The large fibers (Aβ), located dorsomedially in the dorsal root entry zone, reach the dorsal column. Their function is to carry information of the epicritic tactile and the conscious proprioception types to the brainstem lemniscal pathways.

The neurotransmitters released by afferents are mainly excitatory amino-acids (glutamate, aspartate). Only the neurotransmitters released by small-diameter afferents projecting onto the superficial laminae I and II are inhibitory (γ-aminobutyric acid [GABA], glycine). The lamina I neurons receive only glycinergic synaptic inhibition, whereas about half of the lamina II neurons receive pure GABAergic, and the rest receive mixed GABAergic and glycinergic inhibition.

3.1.3 System of Spinal Interneurons

The interneurons of the spinal cord, called propriospinal interneurons, constitute three types. Most have short nerve fibers, some have intermediate, and some have long nerve fibers. Their cell bodies are located in all laminae of the gray matter. However, the interneurons located in the intermediate zone (VII and VIII laminae) control particularly the intersegmental spinal reflexes. The axons of short interneurons travel to the dorso- and ventrolateral tracts on 4–8 adjacent metameres, to project predominantly onto the motoneurons of the flexor muscles in the lateral part of the lamina IX. The intermediate interneurons send their axons via the ventrolateral tract on the lamina IX of even larger adjacent metameres, particularly on the columns of the motoneurons of the extensor muscles.

All of these interneurons are targets of converging information from peripheral origin but also from the suprasegmental descending pathways. After processing this information, the interneurons send a modulatory resulting command, inhibitory or facilitatory, on the pool of motoneurons. Physiologically, there are several types of interneurons. The interneurons of the autogenic inhibition reflex, activated by IB afferents, are located in the lateral part of laminae V and VI. The interneurons that support the reflex reciprocal IA fibers are in the lamina VII. The interneurons involved in the reflexes of flexion are located in the dorsolateral portion of the lamina VII. On the other hand, the Renshaw cells, which are the interneurons of the recurrent inhibition of alpha motoneurons, are located in the most ventral part of the lamina VII.

The inhibitory interneurons have glycine as their predominant neurotransmitter. Most of other interneurons are GABAergic and enkephalinergic. Renshaw cells are mainly glycinergic and in some cases GABAergic. They are activated by the recurrent motoneuron fibers using acetylcholine. They in turn have an inhibitory (hyperpolarizing) action on the same alpha or gamma motoneurons. These Renshaw interneurons are themselves modulated by afferent fibers and descending pathways of supraspinal origin. Another population of GABAergic interneurons acts through a presynaptic, axono-axonal, inhibition of afferent fibers. Receptors may be either GABA-A (coupled to a transmembrane Cl^- channel benzodiazepine agonist) or GABA-B (K^+ channel baclofen agonist). The activated GABA-A and GABA-B receptors lead to membrane hyperpolarization and thus reduce motoneuron excitability. These inhibitory interneurons can be activated either by primary afferents or by descending monoaminergic pathways. These activate receptors of type alpha-2 (for noradrenergic pathways) and type 5-HT1 (for serotonergic pathways). The enkephalinergic interneurons are located in large numbers in the superficial laminae of the dorsal horn and exert an inhibitory effect specifically on nociceptive transmission via opioid receptors mu, delta, and kappa.

3.1.4 Ascending Pathways

The spinocerebellar tracts are essentially secondary neurons that consist of axons from the Clarke and Betcherew nuclei of lamina VI and also of laminae IV and IX. These ascending tracts travel the lateral column and they are differentiated into a ventral bundle of proprioceptive contralateral fibers carrying information from the limbs (fasciculus of Gowers) and a dorsal bundle of ipsilateral fibers carrying information from the trunk (fasciculus of Flechsig). The ventral column harbors the spinoreticular tract that originates from the deep layers of laminae VII, VIII, and X with ipsi- and contralateral projections. This tract plays a role not only in the nociception but also in the field of the motor control, through the reticular formation.

3.2 Supraspinal Descending Pathways

3.2.1 Corticospinal System

In large areas of the frontoparietal cortex (e.g., Brodmann areas 4, 3a, 3b, 1, 2, 5, SII, supplementary motor area), fibers originate which are called corticospinal fibers and constitute the axons of neurons located in layer V, the internal pyramid layer, of those cortical areas.

The majority of the corticospinal fibers decussate in the medullary pyramids and descend in the medial part of the lateral column. They project onto the alpha motoneurons in the ventral horn. A minority of fibers remain ipsilateral and descend in the ventral column before crossing the midline at the level of their metameric projection onto the motoneurons. Most of these corticospinal fibers end in the ventral horn, but some end also on laminae IV to IX spreading over the dorsal horn and intermediate zone. The fibers of parietal origin project preferentially on the dorsal horn (laminae IV–VI), whilst the fibers from the motor cortex project preferentially on the interneurons of the intermediate zone and on the ventral horn.

3.2.2 Descending Lateral System

The descending lateral system includes the rubrospinal and the reticulospinal pathways coming from the lateral pontine and medullary reticular formation (gigantocellular nucleus). These pathways are regrouped in the dorsolateral column and project contralaterally to lamina I and the lateral part of laminae V, VI, VII, and IX.

3.3 Importance of the Reticular Formation

Most patients affected with excessive spasticity, particularly children with cerebral palsy, are hampered by additional manifestations linked to overreactivity that strongly aggravates their disability. These manifestations consist, among others, of startle responses to even minor physical or psychological irritations, of parasite motor reactions, incongruous movements to any close or remote stimuli.

The whole central nervous system is involved in those manifestations not only via the propriospinal interneuron network but also, and to a significant extent, through the reticular formation (RF) and its widespread connections.

The RF is composed of widely spaced neurons loosely arranged into nuclear groups throughout the entire brainstem tegmentum. The huge dendritic trees and the highly branched afferent and efferent network of axons that separate the RF perikarya cause its "reticular" appearance in microscopic sections.

The RF extends continuously throughout the entire length of the tegmentum. It fills all of the space not occupied by cranial nerve nuclei, supplementary sensory and motor nuclei, and long and short tracts. The medullocervical junction is generally regarded as its caudal limit. From the anatomic point of view the rostral limit of the RF is at the midbrain–diencephalon junction, but functionally it represents a continuum between spinal cord and diencephalic and cerebral connections.

The RF has the most heterogeneous connections of any single part of the central nervous system. Stated epigrammatically, the RF receives impulses from and sends impulses to all of the central nervous system; thus, it influences all mental, motor, and sensory functions. Physiologically, RF neurons are characterized by recruitment, divergence, and afterdischarge. The RF is particularly sensitive to general anesthetics and certain psychoactive drugs that have much less effect on the lemniscal and other specific afferent sensory systems.

3.3.1 RF Afferents

The RF receives collaterals from most ascending or descending pathways through the brainstem, regardless of the location of a pathway's origin, in the spinal cord or in the brain, and of the pathway's function, visceral or somatic, motor or sensory.

Afferents tend to synapse in the lateral, parvicellular nuclei, which then relay to the gigantocellular medial nuclei that disperse the RF efferents. An exception is the medial lemniscus. Its fibers that relay discriminative sensations from the dorsal columns apparently do not send collateral branches to the RF; but the lateral spinothalamic and trigeminothalamic tracts, which join the medial lemniscus after its origin, send collateral branches to the RF. Also the spinoreticular tracts strongly project on the RF.

The afferent fibers that bypass the RF are the discriminative or one-to-one systems designed to preserve the topographic order of the information transmitted. They include the dorsal column pathway through the medial lemniscus, the retino-geniculo-calcarine tract, and the tonotopic fibers of the auditory system. Auditory and optic pathways reach the RF as inferred from the prompt startle response to loud sound or a sudden bright light, but the one-to-one component of these systems bypasses the RF.

3.3.2 Specific Efferent RF Pathways

The efferent pathways are the reticulobulbar and the reticulospinal tracts with their specific neurotransmitter pathways. The reticulobulbar tracts run to all cranial nerve nuclei. The reticulospinal tracts run within the ventrolateral columns of the spinal cord. These tracts arise from the medial RF nuclei and include the pontine and medullary reticulospinal tracts.

The pontine reticulospinal tracts arise from the pontine reticular nuclei. After descending in the medial longitudinal fasciculus, they end in the laminae VII and VIII at all cord levels and overlap extensively with the termination fields of the vestibular nuclei. These pathways act on the axial muscles, particularly those of the neck, to mediate postural reflexes and muscle tone.

The medullary reticulospinal tract arises from the nucleus reticularis gigantocellularis and synapses at all cord levels in the laminae VII and IX. Their field of termination overlaps with the terminals of the corticospinal and rubrospinal tracts.

Whereas a minority of reticulospinal axons ends on the ventral motoneurons, most end on internuncial neurons of the laminae VII to IX.

Conclusion

Strictly, spasticity corresponds to the exaggeration of the myotatic reflex and is linked to spinal hyperexcitability. This hyperexcitability results from a loss of inhibitory control from the supraspinal descending pathways (Fig. 3.3).

Spasticity is part of a wide and diverse impairment in the motor system function, as summarized in this chapter (Fig. 3.4).

Spinal plasticity after pathological process occurs also and plays a role. It can be summarized according to the two following mechanisms: phenomena of axonal growth (collateral sprouting) from intact nerve fibers in the direction of synaptic sites vacated by the degeneration of lesioned nerve fibers, and to a lesser extent, a phenomenon of hypersensitivity of neuronal receptors, compensating for the loss of presynaptic afferents.

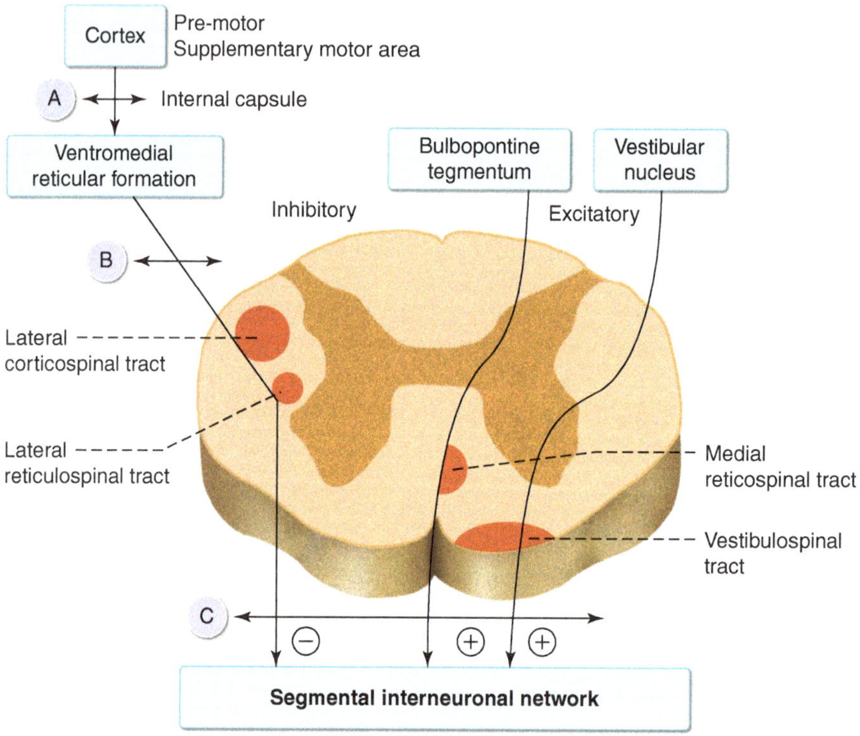

Fig. 3.3 Major descending systems exerting supraspinal control. The anatomical relations and the differences with respect to cortical control between the inhibitory and excitatory descending systems indicate that anatomical location of the upper motor neuron lesion plays a significant role in the determination of the resulting clinical pattern. *A:* Lesion affecting the corticospinal tract and the corticoreticular tract, which are facilitating structures of the main inhibitory system, namely the lateral reticulospinal tract. *B:* Incomplete spinal cord lesion affecting the corticospinal fibers and the lateral reticulospinal tract. *C:* Complete spinal cord lesion affecting the corticospinal fibers, together with the lateral reticulospinal fibers, and the excitatory pathways, namely the medial reticulospinal tract and the vestibulospinal tract. Plus symbol indicates excitatory pathway; minus symbol indicates inhibitory pathway. The excitatory pathways have inhibitory effects on flexor reflexes

Fig. 3.4 Schematic representation of pathophysiology leading to impaired function in the upper motor neuron lesion (Modified from Sheean G (2008) Neurophysiology of spasticity. In: Barnes MP, Johnson GR (eds) Upper motor neurone syndrome and spasticity – clinical management and neurophysiology, 2nd edn. Cambridge University Press, Cambridge, p 27)

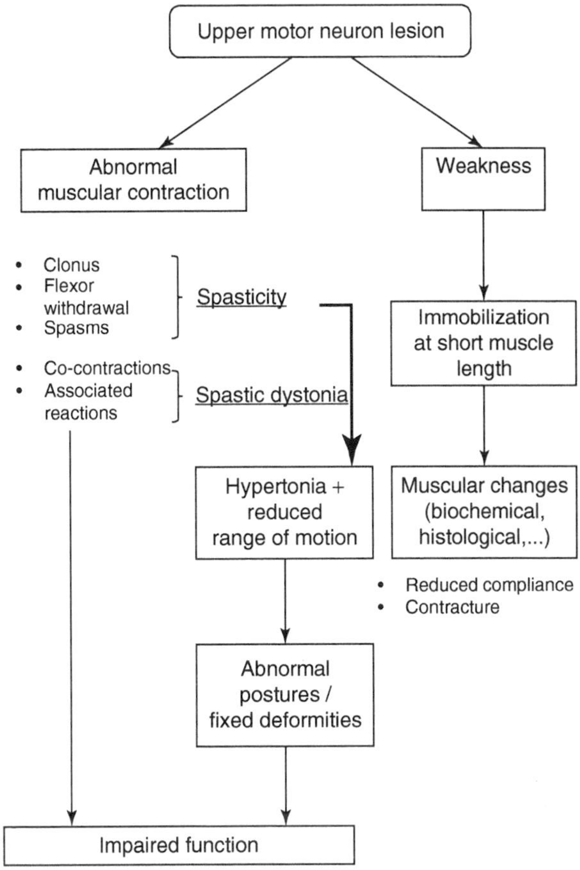

Part II

Adults

4 Evaluation of Spasticity in Adults

Often preferable to flaccid paralysis, spasticity must not be considered a disease that must be treated at all cost. It needs to be reduced only when it interferes with the patient's residual functional capacities. The aims of evaluation are to recognize the spastic components among the other various neurologic disorders that contribute to disability and to establish the extent to which spasticity is harmful in each examined patient.

Patients do not consult because of spasticity; they come complaining about stiffness and deformities (Figs. 4.1 and 4.2), limitations in functional capabilities, discomfort, or pain. The clinician must try to understand what patients mean by their terms.

"Stiffness" is a useful term because it is widely understood by both clinicians and patients. In any discussion on spasticity management, an agreed terminology is important in recognizing two principal components of muscle stiffness. The first is a dynamic shortening of muscles which is caused by **spasticity**. Such patients exhibit hyperreflexia, clonus, and a velocity-dependent resistance to passive joint motion. The second is a fixed shortening of muscles which is described as contracture. **Contractures** are much less velocity-dependent and remain present under local blocks or anesthesia.

When an agonist muscle is involved in a voluntary effort, contraction of antagonist muscles may occur simultaneously, resulting in the phenomenon of co-contraction. **Co-contraction** of an antagonist muscle may act as a restraining force during movement. This phenomenon can be confused with spasticity. Co-contraction is characterized by simultaneous activation of agonist and antagonist muscles during voluntary movement.

Synkinesis (from the Greek words "syn", plus or additional, and "kinesis", motion) is a term used to describe the associated additional postural reactions deprived of voluntary control. Synkinesis refers to involuntary activity in one limb that is associated with a voluntary movement effort made by other limbs. This phenomenon may be due to disinhibited spread of voluntary motor activity into a spastic limb and is dependent on the extent of voluntary effort made.

Spasticity and dystonia have to be distinguished one from another. **Dystonia** causes a sustained involuntary movement. Spasticity and dystonia are two symptoms with a completely different pathophysiology: a lesion of the basal ganglia results in dystonia

M. Sindou et al., *Neurosurgery for Spasticity*,
DOI 10.1007/978-3-7091-1771-2_4, © Springer-Verlag Wien 2014

Clinical pattern			Muscles involved	Nerve(s)	Roots / segments of origin
Name	Figure	Description			
Flexed hip	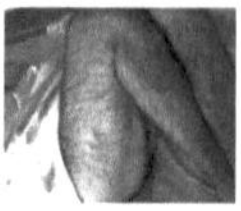	Sustained hip flexion that interferes with positioning. Shortened contralateral step. When bilateral: crouched gait pattern	• Psoas/Iliacus • Rectus femoris	Branch of lumbar plexus Femoral	L2–L3 L3–L4
Adducted thigh	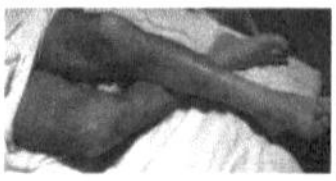	Unilateral or bilateral scissoring thighs	• Adductor group (longus, brevis, magnus) • Gracilis • Obturator externus • Pectineus	Obturator	L2–L3
Extended knee	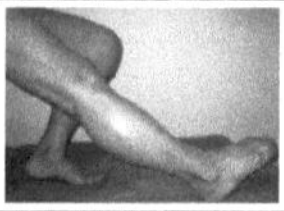	Knee remaining extended. The limb becomes functionally longer	Quadriceps group (rectus femoris, vastus intermedius, vastus medialis and lateralis)	Femoral	L3–L4
Flexed knee	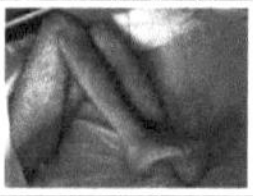	Knee that remains flexed	Hamstrings • Biceps femoris • Semitendinosus • Semimembranosus	Sciatic	L5–S2
Equino-varus foot	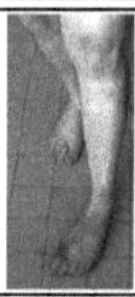	The most common pathologic posture in the lower extremity. Presents as the foot and ankle turned down and in	Equinus: • Gastrocnemius • Soleus • Popliteal Varus: • Tibialis posterior	Tibial	S1
Claw toes	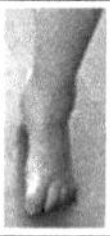	Toes in permanent flexion. Clawing – like may co-exist with equino-varus foot	• Flexor digitorum longus/brevis • Flexor hallucis longus	Tibial	S1–S2
Striatal toe (hitchhiker's great toe)	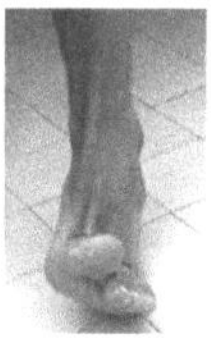	Persistent hyperextension of great toe	Extensor hallucis longus	Peroneal	L4–L5

Fig. 4.1 Clinical patterns of characteristic deformities in patients with spasticity of the lower limbs describing the main involved muscle groups, nerve(s) and roots

and a lesion of the corticospinal tracts results in spasticity. Given the anatomical proximity of these two structures, both can be injured by the same pathological process. For instance, a subcortical hemorrhagic lesion may affect both the internal capsule and the basal ganglia and therefore induce both spasticity and dystonia.

4.1 Common Clinical Patterns of Abnormal Postures in Spasticity

The generally accepted definition of spasticity is the one proposed by Lance in 1980 [1]: "Spasticity is a motor disorder characterized by a velocity-dependent increase in tonic stretch reflexes ('muscle tone'), with exaggerated tendon jerk,

Clinical pattern			Muscles involved	Nerve(s)	Roots / segments of origin
Name	Figure	Description			
Adducted /internally rotated shoulder	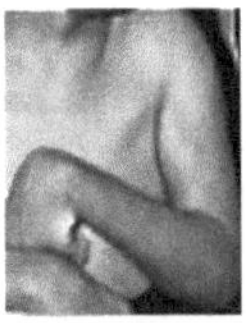	Arm held tightly against the chest wall and shoulder with internal rotation	• Pectoralis major • Teres major	Lateral and Medial thoracic Inferior Subscapular	C5–C6 and C7–C8 C5–C8
Flexed elbow	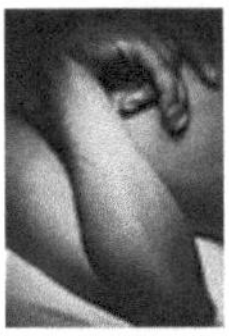	Persistent elbow flexion	• Coraco-brachialis • Biceps • Brachialis	Musculocutaneous	C5–C6
Pronated forearm	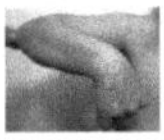	Forearm fully "pronated"	• Pronator quadratus • Pronator teres	Median	C6–C7
Flexed wrist	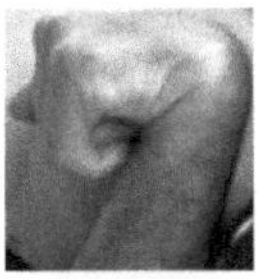	Wrist flexed, in neutral position, radial or ulnar deviation	• Flexor carpi radialis • Palmaris longus • Flexor carpi ulnaris	Median Ulnar	C6–C7 C8–T1
Clenched fist	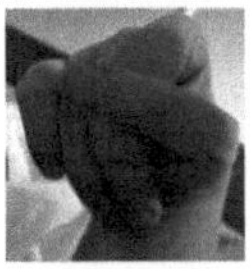	Fingers flexed into the palm	• Flexor digitorum sup. • Flexor digitorum prof.	Median	C7–C8
Thumb in palm	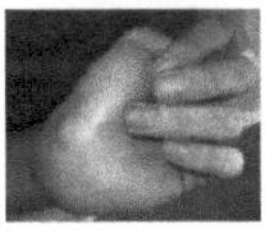	Thumb is pulled into the palm	• Flexor pollicis longus • Adductor pollicis • Opponens	Median Ulnar	C7–C8 C8–T1
"Swan neck"	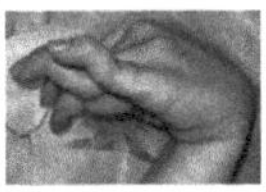	Permanent flexion of distal inter-phalangeal joints of fingers	• Lumbricals (1–2) + Interossei • Lumbricals (3–4) + Interossei	Median Ulnar	C7–T1 C8–T1

Fig. 4.2 Clinical patterns in characteristic deformities of patients with spasticity of the upper limbs describing the main involved muscle groups, nerve(s) and roots

resulting from hyperexcitability of the stretch reflex, as one of the components of the upper motor neuron syndrome."

In practice, clinicians do not always use this definition and tend to assess spasticity schematically in two different ways, thereby creating a certain degree of confusion [2]. They either use Lance's definition, reserving the term spasticity exclusively for exaggeration of the tonic stretch reflex, or they define spasticity by all of the positive signs of the upper motor neuron syndrome.

The intensity of spasticity may vary over time. In case of a recent and sudden modification of spasticity, the clinical examination must exclude the presence of an irritating factor (e.g., urinary tract infection, bladder stones, pressure ulcer, ingrown toenail, altered bowel habit), which must be treated before any treatment of spasticity is considered.

The development of typical patterns of deformity is secondary to agonist muscle weakness, antagonist muscle spasticity, and changes in the characteristics of stiffness in spastic muscles. These patterns are commonly associated with complaints of disfigurement and pain.

4.1.1 Lower Limb

Characteristic clinical patterns and abnormal postures of the lower limb are described in Fig. 4.1.

4.1.1.1 Hip Flexion

Muscles that potentially contribute to an excessively flexed hip include the iliopsoas, the rectus femoris, and the pectineus. The adductor longus and brevis may also contribute to hip flexion.

Chronic flexion posturing leads to flexion contracture and may also contribute to knee flexion deformity. Excessive hip flexion during the stance phase of gait interferes with limb advancement and results in a shortened contralateral step. Patients with bilateral muscle overactivity of the hip flexors may walk with a crouched gait pattern. The hips remain flexed throughout swing and stance. Crouched gait resulting from hip flexion can lead to compensatory knee flexion and continuous use of quadriceps, hip extensors, and calf muscles to maintain balance with increased effort and fatigue.

4.1.1.2 Adducted Thighs

Muscles that potentially contribute to an adducted thigh include the adductor longus and brevis, the adductor magnus, the gracilis, and also iliopsoas and pectineus.

The patient presents with unilateral or bilateral scissoring thighs. Severe hip adduction interferes with limb clearance and advancement during the swing phase of gait. The base of support is narrow with potential impairment in balance that usually requires an upper-extremity assistive device.

4.1.1.3 Extended Knee

Muscles that potentially contribute to a stiff – extended – knee include rectus femoris, vastus intermedius, and vastus medialis and lateralis.

The stiff knee typically presents as a gait deviation with the knee remaining extended through most of the gait cycle, therefore the limb becomes functionally longer. A stiff knee might fail to relax while the patient is seated and also requires elevated leg support. Standing and transfers are problematic.

4.1.1.4 Flexed Knee

Muscles that potentially contribute to a flexed knee include the medial and lateral hamstrings. Weakness of the quadriceps or the gastrocnemius exacerbates this condition.

The patient presents with a knee that remains flexed throughout the swing and stance phases of gait. A flexed knee during the stance phase requires compensatory ipsilateral hip flexion and might also induce contralateral hip and knee flexion (crouch gait pattern). Stretching of overactive hamstrings can be painful. Sitting and wheelchair positioning are hampered. During standing transfers, body weight support is difficult because the body's weight line causes the knees to flex even more, making the patient prone to collapse. Overactive hamstrings can flex the knees or act posterior to the hip joints, causing the trunk to extend. As a result, seated patients with flexed knee tend to slide forward in their wheelchairs.

4.1.1.5 Equinovarus Foot

Muscles that can potentially contribute to an equinovarus foot include the soleus, the medial and lateral gastrocnemius, the tibialis posterior, and the long toe flexors. The tibialis anterior, extensor hallucis longus, and peroneus longus may also indirectly contribute.

Equinovarus foot, the most common pathologic posture seen in the lower extremity, presents as the foot and ankle turned downwards and inwards. Toe clawing may coexist. Dorsiflexion motion is limited during early and mid-stance and prevents forward progression of the tibia over the stationary foot, resulting in hyperextension thrust and even more hyperextended position of the knee and dysrhythmic and restrained forward progression of body mass. Equinovarus with toe clawing results in an inadequate base of support that leads to unstable gait.

4.1.1.6 Striatal Toe

An overactive extensor hallucis longus contributes to a striatal toe (hitchhiker's great toe or permanent Babinski sign). Persistent hyperextension can be seen in isolation or with some degree of equinovarus foot deformity. Patients complain of pain at the tip of the great toe and under the first metatarsal head during the stance phase of gait.

4.1.2 Upper Limb

Characteristic clinical patterns and abnormal postures of the upper limb are described in Fig. 4.2.

4.1.2.1 Adducted and Internally Rotated Shoulder

Muscles that potentially contribute to an adducted and internally rotated shoulder include the pectoralis major, the teres major, and also the latissimus dorsi, the anterior deltoid, and the subscapularis.

The patient typically presents with the arm held tightly against the chest wall. The elbow is often flexed and, because of the internal rotation of the shoulder, the hand and forearm are draped on top of the chest anteriorly. Patients complain of shoulder stiffness and painful passive range of motion because the large adductor muscles of the shoulder can generate strong spastic tension when stretched. Pectoralis major, latissimus dorsi, teres major, and long head of triceps are often overactive.

4.1.2.2 Flexed Elbow

Muscles that potentially contribute to the flexed-elbow deformity include the biceps, the brachialis, and the brachioradialis. Secondary contributory muscles may include the extensor carpi radialis and the pronator teres.

The patient typically presents with persistent elbow flexion during sitting, standing, and especially walking. Prolonged elbow flexion posturing is frequently associated with contracture. Stiffness is a frequently reported sensation. Dressing, reaching for objects, and bringing them to the body can be difficult.

4.1.2.3 Pronated Forearm

Muscles that potentially contribute to a pronated forearm include the pronator teres and the pronator quadratus.

The patient typically presents with a forearm that is fully pronated; pronation posturing is more common than supination posturing. The pronated forearm is commonly associated with a flexed elbow. Passive stretching of stiff pronators is often uncomfortable or painful. Overactive pronator muscles inhibit supination.

4.1.2.4 Flexed Wrist

Muscles that potentially contribute to the flexed-wrist deformity include flexor carpi radialis, flexor carpi ulnaris, palmaris longus, flexor digitorum superficialis, and flexor digitorum profundus.

The patient typically presents with a wrist that is flexed, sometimes with radial deviation, sometimes with ulnar deviation. In many cases, a flexed wrist is associated with the clenched-fist deformity. The extrinsic finger flexors cross the wrist anterior to its axis of rotation and therefore act as accessory wrist flexors themselves. Passive stretching of stiff flexors can be uncomfortable or painful. Associated compression of the median nerve can produce carpal tunnel syndrome with hand pain. The flexed wrist may receive contributions from the wrist flexors including palmaris longus and flexor carpi radialis and ulnaris. The superficial and deep finger flexors may also contribute to wrist flexion, as they cross in front of the axis of rotation of the wrist.

4.1.2.5 Clenched Fist

Muscles that potentially contribute to a clenched fist include the flexor digitorum superficialis and the flexor digitorum profundus.

The patient typically presents with fingers flexed into the palm. Many patients have little or no active finger extension. In many cases, the clenched fist is also associated with the thumb-in-palm deformity. Clenched fist associated with overactive flexor digitorum profundus is linked to flexion of the distal interphalangeal joint. Clenched fist associated with overactive flexor digitorum superficialis is linked to proximal interphalangeal joint flexion and distal interphalangeal joint extension.

4.1.2.6 Thumb in Palm

Muscles that potentially contribute to the thumb-in-palm deformity include flexor pollicis longus, flexor pollicis brevis, opponens, adductor pollicis, and first dorsal interosseous. The patient's thumb is pulled into the palm. Flexor pollicis longus, flexor pollicis brevis, adductor pollicis, and first dorsal interosseous may contribute to closing off access to the webspace.

4.2 Examination

4.2.1 Lower Limb

4.2.1.1 Walking Patient

Gait is studied under conditions that are natural for patients, i.e., with bare feet and then with shoes, using their usual walking aids, e.g., orthopedic shoes or anti-foot-drop or anti-recurvatum splint.

Gait can be described precisely as it is an alternating automatic motor activity with a 180° phase difference between the two legs, during which the stance phase is longer than the swing phase or transfer phase (Fig. 4.3).

A quantified gait analysis is the only investigation providing a complete, objective [3], and reproducible [4, 5] analysis of the body during movement. Kinematic parameters (analysis of joint displacement by an optoelectronic system), kinetic parameters (analysis of the forces developed by ground force platforms), and electromyographic parameters with surface electrodes are measured during motion. This examination provides an objective description of gait that helps to understand and quantify abnormalities (Figs. 4.4 and 4.5).

4.2.1.2 Nonwalking Patient

Evaluation has to consider all activities of daily life: sitting in a wheelchair, at rest, during movements, and during transfers. In addition, personal hygiene, dressing especially of the lower limbs (pants) and feet (socks and shoes), catheterizations, and sexual performance have to be considered.

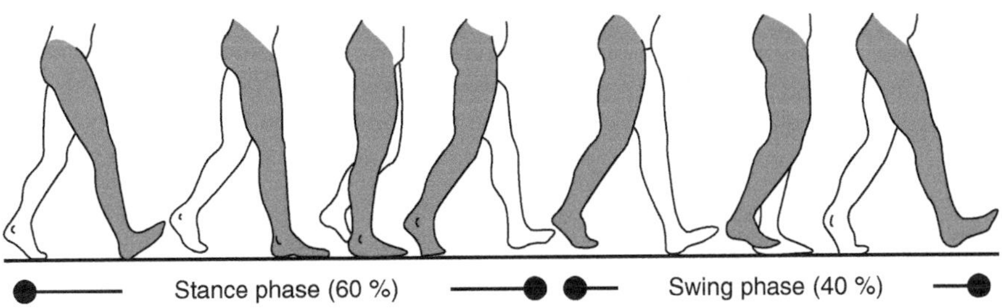

Fig. 4.3 Scheme of normal gait cycle. The relevant information can be captured during one complete gait cycle, which is the time between successive foot contacts of the same limb. Each cycle begins at initial contact with a stance phase and proceeds through a swing phase until the cycle ends with the limb's next initial contact. Stance phase accounts for approximately 60 % and swing phase for 40 % of a single gait cycle

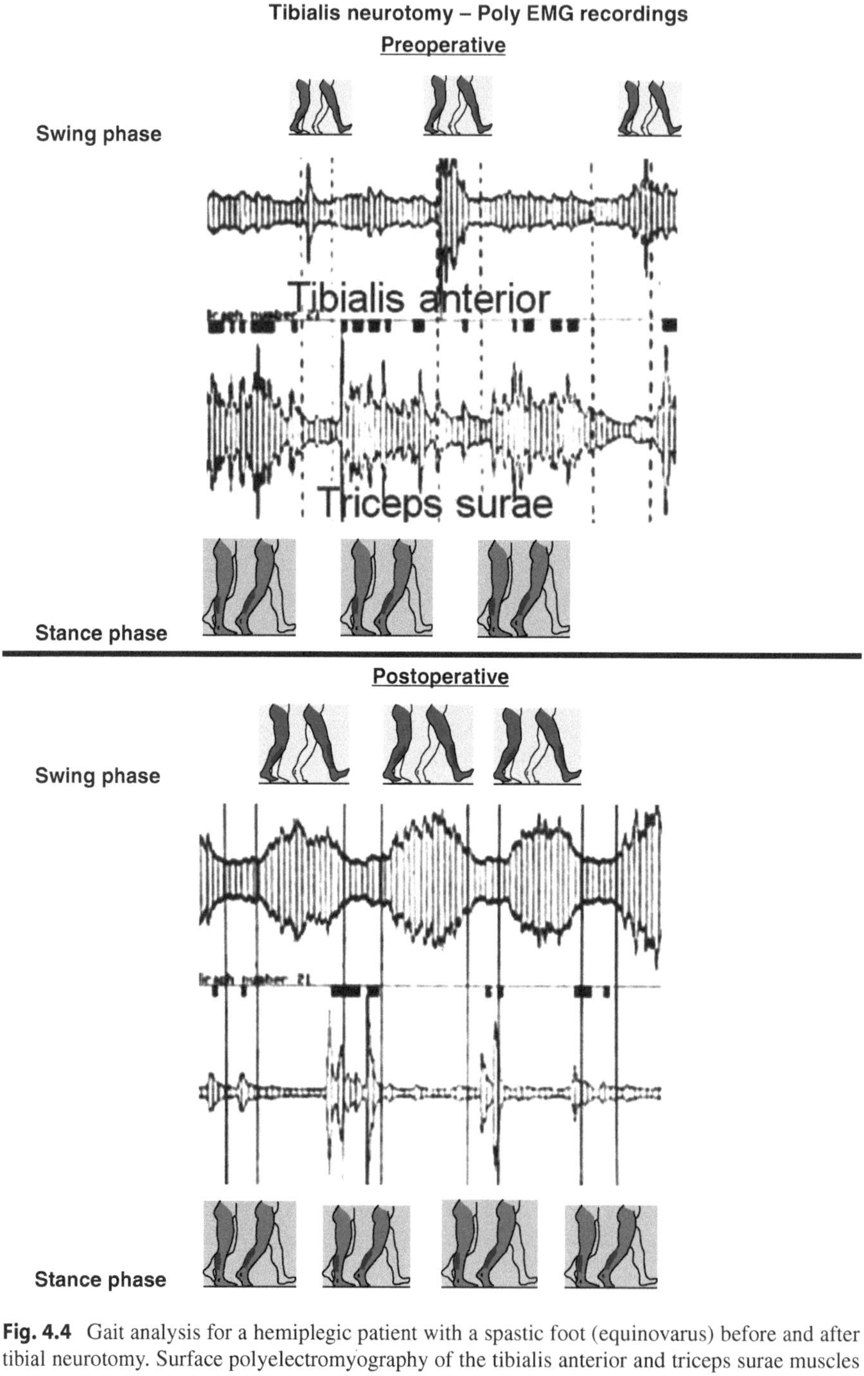

Fig. 4.4 Gait analysis for a hemiplegic patient with a spastic foot (equinovarus) before and after tibial neurotomy. Surface polyelectromyography of the tibialis anterior and triceps surae muscles on the spastic leg during walking, evaluating the change between pre- and postoperative state in stance and swing phase. Preoperative recordings show desynchronized activities of the triceps surae, with abnormal co-contractions of antagonist muscles: triceps surae and tibialis anterior. After tibial neurotomy, there is a reappearance of muscular activity in the tibialis anterior muscle, a clear decrease in triceps surae activity, and normal alternation of contractions of these muscles, i.e., the triceps surae at the end of the stance phase and the tibialis anterior during the swing phase

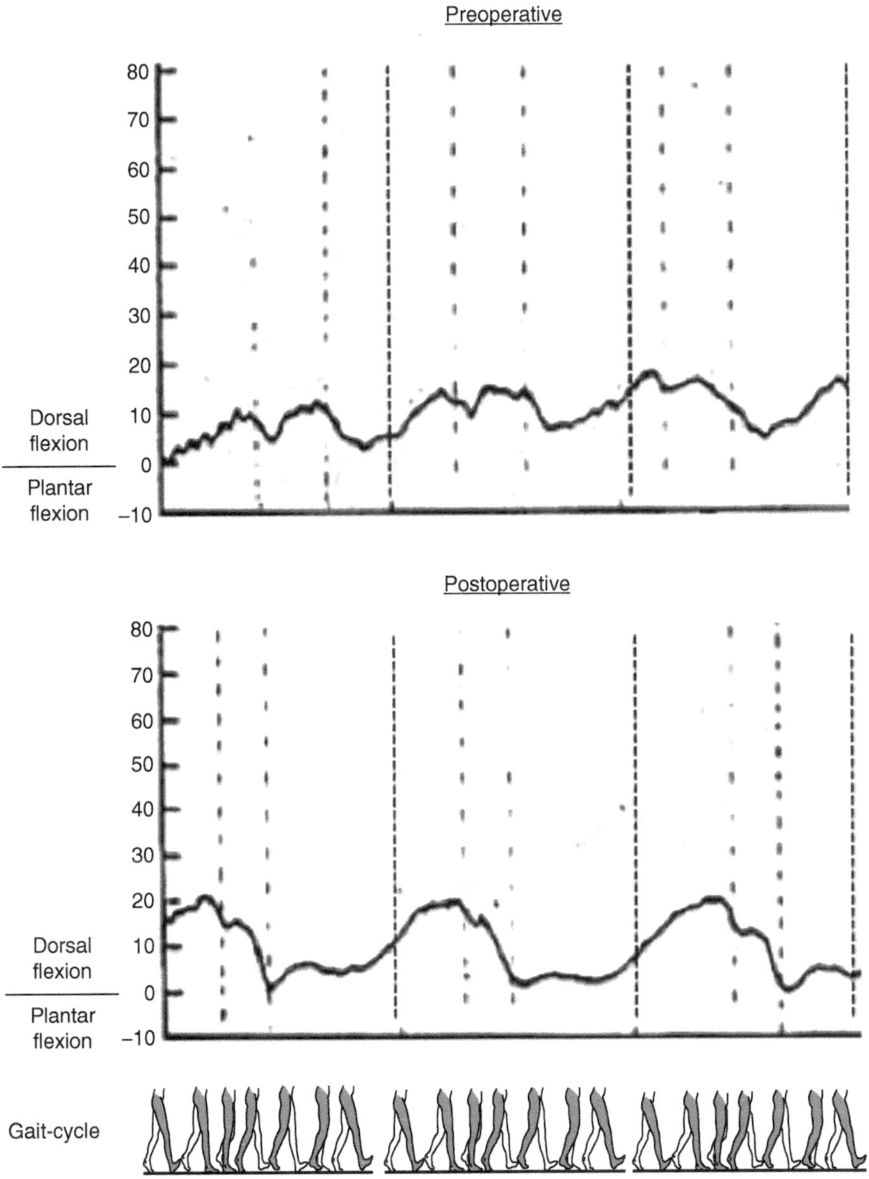

Fig. 4.5 Gait analysis in a hemiplegic patient with spastic foot (equinovarus) before and after tibial neurotomy. Three-dimensional movement analysis of the ankle flexion–extension amplitude during gait with the Vicon system. Preoperatively the amplitude of the spastic ankle was limited to 18° of dorsal flexion. After tibial neurotomy, dorsal flexion increased to 32°. Thus, the tonic balance of the ankle was established by the neurotomy; consequently motor function and gait improved

4.2.2 Upper Limb

The automatic activities of the upper limb have to be examined during gait, from loss of swing to triple flexion, even to dystonic rotation-adduction. The range of motion has to be quantified for abduction, anteflexion, and retroflexion of the shoulder, flexion and extension of the elbow and wrist, and the ability of opening the hand and fingers. Finally, the activities that can be performed by the deficient limb should be evaluated: paperweight hand, temporary use of a humerothoracic grip, flexion of the elbow, hand grasp, also dressing, eating, and washing.

4.2.3 Dynamic Gait Analysis

Modern dynamic gait analysis, together with functional assessment scales, is a key investigation to obtain objective and reproducible data for the planning of treatments and the evaluation of the outcomes of interventions [6] (Luauté J, 2012, Dynamic gait analysis for exploring spasticity. Physical medicine and rehabilitation in spasticity – Teaching program of Lyon University1, personal communication). Dynamic gait analysis includes recordings of kinematics, kinetics, and electrical muscle activity during motion (Fig. 4.6).

Kinematics explores the spatial movement of the body: segment position, joint position, joint motion. Displacement of the markers is captured by an optoelectronic system with multiple cameras (Fig. 4.7).

Kinetics explores the mechanisms that cause movement: ground reaction forces, joint moments, and joint powers. Mechanic constraints are studied with a force platform that measures the ground reaction force generated by a body standing or moving on it. Kinetics helps to understand the pathogenesis of gait problems (Fig. 4.8).

Polyelectromyography recordings are made with surface electrodes (less common with needle electrodes) and depict any decrease in activity of weak muscles and hyperactivity of spastic muscles and co-contractions between agonist and antagonist muscles (Fig. 4.9).

Motion analysis may also be carried out at the upper limb, on the same principles as for gait. Such exploration can help to study capacities of hand prehension and transport (Fig. 4.10).

Dynamic gait analysis has substantial limitations. It can be done only with patients able to walk autonomously over of a distance of at least 20 m, without major equilibrium disturbances and without assistive devices. Practically, kinematics easily explores abnormalities in the sagittal plane (equinus of foot, hyperextended position of knee, flexion of hip), but does much less reliably so for abnormalities in the frontal plane.

Dynamic gait analysis provides useful informations to plan treatment. It helps to verify and characterize spasticity among deformities of a patient's body and define underlying mechanisms. It also helps to establish whether spasticity is harmful or useful and, if harmful, to determine the actually harmful component(s) (Fig. 4.11).

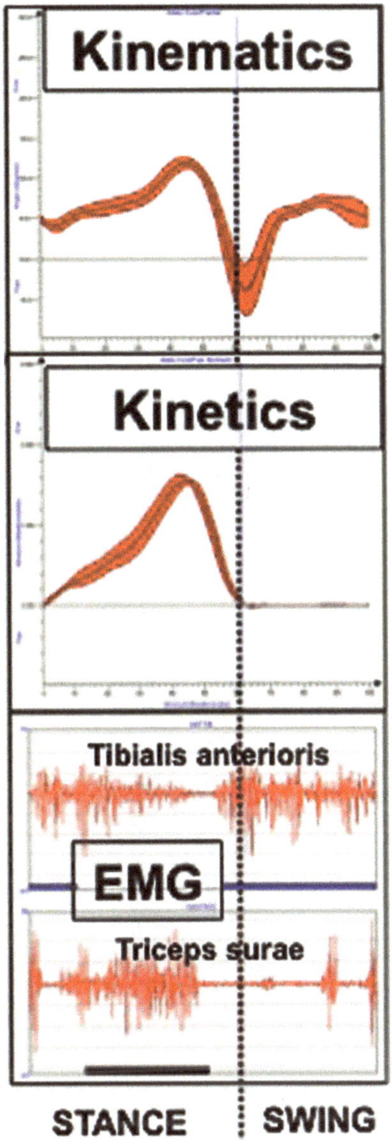

Fig. 4.6 Dynamic gait analysis at level of ankle, including kinematics, kinetics, and electric muscle activity in tibialis anterioris and triceps surae (Courtesy of J. Luauté, University Lyon 1)

Dynamic gait analysis under anesthetic blocks is of prime importance to predict the effects of a possible intervention (e.g., botulinum toxin injections, peripheral neurotomies, dorsal rhizotomies, intrathecal baclofen, orthopedic surgery) (Fig. 4.12). Dynamic gait analysis is nowadays a prerequisite to evaluate the benefits or detriments of interventions and make a postoperative quantitative appraisal of their effects.

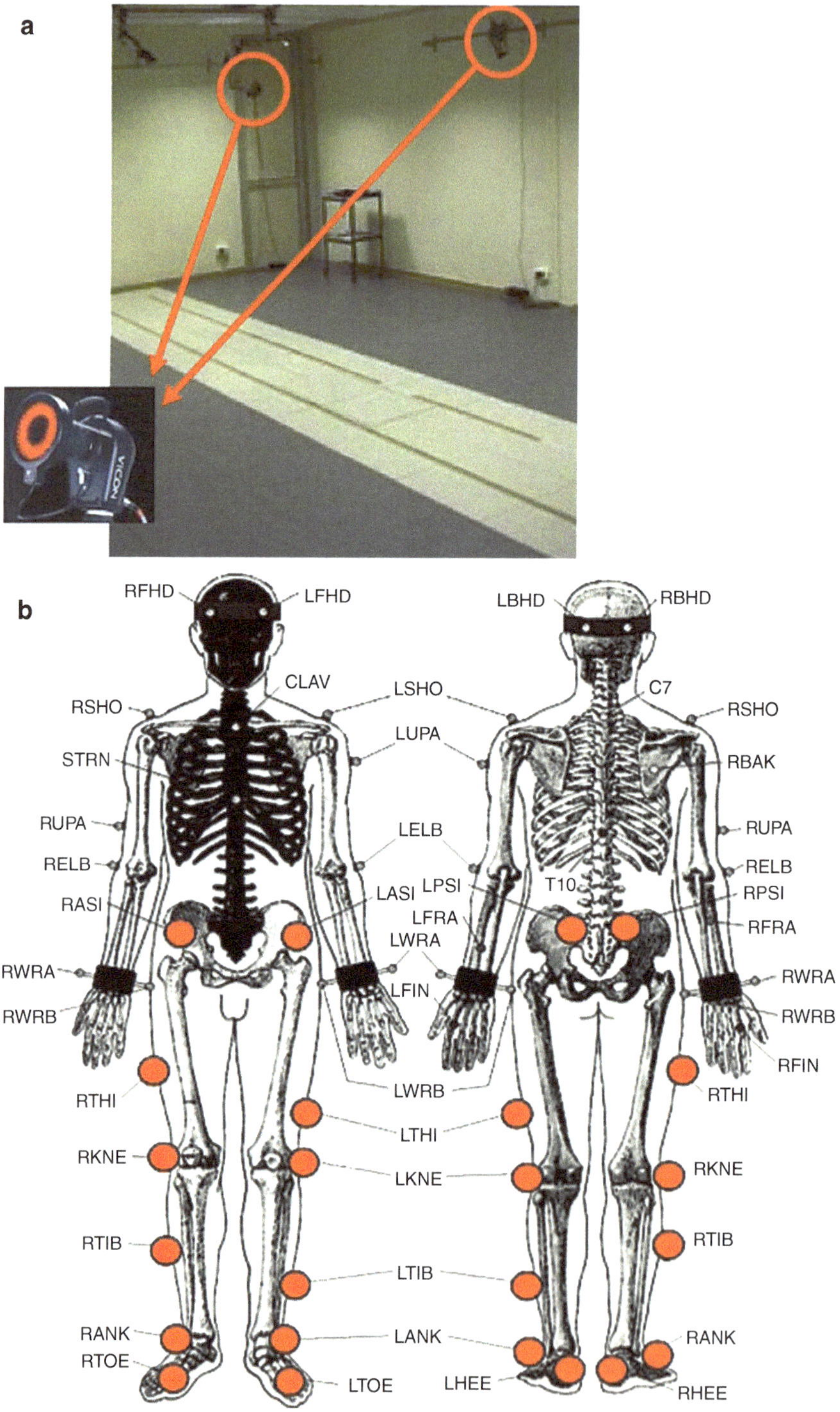
a
VICON
b
RFHD
LFHD
LBHD
RBHD
CLAV
LSHO
C7
RSHO
RSHO
LUPA
STRN
RBAK
RUPA
RUPA
LELB
RELB
RELB
LASI
LPSI
T10
RPSI
RASI
LFRA
RFRA
LWRA
RWRA
RWRA
LFIN
RWRB
RWRB
RFIN
RTHI
LWRB
RTHI
LTHI
RKNE
LKNE
RKNE
RTIB
RTIB
LTIB
RANK
LANK
RANK
RTOE
LTOE
LHEE
RHEE

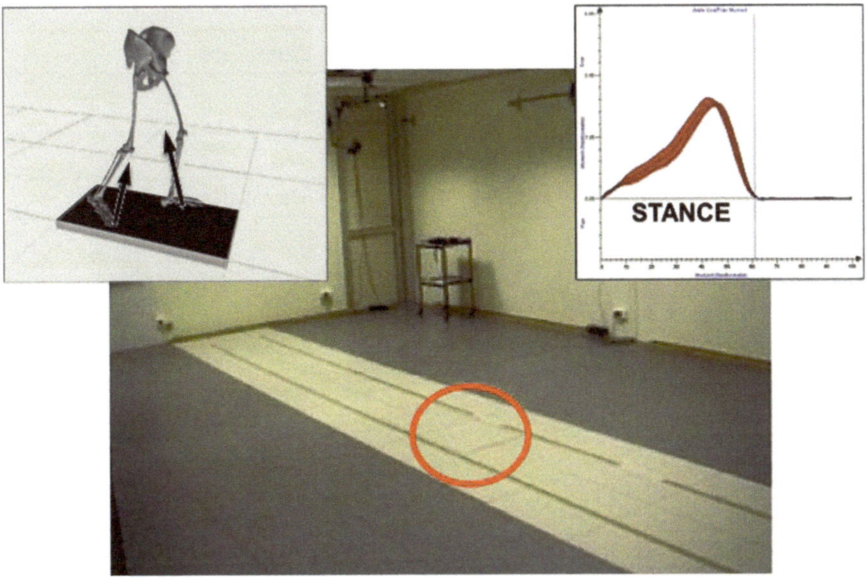

Fig. 4.8 Kinetics studies constraint mechanics with a ground force platform. The circle indicates the squared piece of platform with special sensors. The platform measures the force of reaction of the ground (left upper inset) during the stance phase of a walk (Kinetics - right upper inset)

4.3 Clinical Diagnosis and Evaluation

4.3.1 Clinical Characterization of Spasticity

Spasticity is a sign demonstrated by clinical examination during passive mobilization of limb segments.

Resistance to passive mobilization of the joint detects **exaggeration of the tonic stretch reflex**. The intensity of the resistance is proportional to the rate of stretching. This resistance is "elastic" and contrasts to the "plastic" resistance of extrapyramidal hypertonia, in which the limb remains in the position at which mobilization was stopped.

Stretching a limb segment can also trigger a triple flexion. A **triple flexion**, that is, limb withdrawal, may also be a response to stimulation of cutaneous or articular nociceptive or even nonnociceptive afferents. These responses are related to disinhibition of polysynaptic reflexes. They are particularly frequent after spinal cord injuries or in patient affected with a paraplegic form of multiple sclerosis.

Fig. 4.7 Trajectory analysis of hip, knee, and ankle is possible due to a set of cameras which record the position XYZ of markers in the determined space. One of the principles is to use cameras which send an infrared signal to retroreflective markers and to reconstruct the position of each limb segment and the evolution of the position during the motion cycle in the form of trajectories. (**a**) Room of the laboratory for dynamic gait analysis, (**b**) positions of markers for hip, knee, and foot motion study

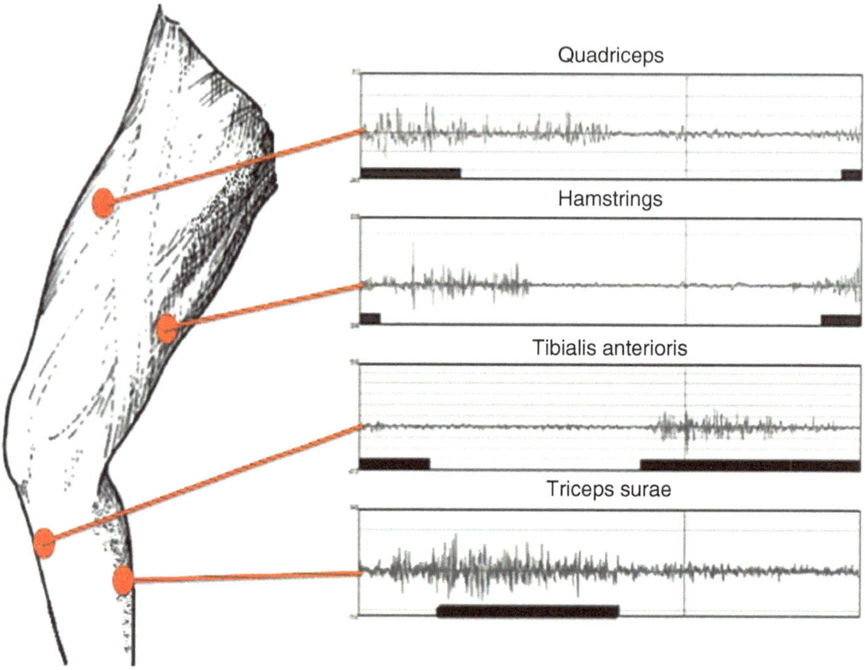

Fig. 4.9 Polyelectromyography recorded with surface electrodes during a walk (Courtesy of J. Luauté, University Lyon 1)

Stretching can trigger **clonus**, which also corresponds to an exaggerated stretch reflex. In the lower limbs it is often observed at the ankle, sometimes in the quadriceps, and may interfere with standing or gait. In the upper limb, clonus can be observed in the wrist and fingers.

Exaggeration of the stretch reflex is quantified by the **Ashworth scale** (Table 4.1) [7]. **Bohannon** [8] modified this scale in 1987 to evaluate flexion spasticity in the elbow of hemiplegic patients (Table 4.2).

The **Tardieu scale**, mostly used to quantify spasticity associated with cerebral palsy, integrates the concept of velocity-related variations and considers the clonus (Table 4.3). Its interobserver reliability is higher than that of the Ashworth scale [9].

Tendon hyperreflexia is caused by hyperexcitability of the stretch reflex arc. In spasticity, tendon reflexes are very brisk, diffuse, or even polykinetic. They can be absent in paraplegic patients with triple flexion due to tendon contractures. Tendon hyperreflexia is quantified by an intensity scale (Table 4.4).

4.3.2 Assessment of Range of Motion

The complete assessment includes goniometric measurements in supine and prone positions. Measurement of range motion can be performed without or with the help

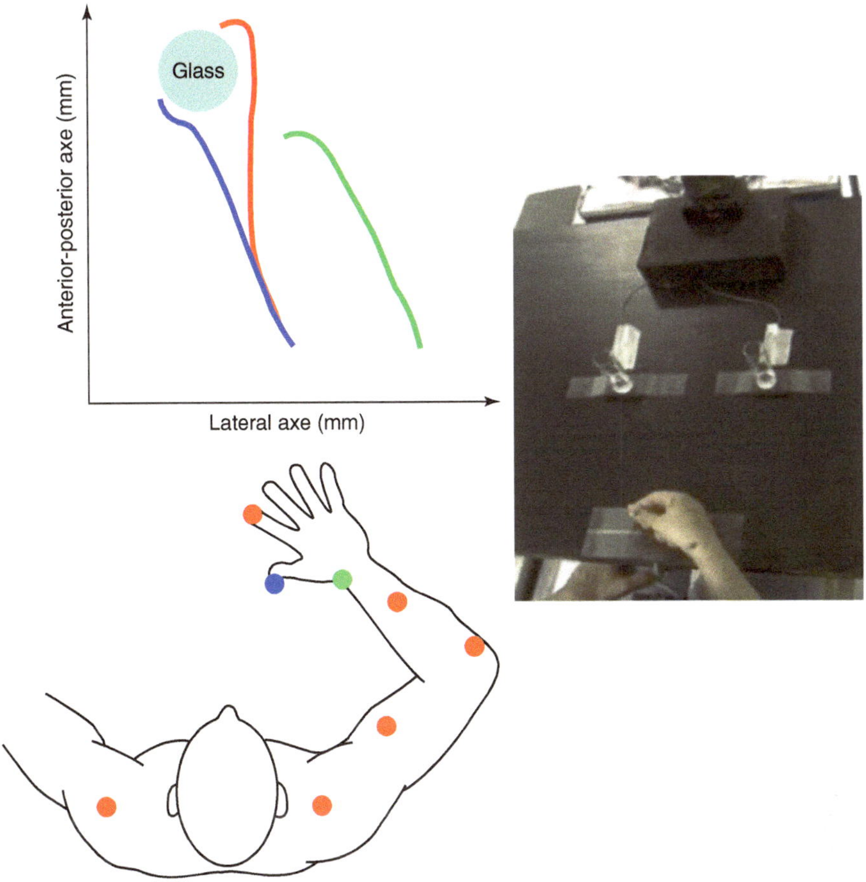

Fig. 4.10 Motion analysis at upper limb by the same technique as for gait. Markers are attached to upper limb, recording captures prehension of a glass (Courtesy of J. Luauté, University Lyon 1)

of a goniometer, the latter offering more precise estimation. The examination should have a rational sequence that requires minimal effort from the patient. After a single turn of the patient, the measurements in supine position are followed by the tests in prone position.

The measurement of passive range of motion determines the angle of arrest upon slow stretch of the muscle group assessed, which provides insight on soft-tissue length and extensibility. Each muscle group is first evaluated by very slow but powerful stretching.

For examination of the passive motion, any displacement from the rest position should be made with the maximal possible stretch but at slow speed in order to avoid any spastic involvement by retriggering the myotatic response. Moreover, excessive manipulations could cause microhemorrhages and subsequent chronic microcalcifications which would increase musculotendinous retractions as well as

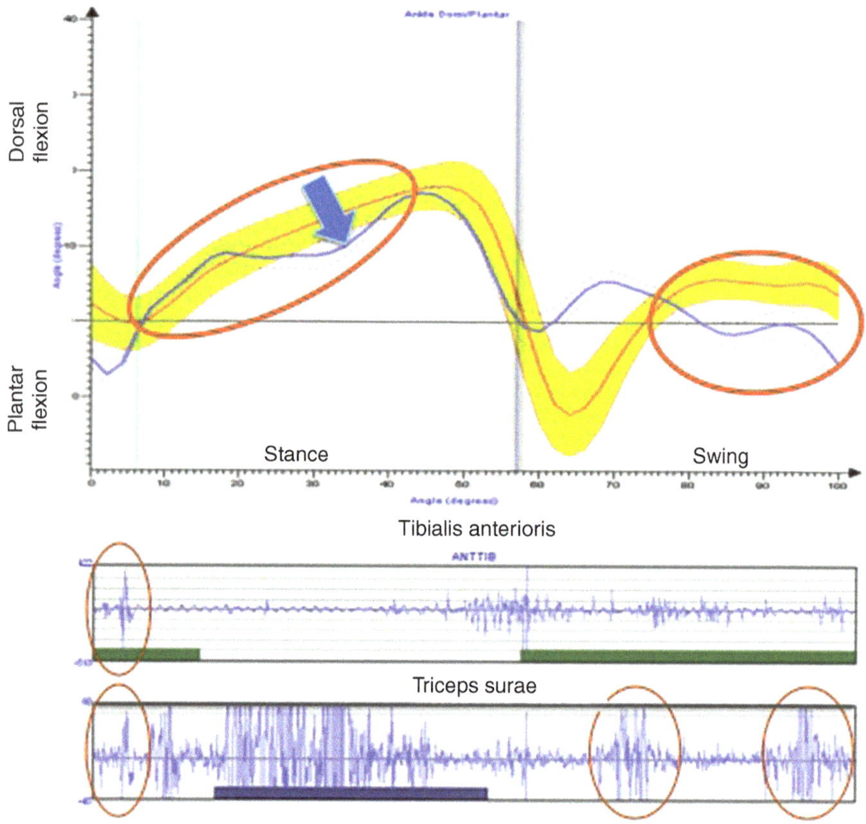

Fig. 4.11 Spastic foot. Ankle kinematics and electromyography of activity of tibialis anterioris and triceps surae. (**a**) Kinematics (*blue curve*) shows excessive plantar flexion at beginning of stance phase and slump of dorsal flexion during stance (*arrow*) and flattening of curve during swing phase (*yellow curve*, normal ankle motion). (**b**) Electromyography shows prolonged hyperactivity in triceps surae in stance phase and weak activity in tibialis anterioris, and intense activity in triceps surae in swing phase (Courtesy of J. Luauté, University Lyon 1)

capsular calcifications and subsequent ankylosis. The angle at which soft-tissue resistance is no longer overcome by the clinician is defined as the passive range of motion in the muscle group assessed. The stretching maneuver is ceased when the clinician appreciates that muscular and articular integrity is threatened or if pain occurs during examination.

If differentiation between permanent contracture and severe spastic posture is uncertain but such distinction becomes critical for therapeutic decisions, complementary techniques may be applied. They include a motor nerve block with local anesthetic, injections of botulinum toxin, or even the assessment of the passive range of motion under general anesthesia and relaxant agents.

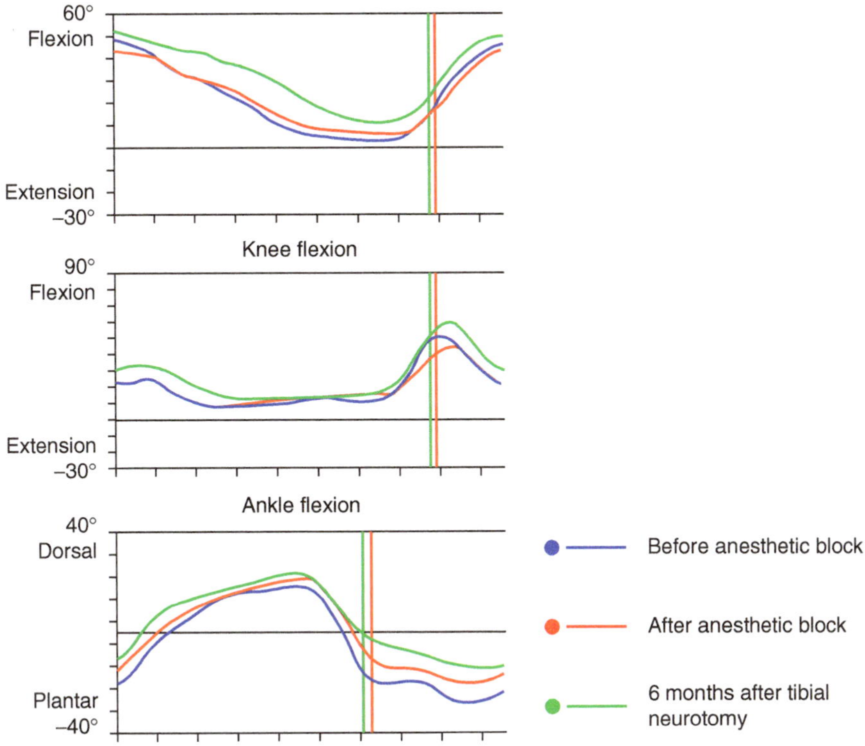

Fig. 4.12 Kinematic recordings of lower-limb motion in a hemiplegic patient before (*blue curve*) and after anesthetic block with bupivacaine of the tibial nerve (*red curve*) to predict the effect of a tibial neurotomy and 6 months after the completed neurotomy (*green curve*). Note improvement under anesthetic block and even more improvement after tibial neurotomy, particularly in ankle recording

In addition, it is very useful to evaluate the **active range of motion**. For each passive movement, the clinician asks the patient to perform an active movement against the muscle group evaluated, as far as possible until the active force produced by the agonist muscle group is neutralized by the combination of passive resistance and spastic formation coming from the stretched antagonist. The maximal range of active motion is thus obtained. Then the difference between the passive and the active range of motion is determined, which expresses the ability for potential therapeutic benefit up to the limit of possible contractures (Fig. 4.13).

One must keep in mind that the value of a range of motion assessment is only a static evaluation after a slow and passive solicitation. The assessment can take a dynamic character if the patient performs the same active movement over the maximal range as measured above, returns to the starting position, and then repeats the movement, as many times as possible over a set duration (alternating movement frequency).

Table 4.1 Ashworth scale for evaluation of spasticity in lower limbs

Criterion	Score
No increase in tone	0
Slight increase in tone giving a "catch" when limb is moved during flexion or extension	1
More marked increase in tone but limb easily flexed	2
Considerable increase in tone – passive movement difficult	3
Limb rigid during flexion or extension	4

The scale rates the exaggeration of the stretch reflex

Table 4.2 Bohannon scale for quantification of spasticity in upper limbs, namely, the elbow

Criterion	Score
No increase in muscle tone	0
No increase in muscle tone, manifested by a "catch" and release or by minimal resistance at end of range of motion when affected	1
Slight increase in muscle tone, manifested by a "catch" followed by minimal resistance throughout the remainder (less than half) of range motion	1+
More marked increase in muscle tone through most of range motion, but affected part(s) easily moved	2
Considerable increase in muscle tone, passive movement difficult	3
Affected part(s) rigid during flexion or extension	4

The scale is a modification of Ashworth scale

Table 4.3 Tardieu scale for evaluation of spasticity associated with cerebral palsy

Criterion	Symbol or score
Speeds at which affected part(s) are passively moved:	
As slow as possible	V1
Intermediate speed	V2
As rapid as possible	V3
Parameters measured:	
Type of muscle reaction	X
Angle at which muscle reaction occurs	Y
Types of muscle reaction:	
No increase in muscle tone throughout the range of motion	0
Slight increase in muscle tone without any "catch" at a particular angle	1
"Catch" interrupting the movement at a particular angle, followed by muscular release	2
Exhaustible clonus (less than 10 s for a permanent stretch) appearing at a particular angle	3
Inexhaustible clonus (more than 10 s for a permanent stretch), appearing at a particular angle	4

Table 4.4 Scale for evaluation of intensity of tendon hyperreflexia

Tendon reflex	Score
Absent	0
Present but weak	1
Normal	2
Brisk	3

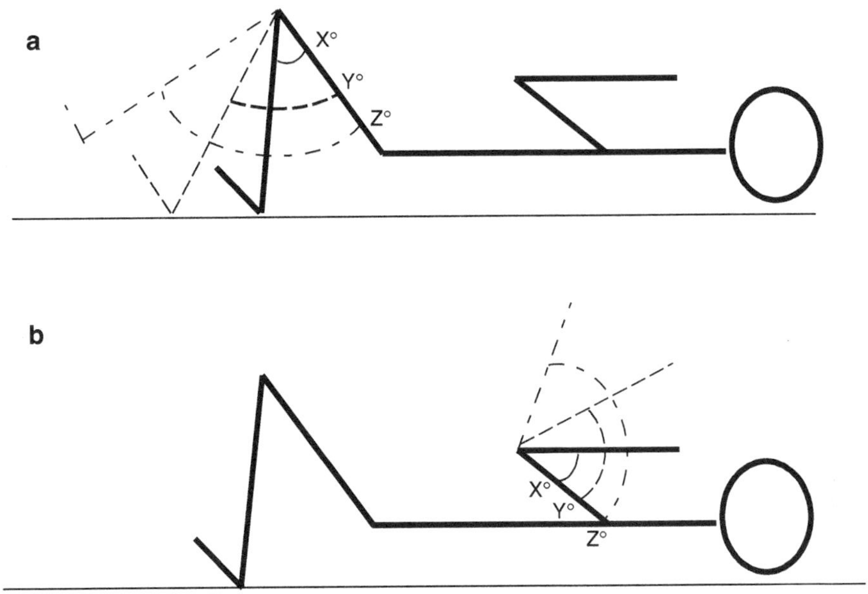

Fig. 4.13 Range of motion assessment for spastic patients in supine position. *X°* Angle of active range of motion, *Y°* angle of passive range of motion under slow stretching, *Z°* angle of range of motion after motor nerve block, botulinum toxin injection, or general anesthesia with relaxants. (**a**) Lower limb, (**b**) upper limb

4.3.3 Retractions and Contractures

Spastic reflex contraction, associated with a deficit of antagonist muscles, predisposes to muscle retraction. When retraction predominates over spasticity, a reduction of spasticity will not be sufficient to improve the patient's functional ability (Fig. 4.14). Patients with central neurological lesions are immobilized, which offers sufficient cause for muscle retraction.

4.3.4 Electrophysiological Diagnosis

The diagnosis of spasticity is clinical. However, it may be useful to complete the clinical evaluation by electrophysiological recordings, especially to quantify the effect of treatments.

The **H reflex**, first described by Hoffman in 1918 [10], is commonly measured in the soleus component of the triceps surae. It can also be recorded at rest in the quadriceps on the anterior aspect of the thigh or in the flexor carpi radialis on the anterior aspect of the forearm. The stretch reflex is studied by recording the muscle response to tendon percussion, the **T reflex**. The amplitude of the reflex response depends on the gain of the primary neuromuscular spindle nerve endings. In contrast, the reflex

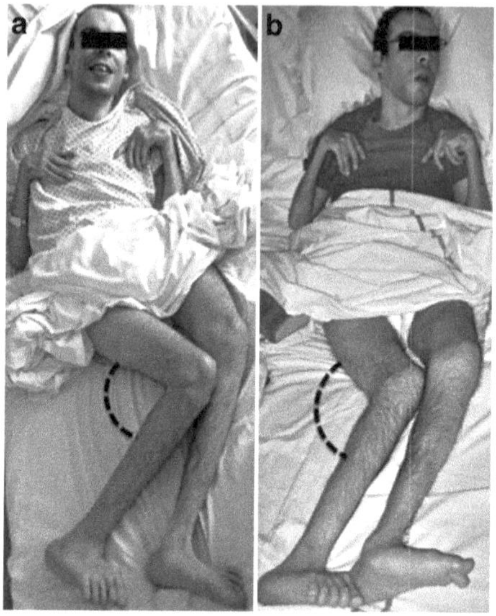

Fig. 4.14 Tetraplegic adult patient with cerebral palsy shows irreducible contractures and deformities. Bed rest before (**a**) and after (**b**) neurosurgical intervention for spasticity (lumbar microsurgical lesion in the dorsal root entry zone at the lumbosacral spinal cord segments). After surgery, retractions and contractures still remain. However, there is a notable increase of the angles of (passive) range of motion of both lower limbs (*dotted lines*) due to decrease of spasticity

is obtained by direct stimulation of proprioceptive fibers. The difference between these two types of reflex can be used to evaluate the control of the spindle system (i.e., the gamma motoneuron activity) [11].

Ib inhibition can be studied by various protocols of double-shock conditioning the reflex. For example, the reflex of the soleus can be conditioned by stimulation applied to the nerve to the medial head of the gastrocnemius with an interstimulus interval of 6 ms. In conditioned reflex protocols, Ib inhibition lasts less than 10 ms [12].

4.3.4.1 H Reflex

The H reflex is the electrically elicited equivalent of the tendon jerk (myotatic reflex), both being mediated through activation of motoneurons by the primary spindle afferents (Fig. 4.15). For normal adults, studies of the H reflex are restricted mostly to the soleus and the flexor carpi radialis muscles. For upper motor neuron lesions, the H reflex may be elicited in muscles where normally it is rarely seen (e.g., intrinsic hand muscles, tibialis anterior, peroneal muscles).

Since the electrical stimulus is easier to control than the mechanical, the H reflex is more extensively used in studies of spasticity. However, there are only a few accessible sites where the H reflex can be elicited, and this is a disadvantage in comparison to the tendon jerk. This quantitative approach is one of the methods used to assess spasticity as an entity that involves the hyperreactivity of spinal reflex and the peripheral changes within the muscles themselves.

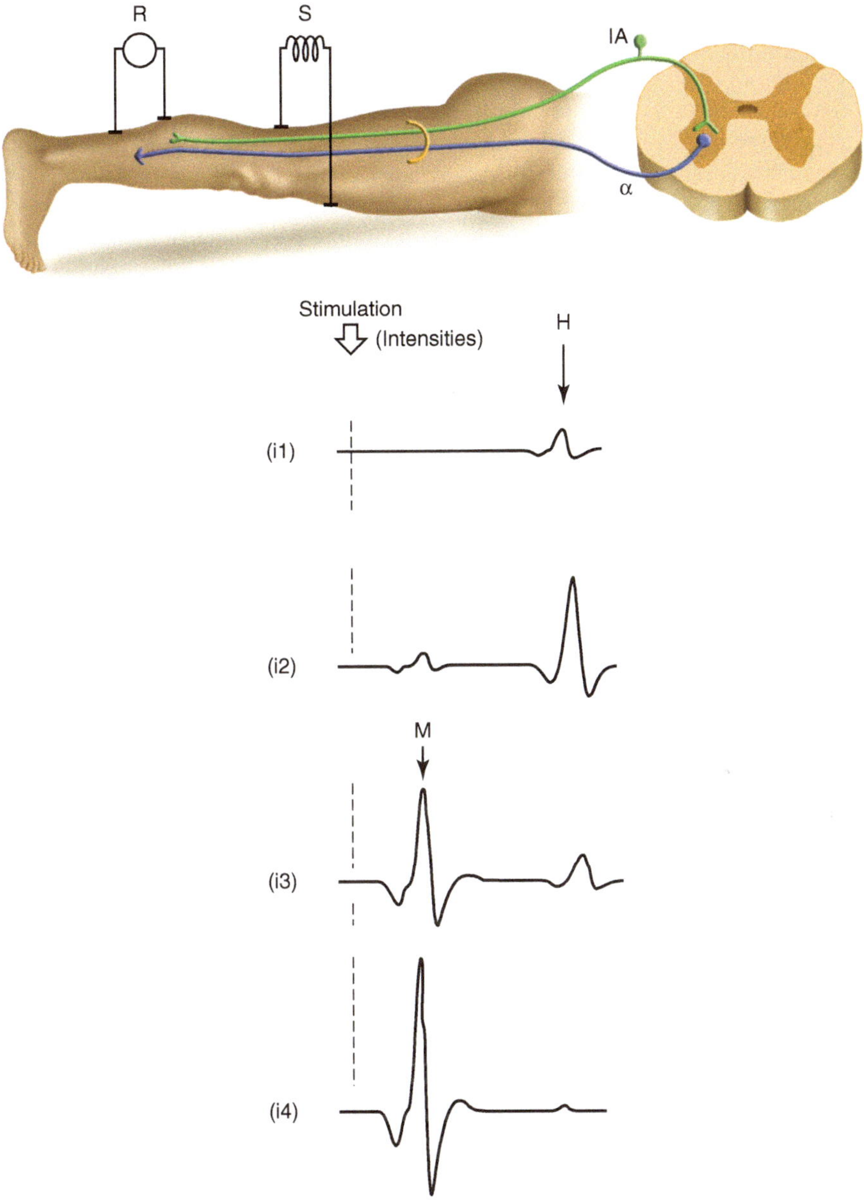

Fig. 4.15 Method of recording the *H* reflex, which explores the monosynaptic pathways (IA afferent fiber to alpha motoneuron). Stimulation (*S*) of tibial nerve at popliteal fossa and recording (*R*) of motor response of soleus muscle. Increasing the stimulation intensities results in the occurrence of the H reflex (*i1*, *i2*). When stimulation intensities continue to increase, the H reflex disappears, by collision with the recruitment of motor fibers that is manifested by the increasing amplitude of direct motor response (*M*; *i3*, *i4*)

4.3.4.2 H_{max}/M_{max} Ratio

The H_{max}/M_{max} ratio as the ratio of maximal amplitudes of the H reflex and the M response is a good indicator of spasticity, especially in the soleus muscle (Fig. 4.15). Electrical stimulation of the tibial nerve gives first a short-latency (6 ms) response, designated M, which is the muscle response to motor nerve stimulation, and a second one with longer latency (30 ms), designated H, which is the 1A monosynaptic reflex (Hoffman). When the intensity of stimulation is increased, first the H and later the M waves reach a maximum. Electrophysiological recording of the H reflex and determination of the ratio of the maximum amplitude of this reflex response (H_{max}) to the maximum amplitude of the direct motor response (M_{max}) measures the excitable fraction of the spinal cord motoneuron pool participating in the myotatic reflex. The ratio H_{max}/M_{max} is considered to accurately reflect the excitability of the motoneuron pool of the muscle recorded. This ratio is normally 0.5. An increase in the ratio greater than 0.5 indicates that more than half of the motoneuron pool is excited by stimulation of afferents derived from this muscle. In spastic cases the ratio rises up to 0.8 due to hyperexcitability of alpha motoneurons. Motoneurons that discharge in the H reflex undergo excitability changes which last for up to 5 s.

4.3.4.3 H-Wave Excitability Curve

The nature and the degree of changes in excitability may be assessed by measuring the H-wave excitability curve (or H-wave recovery curve). This curve is constructed by introducing a conditioning stimulus at various intervals preceding a test stimulus [13]. For normal adults, two electrical shocks applied on the tibial nerve need to be separated by at least 100–150 ms, to give identical H responses. For spastic patients, this delay is shorter and the second H reflex reaches a higher amplitude than the first one. This means that the late period of facilitation begins earlier and is enhanced in spastic patients.

When performing dorsal rhizotomy for spasticity, some authors base the selection of the dorsal roots to be cut on the detection by intraoperative monitoring of the roots harboring “abnormal responses”. The method consists of the intraoperative study of the H-reflex recovery curve. An increased H_2/H_1 ratio (the ratio of the second to the first H curve) indicates involvement in the spastic process. When a pair of stimuli with a varying interstimulus interval is applied to the posterior tibial nerve (as most frequently done in current practice), and the ratio of the amplitudes of the initial and subsequent H responses (H_2/H_1) is plotted against the interstimulus interval, the H-reflex recovery curve can be measured. Patients with upper motor neuron lesion, namely, patients with cerebral palsy, exhibit more rapid and complete recovery with less late inhibition than normal, due to increased excitability of the motor neuron and reduced presynaptic inhibition.

In intraoperative conditions, stimulation can be delivered to the dorsal root proximal to the ganglion. All dorsal roots can be explored, the recording electrodes (preferably a surface electrode) being placed over the appropriate muscle group innervated by its corresponding root [14, 15]. The technique was described in detail by Nishida and Storrs [14, 15]. Each root and rootlet was stimulated at a rate of 1, 2, 5, 10, 20, and 50 Hz, and the ratio of subsequent H (i.e., H_2) to H_1 was determined at each rate of stimulation. Those roots and rootlets considered normal had a ratio of less than 50 % at all frequencies tested. Those considered abnormal had a ratio of more than 50 % or at times over 100 % at any frequency. Other criteria of abnormality which were clinically observed were sustained tonic or clonic contraction that persisted following cessation of stimulation and/or the spread of contractions to other muscle groups outside the stimulated myotome.

4.4 Functional Disability Attributed to Spasticity

After the diagnosis of spasticity has been established, the next important step is to demonstrate that this symptom interferes with the patient's motor capacities and that reduction of this symptom by treatment could offer actually a true improvement.

The Oswestry scale quantifies disability (Table 4.5). The Global Functional Disability scale of Lyon University (Table 4.6) evaluates the global functional capability of spastic paraplegic patients. It quantifies five components which are part of the patient's everyday life and are directly influenced by spasticity and resulting abnormal postures and articular limitations. The score ranges from 0 to

Table 4.5 Oswestry scale for quantification of functional disability

Criterion	Score
Solely spastic No willed movement; tonic reflexes or spinal reflexes present	0
Very severe spasticity Movement very poor, total spastic synergy in one pattern only (i.e., only total extension if limb is passively flexed or only total flexion from an extended position)	1
Severe spasticity Movement poor, marked total spastic synergy but during both flexion and extension patterns (i.e., patient can flex extended limb and extend flexed limb, with or without some isolated proximal control)	2
Moderate spasticity Movement fair, spasticity synergy, but some isolated control in a small range of movement at a distal joint (ankle or wrist)	3
Mild spasticity Movement good with isolated distal control possible in good range; spastic synergy still apparent on reinforcement by resistance to the movement or by effort exerted in another part of body	4
No spasticity Movement normal; no spastic synergy	5

Table 4.6 Global Functional Disability scale of Lyon University for paraplegic patients with spasticity in lower limbs

Criterion	Score
Pain:	
Absent	0
Rare and mild; no disability	1
Frequent; minimal disability	2
Marked and frequent; marked disability	3
Permanent and severe	4
Spasms:	
Absent	0
Rare and mild spasms only during mobilization; no disability	1
Frequent, spontaneous but moderate spasms; some disability	2
Frequent, spontaneous and marked spasms; marked disability	3
Almost constant and severe spasms; severe disability, major problems for sitting and lying	4
Sitting position:	
Normal	0
Mild difficulty	1
Moderate difficulty	2
Severe difficulty, patient has to be tied down in position	3
Impossible	4
Body transfer:	
Normal	0
Mild difficulty	1
Moderate difficulty	2
Marked difficulty, needs one person helping	3
Severe difficulty, needs two persons helping	4
Washing and dressing:	
Normal	0
Mild difficulty	1
Moderate difficulty	2
Marked difficulty, needs one person helping	3
Severe difficulty, needs two persons helping	4

A score of 10 out of 20 corresponds to a functional disability indicating neurosurgery to be considered for spasticity

4 for each component, with a total of 20 out of 20 denoting a bedridden and totally dependent patient. A score of 10 out of 20 corresponds to the threshold between a minimally acceptable condition and an unacceptable condition. It was reproducibly identified as the lowest value at which surgery should be considered [16–19].

Similar global functional disability scales have been designed at Lyon University for hemiplegic patients with spasticity in lower limb (Table 4.7) or upper limb (Table 4.8).

Table 4.7 Global Functional Disability scale of Lyon University for hemiplegic patients with spasticity in lower limb

Criterion	Score
Pain:	
Absent	0
Rare and mild; not generating (by itself) reduction in use	1
Mild but frequent; generating some reduction in use	2
Marked and frequent; generating significant reduction in use	3
Permanent and severe; making (by itself) any use impossible	4
Passive mobilization (of knee):	
Normal amplitude of range of motion	0
Moderate limitation for <25 % of range of motion	1
Significant limitation for 25–50 % of range of motion	2
Marked limitation for >50 % of range of motion	3
Totally fixed	4
Sitting position:	
Normal	0
Mild difficulty	1
Moderate to marked difficulty; causing reduction of sitting periods	2
Severe difficulty; patient has to be tied down in position	3
Impossible	4
Walking:	
Normal	0
Mild difficulty; somewhat limited reach	1
Moderate difficulty; needs splint	2
Marked difficulty; needs splint and cane, but autonomous	3
Nonambulatory; needs wheelchair for transfers	4
Washing and dressing:	
Normal	0
Mild difficulty	1
Moderate difficulty; still autonomous	2
Marked difficulty; overcome by one person helping	3
Severe difficulty; not overcome by one person helping	4

Clinicians can use three tests to temporarily eliminate the spasticity symptom in order to study its influence on motor function and range of motion as well as the resulting abnormal postures. These are motor blocks by injection of a local anesthetic, botulinum toxin injections, and intrathecal baclofen infusion. For motor blocks, the most commonly used anesthetic molecule is bupivacaine (Fig. 4.16). Onset starts 10 min after injection and the effect lasts 2 h on average. Indication is bothersome for focal spasticity affecting one or several muscle groups (e.g., thigh adductors, varus foot drop, elbow flexors, finger or wrist flexors). The effect of the block is predictive of the effect of a peripheral neurotomy or a lesioning procedure with a nerve-blocking agent, namely, phenol or alcohol. Botulinum toxin injections may be used as a blocking test with a long duration of effect. Blocks give the patient

Table 4.8 Global Functional Disability scale of Lyon University for hemiplegic patients with spasticity in upper limb

Criterion	Score
Pain:	
Absent	0
Rare and mild; not generating (by itself) reduction in use	1
Frequent; generating some reduction in use	2
Marked and frequent; generating significant reduction in use	3
Permanent and severe; making (by itself) any use impossible	4
Passive mobilization (at elbow):	
Normal amplitude of range of motion	0
Moderate limitation for <25 % of range of motion	1
Significant limitation for 25–50 % of range of motion	2
Marked limitation for >50 % of range of motion	3
Totally fixed	4
Active mobilization (at elbow):	
Normal	0
<25 % of range of motion	1
25–50 % of range of motion	2
>50 % of range of motion	3
Totally impossible	4
Function (hand):	
Normal	0
Mild difficulty; but fine prehension still possible	1
Marked difficulty; only gross prehension possible	2
Severe difficulty; passive prehension with help	3
Prehension totally impossible	4
Washing and dressing:	
Normal	0
Mild difficulty	1
Moderate difficulty; still autonomous	2
Marked difficulty; overcome by one person helping	3
Severe difficulty; not overcome by one person helping	4

an idea of the expected effect of the treatment; they are most useful to define the objectives of the envisaged treatment not only for the patient but also for the caregivers [20]. Intrathecal baclofen infusion can be used also as a test. Baclofen, an agonist acting on presynaptic γ-aminobutyric acid-B receptors of the nerve endings of the lA type fibers [21, 22], significantly reduces spasticity and polysynaptic flexion (or extension) reflexes [23, 24]. This test is performed through lumbar puncture or via an access port which delivers the agent directly into the subarachnoid space at the level of the conus medullaris.

A precise assessment and determination of the extent to which spasticity is harmful in the particular examined patient are prerequisites for any therapeutic decision. The aim is to predict the potential benefits and to define the objectives and limits of considered surgical treatments.

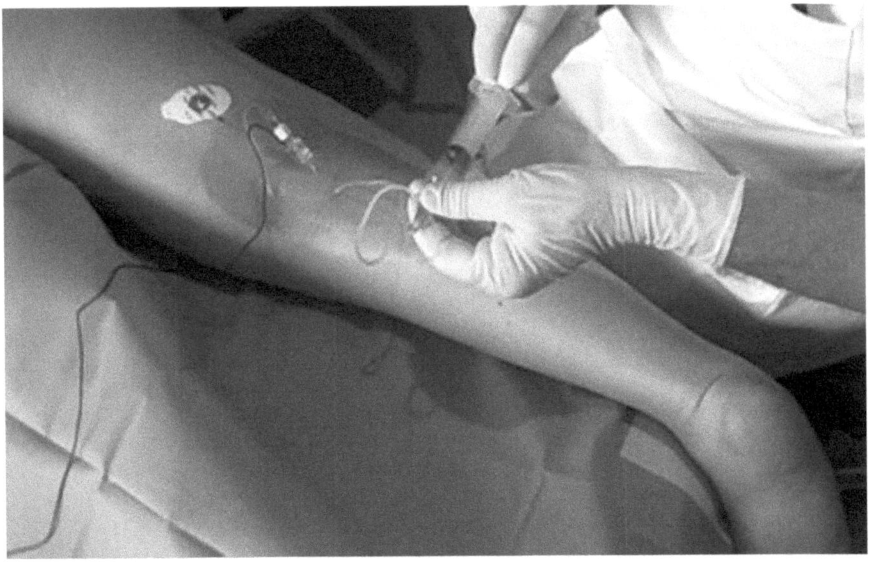

Fig. 4.16 Motor block test with bupivacaine of tibial nerve for right spastic foot to predict the effect of envisaged tibial neurotomy. Nerve was detected by percutaneous electrical stimulation connected to the needle for injection. Note the equino-varus posture of the foot

References

1. Lance JW (1980) Symposium synopsis. In: Feldman RG, Young RR, Koella WP (eds) Spasticity: disordered motor control. Symposia Specialists, Miami, pp 485–494
2. Boisacq-Schepens N (1998) Le contrôle moteur de la marche. Neurochirurgie 44:158–166
3. Johnson GR (2002) Outcome measures of spasticity. Eur J Neurol 9(Suppl 1):10–16; discussion 53–61
4. McGinley JL, Goldie PA, Greenwood KM, Olney SJ (2003) Accuracy and reliability of observational gait analysis data: judgments of push-off in gait after stroke. Phys Ther 83:146–160
5. Subramanian N, Vaughan CL, Peter JC, Arens LJ (1998) Gait before and 10 years after rhizotomy in children with cerebral palsy spasticity. J Neurosurg 88:1014–1019
6. Novachek TF, Gage JR (2007) Orthopedic management of spasticity in cerebral palsy. Childs Nerv Syst 23:1015–1031
7. Ashworth B (1964) Preliminary trial of carisoprodol in multiple sclerosis. Practitioner 192:540–542
8. Bohannon RW, Smith MB (1987) Interpreter reliability of a modified Ashworth scale of muscle spasticity. Phys Ther 67:206–207
9. Gracies JM (2001) Evaluation de la spasticité: rapport de l'echelle de Tardieu. Mot Cereb 22:1–16
10. Hoffmann P (1918) Über die Beziehungen der Sehnenreflexe zur willkürlichen Bewegung und zum Tonus. Z Biol 68:351–370
11. Bishop B, Machover S, Johnston R, Anderson M (1968) A quantitative assessment of gamma-motoneuron contribution to the Achilles tendon reflex in normal subjects. Arch Phys Med Rehabil 49:145–154
12. Pierrot-Deseilligny E, Katz R, Morin C (1979) Evidence of lb inhibition in human subjects. Brain Res 166:176–179

13. Táboríková H, Sax DS (1968) Motoneurone pool and the H-reflex. J Neurol Neurosurg Psychiatry 31:354–361
14. Nishida T, Storrs BB (1991) Electrophysiological monitoring in selective posterior rhizotomy for spasticity: principles, techniques and interpretation of responses. In: Sindou M, Abbott R, Keravel Y (eds) Neurosurgery for spasticity. Springer, Wien/New York, pp 159–163
15. Storrs BB, Nishida T (1988) Use of the 'H' reflex recovery curve in selective posterior rhizotomy. Pediatr Neurosci 14:120–123
16. Sindou M, Millet MF, Mortamais J, Eyssette M (1982) Results of selective posterior rhizotomy in the treatment of painful and spastic paraplegia secondary to multiple sclerosis. Appl Neurophysiol 45:335–340
17. Sindou M, Jeanmonod D (1989) Microsurgical DREZ-otomy for the treatment of spasticity and pain in the lower limbs. Neurosurgery 24:655–670
18. Millet MF, Mortamais J, Sindou M, Eyssette M, Boisson D, Bourret J (1981) Neurochirurgie dans les paraplégiques spastiques et douloureuses de la sclérose en plaques: résultats à moyen terme de la radicellotomie postérieure sélective dans 12 cas. In: Simon L (ed) Actualités en rééducation fonctionelle et réadaptation, ser 6. Masson, Paris, pp 76–85
19. Sindou M, Jeanmonod D, Mertens P, Millet MF (1991) Surgery in the dorsal root entry zone: microsurgical DREZ-otomy (MDT) for the treatment of spasticity. In: Sindou M, Abbott R, Keravel Y (eds) Neurosurgery for spasticity. Springer, Wien/New York, pp 165–182
20. Filipetti P, Decq P (2003) L'apport des blocs anesthésiques dans l'évaluation du patient spastique. Neurochirurgie 49:226–238
21. Jiménez I, Rudomin P, Enriquez M (1991) Differential effects of (−)-baclofen on la and descending monosynaptic EPSPs. Exp Brain Res 85:103–113
22. Stuart GJ, Redman SJ (1992) The role of GABAA and GABAB receptors in presynaptic inhibition of la EPSPs in cat spinal motoneurones. J Physiol 447:675–692
23. Azouvi P, Mane M, Thiebaut JB, Denys P, Remy-Neris O, Bussel B (1996) Intrathecal baclofen administration for control of severe spinal spasticity: functional improvement and long-term follow-up. Arch Phys Med Rehabil 77:35–39
24. Penn R, Kroin JS (1985) Continuous intrathecal Baclofen for severe spasticity. Lancet 2:125–127

Decision-Making for Treatment of Adults with Disabling Spasticity

5

Spasticity should not be treated just because it is present; it should be treated when it is harmful. Indeed, paralyzed patients may make use of spasticity for functional activities. An extensor pattern in the lower limb(s) allows the hemiplegic patient to walk and helps the paraplegic patient in standing transfers. In these scenarios, a "successful" treatment of the spasticity, as measured by reduction in tone and improved range of motion, could well reduce rather than enhance function [1]. Differentiation of reversible abnormal postures from fixed deformities is of prime importance before indicating surgical treatment. Operative methods for a reduction of spasticity can be classified according to their effects being either focal or general and being either permanent or temporary (Fig. 5.1). Anatomical targets are illustrated in Fig. 5.2.

Intrathecal baclofen (ITB) administration is indicated for para- or tetraplegic patients with severe diffuse spasticity, especially from a spinal origin. Because of its reversible effects, this method must be considered before an ablative procedure. However, the range between an excessive hypotonia with loss of strength and an insufficient effect is narrow. An intrathecal test through a temporary access port can be useful before proceeding to permanent implantation.

Neurolesioning techniques are indicated for severe spasticity in the limbs of paraplegic, tetraplegic, or hemiplegic patients. Neurotomies are indicated when spasticity is focalized and corresponds to muscle groups innervated by a single or a small number of peripheral nerve(s). When spasticity globally affects a limb, microsurgery in the dorsal root entry zone may be preferred. When needed, several types of neurodestructive procedures can be combined in the same patient.

In our view, orthopedic surgery should be considered only after spasticity has been reduced by pharmacological treatments and, if necessary, by neurosurgical procedures. The general rule is to tailor treatment to every individual patient. Guidelines for surgical indications are schematized in Figs. 5.3 and 5.4.

M. Sindou et al., *Neurosurgery for Spasticity*,
DOI 10.1007/978-3-7091-1771-2_5, © Springer-Verlag Wien 2014

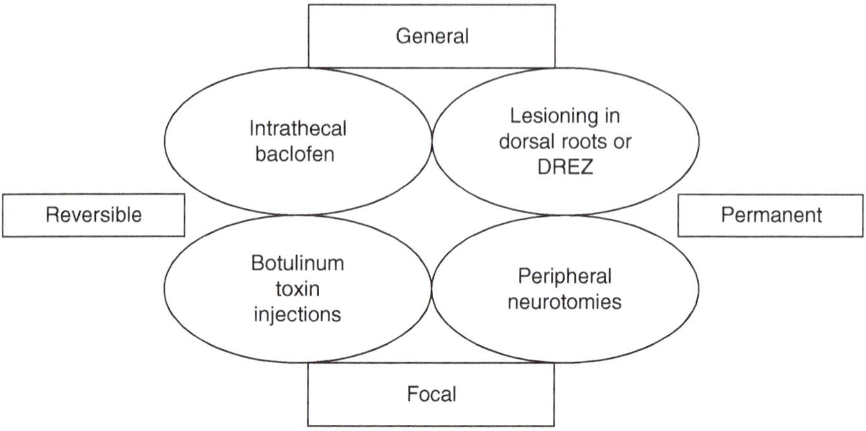

Fig. 5.1 Methods for controlling spasticity, based on whether harmful spasticity is focal or general and whether effect is intended to be permanent or temporary

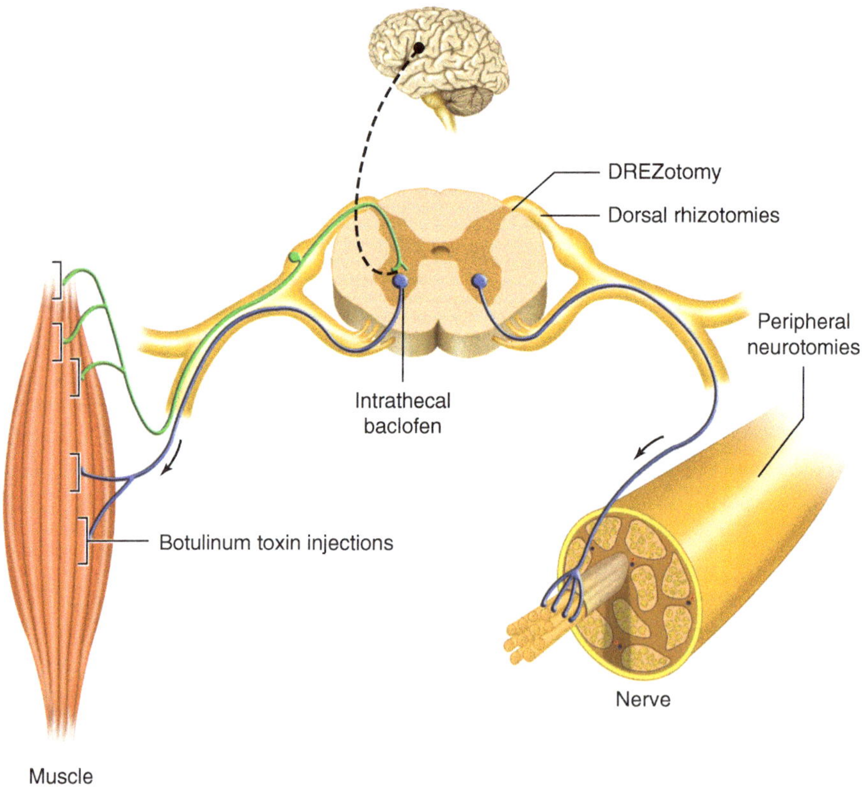

Fig. 5.2 Operative methods for reduction of spasticity and their anatomical targets

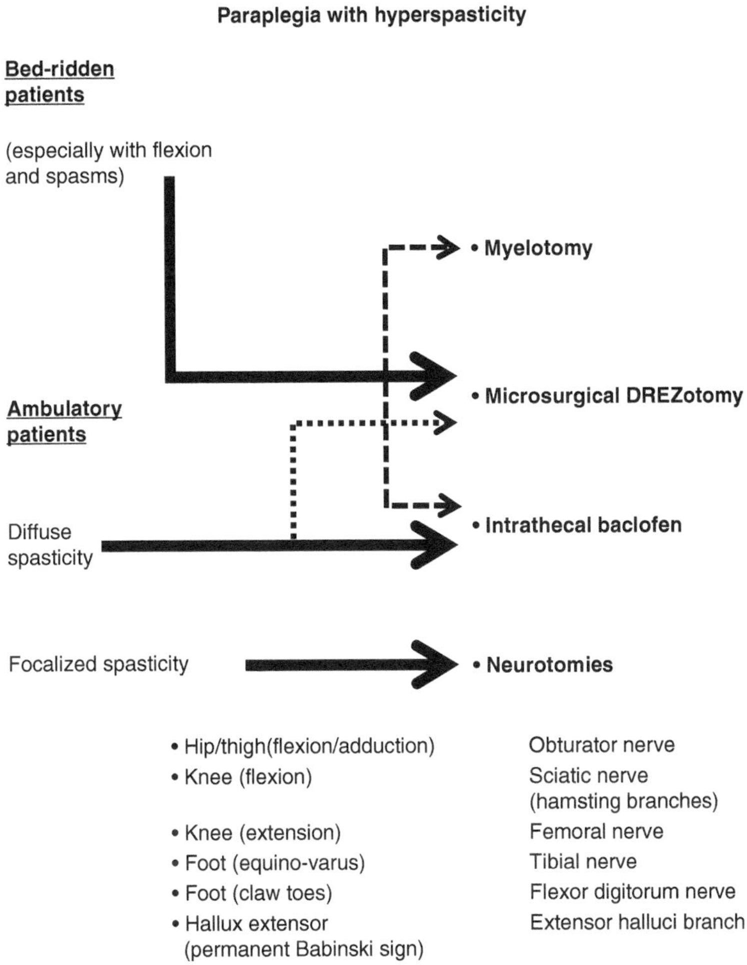

Fig. 5.3 Algorithm for treatment of paraplegic patients with disabling hyperspasticity

5.1 Intrathecal Baclofen Therapy

To overcome the obstacle of poor transfer of baclofen through the blood–central nervous system barrier, Penn and Kroin introduced a new treatment of spasticity: direct spinal intrathecal administration of baclofen [2]. The effectiveness of the method is linked to the presence of high concentrations of γ-aminobutyric acid-B binding sites in the dorsal horn, which allow the necessary dosage to be decreased from an average of 10–90 mg/day orally to an average of 20–800 μg/day intrathecally. The method uses a programmable pump device implanted subcutaneously. The pump consists of a reservoir that contains the drug. It is refilled percutaneously about every 3 months. A programmable pump provides the desired flow. The most appropriate and sophisticated pump is the Synchromed pump from Medtronic Co.

Hemiplegia with hyperspasticity

Upper limb

Diffuse spasticity with proximal predominance	→	**Microsurgical DREZotomy**
Diffuse spasticity with distal predominance	→	**Microsurgical DREZotomy** (with neurotomy of Median + ulnar flexor branches)
Focalized spasticity	→	**Neurotomies**
• Shoulder (internal rotation/adduction)		Brachial plexus branches
• Elbow (flexion)		Musculocutaneous nerve
• Wrist, hand, fingers (pronation/flexion)		Median ± ulnar nerve

Lower limb

Spastic foot: Neurotomy tibial nerve

• With Equinus	Triceps surae
• With Varus	Posterior tibialis
• With Flexion of toes (claw)	Flexor fascicles of toes

Hallux extensor (permanent Babinski sign): Neurotomy of extensor halluci branch

Fig. 5.4 Algorithm for treatment of hemiplegic patients with disabling hyperspasticity

(Minneapolis, MN) [3]. ITB therapy can be preceded by a test to screen for an adequate response to the medication. The common standard procedure is as follows. The patient receives a single trial dose of 50–100 μg of intrathecal baclofen via lumbar puncture or via a temporary intrathecal lumbar catheter connected to a subcutaneous access reservoir. In the absence of a positive response, as indicated by a reduction in the Ashworth score 4–8 h after drug administration, the bolus dose is increased in 25 μg increments up to a maximum bolus of 100 μg. Once a positive response is observed without an unacceptable loss of function, the patient is considered a candidate for pump implantation. However, the bolus dose response is a poor guide to the likely daily infusion rate that the patient will need. Furthermore, the bolus method may produce a harsh and/or exaggerated loss of motor power and muscle tone that patients may interpret as a decrease in their functional status. Such a response could eliminate the indication for pump implantation. Especially for patients who can walk, the bolus test should be replaced by a continuous-infusion test, using an external automatic injection pump connected to a line punctured into the subcutaneous reservoir. The test should last a few days to an entire week so that functional capabilities can be reliably evaluated. The initial postimplantation infusion dose partially depends on the effective screening dose. The most useful criteria for dose adjustment are the effective suppression of the reflexes (i.e., tendon jerk, clonus, spasms, cramps) and decrease in muscle tone. A programmable pump allowing cyclical dose adjustments makes it possible to provide levels that correlate with the daily variability of spastic symptoms.

ITB is particularly indicated for patients with severe spasticity of spinal cord origin [4], especially if spasms are painful, as for patients with advanced multiple sclerosis, or after spinal cord injury when physical therapy and rehabilitation have failed to prevent harmful spasticity from developing. A multicenter study with 205 patients studied doses at 12 months and the safety and efficacy of ITB in the treatment of spasticity of spinal origin. Doses ranged between 167 and 462 μg/day (average, 298 μg). Mean Ashworth scores decreased from 3–4 to 0.5–1.8 [5].

ITB can be also indicated for hyperspasticity related to brain or brainstem lesions. It has also been used to treat cerebral palsy patients [6]. Because the available pump is large, ITB can hardly be performed in children younger than 6 years. Children with associated choreo-athetosis, hypotonia of neck and trunk, obesity, poor motivation and/or severe multiple deformities or combinations thereof are poor candidates for ITB. Adequate doses (i.e., those effectively treating excessive tone while not producing motor weakness) are often difficult to establish for patients with cerebral palsy, especially for those able to walk. Overdosage is a risk of ITB administration and could be irreversible because of the lack of true baclofen antagonists. This remains quite rare if the technique is performed prudently. Other complications include mechanical catheter migration, occlusion or infection; these require revision or removal of the system, respectively. The advantage of ITB is its reversibility. On the other hand, it is expensive, and periodic refilling and reprogramming are necessary. Geographic dependence is another limitation to this conservative therapy.

5.2 Neurolesioning Procedures

When spasticity cannot be controlled by conservative methods, such as ITB or botulinum toxin injections, neurolesioning procedures can be considered. The surgery should be performed so that excessive hypertonia is reduced, without suppressing useful muscular tone or impairing residual motor and sensory functions. Neurolesioning techniques must be selective whatever their target may be: the peripheral nerves, spinal roots, spinal cord, or dorsal root entry zone.

Peripheral neurotomies were first introduced by Stoffel [7] for the treatment of spastic deformities. Later, Gros and coworkers [8] and Sindou and Mertens [9, 10] attempted to make neurotomies more selective by microsurgical dissections and intraoperative electrical stimulation, which allows better identification of the function of the various fascicles constituting the nerves. Selectivity is required to suppress excessive spasticity without weakening motor strength too much and causing severe amyotrophy and trophic ulcers. To achieve this goal, at least 25 % of the motor fibers must be spared. Neurotomies are indicated when harmful spasticity is focal, that is, localized to muscles or muscular groups supplied by a single (or a few) peripheral nerve(s). To help the surgeon decide, anesthetic block of the nerve, in our practice with 3 h of activity of bupivacaine, is useful. The test determines whether articular limitations result from spasticity or from musculotendinous contractures and articular ankyloses. Only spasticity is decreased by the test. The test also gives the patient an idea of what to expect from the operation. Botulinum toxin injections, in addition to their therapeutic value, may act as a "prolonged" test for several weeks or months.

At the lower limbs, neurotomies of the tibial nerve at the popliteal region and of the obturator nerve just below the subpubic canal are the most commonly performed, for the so-called spastic foot and the spastic flexion-adduction hip deformity, respectively. For knee flexor spasticity, neurotomy of the hamstrings branches of the sciatic nerve can be performed at the level of the sciatic trunk through a short skin incision at the buttock. For hyperextension of the first toe (so-called permanent Babinski sign), neurotomy of the branch of the deep peroneal nerve to the hallux extensor can be indicated.

Neurotomies can also be used for spasticity in the upper limb, namely, of the musculocutaneous nerve for the spastic elbow in flexion and of the median (and ulnar) nerve for the spastic hand. The latter procedure consists of sectioning the branches to the forearm pronators, wrist flexors and extrinsic finger flexors. The goal is to open the hand and fingers and to improve prehension. When the fascicular organization of the median and ulnar nerves does not allow accurate differentiation between motor and sensory fascicles at the level of their trunks, the motor branches must be reached after they exit the nerve trunk at the forearm. Special care must be taken to spare the sensory fascicles, in order to avoid painful and dysesthetic manifestations. Sectioning of brachial plexus branches has also been developed to treat the spastic shoulder. Pectoralis major and teres major are the main muscles implicated in this condition. Excessive spasticity of these muscles restrains the abduction and external rotation of the shoulder.

Basically, selective neurotomies not only reduce excessive spasticity and prevent deformity but also improve motor function by rebalancing the tonicity of agonist and antagonist muscles (Fig. 5.5). This is especially true for the spastic foot with equinovarus. Spastic hands are more difficult to treat. A functional benefit in prehension can be achieved only if patients retain residual motor function in the extensor and supinator muscles and also have sufficient residual sensory function. If these conditions are not met, only the patient's comfort and cosmesis can be improved.

Dorsal rhizotomies were developed after Sherrington in 1898 showed that rigidity in decerebrate cats was abolished by section of the dorsal roots, which is achieved by interruption of the afferent input to the monosynaptic stretch and polysynaptic withdrawal reflexes. On this basis, Foerster in 1908 performed dorsal rhizotomies at the lumbosacral level to reduce spasticity in children with cerebral palsy [11]. Its undesired effects on sensory and sphincter functions limited its application. To diminish these disadvantages, attempts were made to perform more limited and more selective rhizotomies, especially for children with cerebral palsy able to walk [12–18]. At some centers, intrathecal chemolysis or percutaneous radiofrequency rhizolysis were preferred to open surgery. Initially performed for the treatment of pain [19], these methods were applied to treat severe spasticity in the lower limbs [20], and also to treat neurogenic detrusor hyperactivity and hyperreflexia [21], in bedridden paraplegic patients [22, 23].

Longitudinal myelotomy was introduced by Bischof [24] and then made more selective by Pourpre [25] and later by Laitinen and Singounas [26]. The method

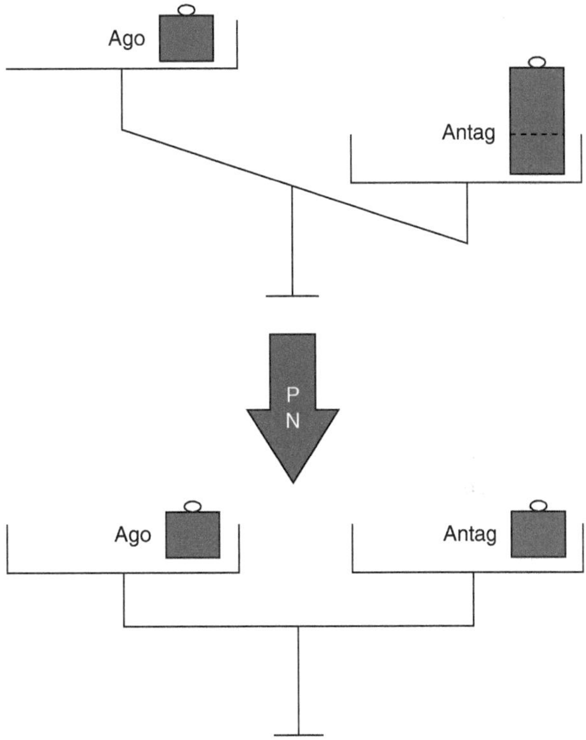

Fig. 5.5 Peripheral neurotomy (*PN*) improves motor function through reduction of excess tone by rebalancing agonist and antagonist muscles

consists in a frontal separation between the dorsal and ventral horns at the lumbosacral enlargement, from T11 to S2. The division is performed from inside the spinal cord after the posterior commissure is incised deep to the ependymal canal. It is indicated for bedridden patients with complete paraplegia, total anesthesia and loss of genitosphincterian functions.

Surgery in the dorsal root entry zone (DREZ) – the first level of central nervous system modulation – was introduced in 1972 to treat topographically limited intractable pain [27]. Because of its inhibitory effects on muscular tone, DREZ lesioning was then applied to patients with regional hyperspasticity [28, 29]. The method termed microsurgical DREZotomy (MDT) intends to interrupt the small caliber (nociceptive) and large myotatic caliber fibers, situated laterally and centrally at the DREZ, respectively. Simultaneously, it attempts to spare part of the medially located large caliber fibers running to the dorsal column. The procedure, which has been described in detail elsewhere [30–33], consists of opening the dorsolateral sulcus ventrally to the rootlet entrance. The incision is 3 mm deep, down to the dorsal horn, following its axis, which is a 35° angle at the cervical level and a 45° angle at the lumbosacral level, according to the respective internal morphology of the spinal cord. Then continuous bipolar microcoagulations – in a dotted manner – are performed at high magnification by the surgical microscope, ventrolaterally at the entry of the rootlets into the dorsolateral sulcus, and into the gray matter of the dorsal horn, along all the spinal cord segments selected as the target for surgery. For patients with paraplegia, the L2–S5 segments are accessed through a T11–L2 laminectomy. For hemiplegic upper limbs, a C4–C7 hemilaminectomy with conservation of the spinous processes is sufficient to reach the C5–T1 segments.

MDT is indicated for severely affected paraplegic patients, especially when they are bedridden as a result of flexion spasms [34], and for hemiplegic patients with irreducible or painful hyperspasticity in the upper limb [35].

Whatever the surgical methods considered, indication for surgery, choice of the most appropriate method and target have to be rigorously discussed by the medico-surgical team within the frame of a multidisciplinary approach.

References

1. Pirpiris M, Graham HK (2001) Management of spasticity in children. In: Barnes MP, Johnson GR (eds) Upper motor neurone syndrome and spasticity. Cambridge University Press, Cambridge, pp 267–305
2. Penn RD, Kroin JS (1985) Continuous intrathecal baclofen for severe spasticity. Lancet 2:125–127
3. Decq P, Keravel Y (1991) Drug pump: technical description, operative procedure and post-operative management. In: Sindou M, Abbott R, Keravel Y (eds) Neurosurgery for spasticity: a multidisciplinary approach. Springer, Wien/New York, pp 97–101
4. Lazorthes Y, Sallerin-Caute B, Verdie JC, Bastide R, Carillo JP (1990) Chronic intrathecal baclofen administration for control of severe spasticity. J Neurosurg 72:393–402
5. Ochs G, Naumann C, Dimitrijevic M, Sindou M (1990) Intrathecal baclofen therapy for spinal origin spasticity: spinal cord injury, spinal cord disease, and multiple sclerosis. Neuromodulation 2:108–119
6. Albright AL, Cervi A, Singletary J (1991) Intrathecal baclofen for spasticity in cerebral palsy. JAMA 265:1418–1422
7. Stoffel A (1913) The treatment of spastic contractures. Am J Orthop Surg 2(10):611–644
8. Gros C, Frèrebeau P, Benezech J, Privat JM (1977) Neurotomie ramiculaire selective. In: Simon L (ed) Actualités en rééducation fonctionnelle et réadaptation, ser 2. Masson, Paris, pp 230–235
9. Sindou M, Mertens P (1988) Selective neurotomy of the tibial nerve for treatment of the spastic foot. Neurosurgery 23:738–744
10. Mertens P, Sindou M (1991) Selective peripheral neurotomies for the treatment of spasticity. In: Sindou M, Abbott R, Keravel Y (eds) Neurosurgery for spasticity: a multidisciplinary approach. Springer, Wien/New York, pp 119–132
11. Foerster O (1913) On the indications and results of the excision of posterior spinal nerve roots in men. Surg Gynecol Obstet 16:463–474
12. Gros C, Ouaknine G, Vlahovitch B, Frèrebeau P (1967) La radicotomie sélective postérieure dans le traitement neurochirurgical de l'hypertonie pyramidale. Neurochirurgie 13:505–518
13. Ouaknine G (1980) Le traitement chirurgical de la spasticité. Union Med Can 109: 1424–1444
14. Gros C (1979) Spasticity: clinical classification and surgical treatment. In: Krayenbühl H, Brihaye J, Loew F, Logue V, Mingrino S, Pertuiset B, Symon L, Troupp H, Yaşargil MG (eds) Advances and technical standards in neurosurgery, vol 6. Springer, Wien/New York, pp 55–97
15. Privat JM, Benezech J, Frèrebeau P, Gros C (1976) Sectorial posterior rhizotomy, a new technique of surgical treatment of spasticity. Acta Neurochir (Wien) 35:181–195
16. Frèrebeau P (1991) Sectorial posterior rhizotomy for the treatment of spasticity in children with cerebral palsy. In: Sindou M, Abbott A, Keravel Y (eds) Neurosurgery for spasticity: a multidisciplinary approach. Springer, Wien/New York, pp 145–147

17. Fraioli B, Guidetti B (1977) Posterior partial rootlet section in the treatment of spasticity. J Neurosurg 46:618–626
18. Fasano VA, Barolat-Romana G, Ivaldi A, Sguazzi A (1976) La radicotomie postérieure fonctionnelle dans le traitement de la spasticité cérébrale: premieres observations sur la stimulation électrique peropératoire des racines postérieures, et leur utilisation dans le choix des racines à sectionner. Neurochirurgie 22:23–34
19. Uematsu S, Udvarhelyi GB, Benson DW, Siebens AA (1974) Percutaneous radiofrequency rhizotomy. Surg Neurol 2:319–325
20. Magid A, Bakheit O (2008) Chemical neurolysis in the management of muscle spasticity. In: Barnes MP, Johnson GR (eds) Upper motor neurone syndrome and spasticity: clinical management and neurophysiology, 2nd edn. Cambridge University Press, Cambridge, pp 150–164
21. Young B, Mulcahy JJ (1980) Percutaneous sacral rhizotomy for neurogenic detrusor hyperreflexia. J Neurosurg 53:85–87
22. Kenmore D (1983) Radiofrequency neurotomy for peripheral pain and spasticity syndromes. Contemp Neurosurg 5:1–6
23. Herz DA, Parsons KC, Pearl L (1983) Percutaneous radiofrequency foraminal rhizotomies. Spine 8:729–732
24. Bischof W (1951) Die longitudinale Myelotomie. Zentralbl Neurochir 11:79–88
25. Pourpre MH (1960) Traitement neurochirurgical des contractures chez les paraplégiques post-traumatiques. Neurochirurgie 6:229–236
26. Laitinen LV, Singounas E (1971) Longitudinal myelotomy in the treatment of spasticity of the legs. J Neurosurg 35:536–540
27. Sindou M (1972) Etude de la jonction radiculo-medullaire postérieure: la radicellotomie postérieure sélective dans la chirurgie de la douleur. Thèse de Médecine, Université de Lyon, Lyon
28. Sindou M, Fischer G, Goutelle A, Schott B, Mansuy L (1974) La radicellotomie postérieure selective dans le traitement de spasticité. Rev Neurol (Paris) 130:201–216
29. Sindou M, Millet MF, Mortamais J, Eyssette M (1982) Results of selective posterior rhizotomy in the treatment of painful and spastic paraplegia secondary to multiple sclerosis. Appl Neurophysiol 45:335–340
30. Sindou M, Jeanmonod D, Mertens P (1991) Surgery in the dorsal root entry zone: microsurgical DREZotomy (MDT) for the treatment of spasticity. In: Sindou M, Abbott R, Keravel Y (eds) Neurosurgery for spasticity: a multidisciplinary approach. Springer, Wien/New York, pp 165–182
31. Sindou M, Mertens P (2009) Surgery in the dorsal root entry zone for spasticity. In: Lozano AM, Gildenberg PL, Tasker RR (eds) Textbook of stereotactic and functional neurosurgery, 2nd edn. Springer, Berlin, pp 1959–1972
32. Sindou M, Mertens P (2011) Surgical interventions for spasticity: ablative surgery for spasticity. In: Winn HR (ed) Youmans neurological surgery, 6th edn. Elsevier Saunders, Philadelphia, pp 1025–1037
33. Sindou M, Mertens P (2012) Surgery for intractable spasticity. In: Quiñones-Hinojosa A (ed) Schmidek and sweet operative neurosurgical techniques: indications, methods, and results, 6th edn. Elsevier Saunders, Philadelphia, pp 1377–1392
34. Sindou M, Jeanmonod D (1989) Microchirurgical DREZ-otomy for the treatment of spasticity and pain in the lower limbs. Neurosurgery 24:655–670
35. Sindou M, Mifsud JJ, Boisson D, Goutelle A (1986) Selective posterior rhizotomy in the dorsal root entry zone for treatment of hyperspasticity and pain in the hemiplegic upper limb. Neurosurgery 18:587–595

Intrathecal Baclofen Therapy

6

Baclofen, a γ-aminobutyric acid-B (GABA-B) receptor agonist, has a direct action on the receptors of the dorsal horn gray matter, where density of GABA-B receptors is high. Baclofen activates GABA-B presynaptic receptors that inhibit the release of excitatory neurotransmitters of the dorsal horn, particularly aspartate and glutamate. The excitability of monosynaptic and polysynaptic reflexes of the spinal cord becomes thereby reduced. Given orally, baclofen has a weak capacity to penetrate the blood–central nervous system barrier. After oral administration the drug is absorbed by more than 80 % through the intestinal mucosa [1]; the plasmatic concentration is maximal within 90–120 min; most is eliminated by urinary excretion [2]. Failure of oral medication to produce sufficient reduction of spasticity is due to the poor passage of the drug across the blood–central nervous system barrier [3]. In animal experiments, the concentration in the cerebrospinal fluid (CSF) was less than one-tenth of that in the plasma level [4]. Systemic delivery would produce the same concentrations along the spinal cord and would be distributed equally to the brain, and the consequences would be somnolence or even coma. To circumvent this problem, Penn and Kroin introduced and developed the method of delivering baclofen intrathecally by subarachnoid lumbar infusion [5, 6].

The development of pumps that can be implanted and programmed, such as the Synchromed model (Medtronic, Inc., Minneapolis, MN), enables the method to be used for handicapped patients, not only for adults but also, with the smaller pump, for children with cerebral palsy. Implanted programmable pumps with a catheter in the lumbar subarachnoid space not only deliver baclofen regionally but also provide the means for achieving constant levels all day long. The level can be adjusted to allow precise therapeutic effects.

6.1 Physiologic and Pharmacokinetic Effects of Baclofen

Baclofen is a lipophilic GABA-B receptor agonist that only partially permeates from blood to nervous system. Baclofen affects the type B receptor, which is a transmembrane protein that controls calcium and potassium channels (Fig. 6.1). By activation of the GABA-B receptors, which decreases the influx of calcium into the

M. Sindou et al., *Neurosurgery for Spasticity*,
DOI 10.1007/978-3-7091-1771-2_6, © Springer-Verlag Wien 2014

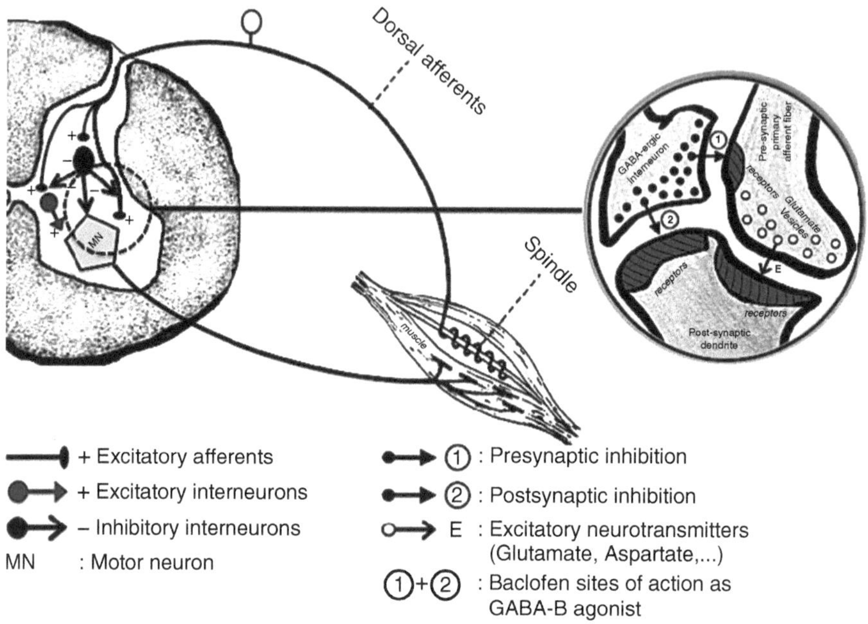

Fig. 6.1 Baclofen as a γ-aminobutyric acid (*GABA*) agonist. Baclofen affects only the B type receptor in the spinal cord, which is a transmembrane protein. Baclofen produces a profound reduction in monosynaptic and polysynaptic spinal reflexes

presynaptic terminals of the afferent fibers, baclofen reduces the release of the excitatory transmitters and thereby produces a decrease in monosynaptic and polysynaptic spinal reflexes. Baclofen also affects the postsynaptic membrane by increasing potassium influx and thus raises the membrane potential and inhibits neuronal firing. Intrathecal baclofen given to normal patients does not significantly decrease strength, but the same dose given to a spastic patient markedly decreases muscle tone and spasticity. The reason that baclofen is so effective in reducing spasticity is that the same changes in the spinal cord that produce spasticity enhance the sensitivity to baclofen as pointed out by Penn and Corcos [7].

When a bolus of baclofen is delivered into the lumbar subarachnoid space, it mixes rapidly with lumbar CSF and is gradually carried upward along the spinal cord. In 3–6 h it reaches the brainstem and then the convexities, where it is eliminated into the systemic circulation at the arachnoid granulations [8]. Bolus administration leads to transient but very high drug levels at the spinal cord and later at the brainstem. Half-life of a bolus of baclofen in cerebrospinal fluid is variable among individuals, ranging from 1 to 5 h [9, 10].

When baclofen is delivered in a continuous mode, pharmacokinetics is different. A steady-state concentration is reached in CSF after 12–18 h. In their investigations with 14 patients who underwent continuous intrathecal baclofen (ITB) infusion, Muller et al. [11] showed that the concentration in CSF was in the range of 130–950 ng/ml for an infused dose of 50–1200 μg/24 h and was proportional to the infusion rate. It is noteworthy that the concentration in plasma of the same patients was found to be between 0 and 5 ng, which is almost negligible. In a more recent study of children with cerebral palsy who received continuously ITB with doses of 77–400 μg/day, Albright and Shultz [12] found that plasma level was at the limit of detection, that is, 10 ng/ml, in all patients. Further, in a study of the distribution of concentration along the spinal cord, using indium 111 to measure CSF dynamics, Kroin et al. [8] showed for patients with ITB that in steady state the concentration of baclofen decreased linearly to one quarter, from lumbar to high cervical CSF space.

The practical consequences of the above pharmacokinetics have been very clearly described by Penn and Corcos [7, p.1045] as follows: "(1) Bolus administrarion produces immediate and extremely high transient levels in the spinal cord. Several hours later Baclofen reaches the brainstem and causes side-effects such as light-headedness and drowsiness. (2) Slow, constant delivery with a drug pump produces levels of drug proportional to the delivery rate. (3) A change in delivery rate takes at least 12 h to reach new steady-state levels in cerebrospinal fluid. Therefore infusion rates should not be adjusted more than twice daily. (4) A constant infusion into the lumbar space distributes Baclofen along the cord so that the concentration decreases linearly with distance and is about one quarter as high at the brainstem as it is at the point of infusion. Fewer brainstem effects are likely to occur if a constant infusion is administered and the infusion is directed into the lumbar intrathecal space. (5) Diffusion of Baclofen from CSF to (intraparenchymal) spinal cord receptors is a slow process accounting for approximately 1 h of delay. A single bolus dose may reduce spasticity for 4–12 h. When giving medication intrathecally, the physician must be aware that clinical effects on spasticity, and also eventual harmful side-effects on brainstem (respiratory depression, coma, …) are slow to appear, but equally slow to clear because the cord acts as a reservoir after it is loaded."

6.2 Implanted Programmable Pump

An implanted programmable pump connected to a catheter inserted in the lumbar subarachnoidal space allows delivering the drug regionally at a constant pharmacological level. The most frequently used implanted programmable pump is the Synchromed II (with reservoir volume of 20 or 40 ml) manufactured by Medtronic, Inc. (Fig. 6.2). It is a battery-powered device that stores the drug and dispenses it according to instructions set by the programmer (Fig. 6.3).

Each pump contains a collapsible drug reservoir, microprocessor-based circuitry, lithium thionyl-chloride battery, antenna, acoustic transducer, peristaltic pump, bioretentive filter through which the drug passes as it leaves the drug reservoir and a fill port with a self-sealing septum and needle stop (Fig. 6.4, Table 6.1).

The pump has three sealed chambers: one contains the drug reservoir, the second a hybrid electronic module and battery, and the third a peristaltic pump. The peristaltic positive-displacement pump forces the drug from the reservoir through a bacterial filter and administration site. The pump is driven by an integral step motor, which is

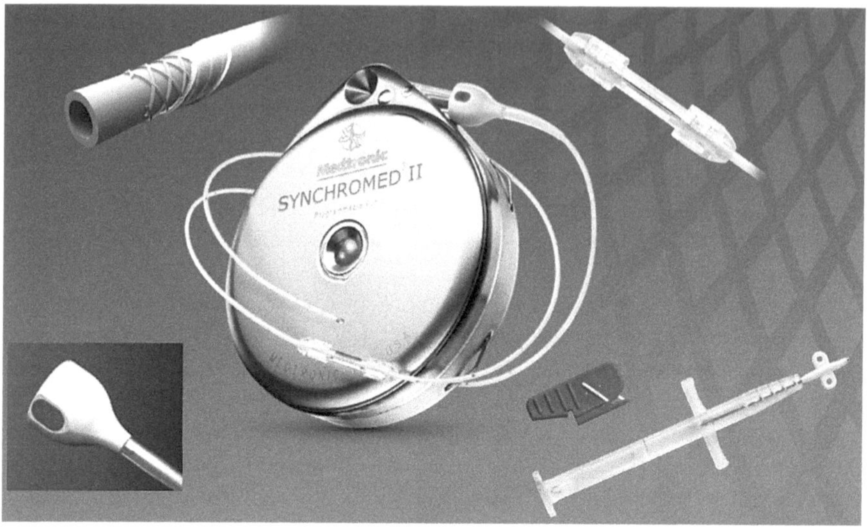

Fig. 6.2 SynchroMed II programmable implanted infusion pump manufactured by Medtronic, Inc., together with intrathecal subarachnoidal catheter system (of the Ascenda type in this picture)

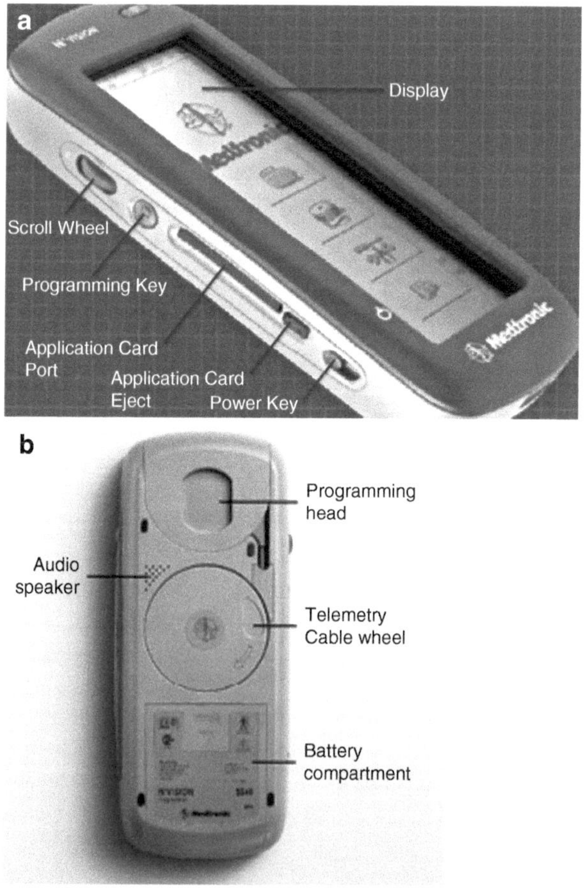

Fig. 6.3 Hand-held programmer for use adjustment and refill. (**a**) Front and left side. (**b**) Rear. The N'Vision model 8840 clinician programmer is a portable device that offers a single programming platform for the implantable Synchromed pump. The programmer is equiped with a touchscreen display for data entry, telemetry module for device programming, and an infrared port through which communications can be established with compatible printers

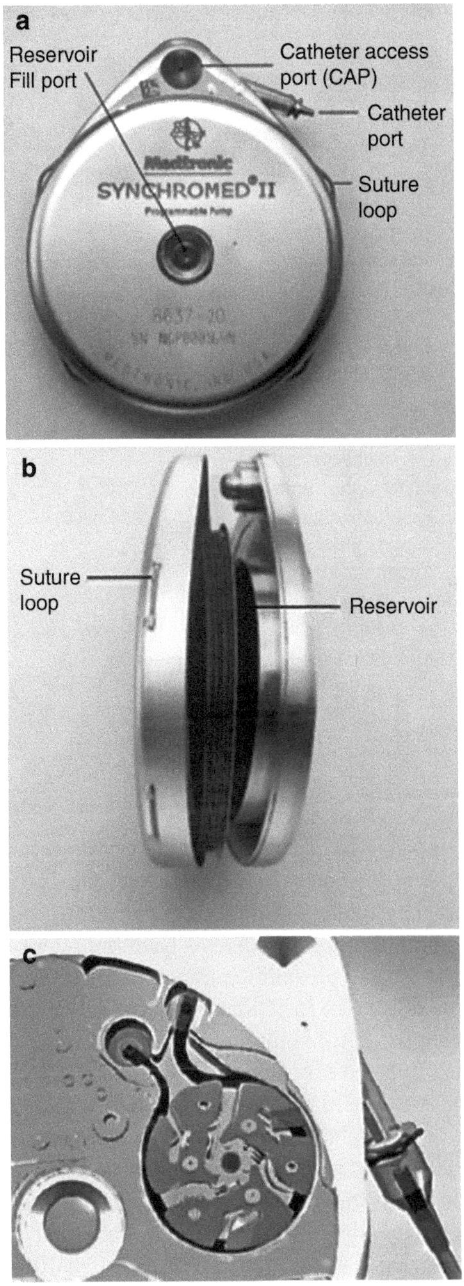

Fig. 6.4 (**a**) SynchroMed II model 8637 pump is available with two reservoir sizes: 20 and 40 ml. The pump precisely delivers a prescription according to instructions programmed by the clinician. The catheter access port allows direct access to the catheter and CSF. The pump has suture loops that can be used to anchor the pump in the "subcutaneous pocket". (**b**) Pump side view. Drug is held in the pump reservoir, which is constructed with a bellows design that allows the reservoir to expand or contract according to the drug volume. (**c**) Pump rollers. The battery-powered electronics and motor cause the roller arm in the peristaltic pump to rotate, precisely pushing the programmed dose out through the catheter port and into the catheter. A valve protects the pump reservoir from being overfilled or overpressurized

Table 6.1 Specifications of Synchromed II ITB pump models

	Specification for model	
Characteristic	8637-20	8637-40
External properties:		
Thickness (mm)	19.5	26.0
Weight (empty/full; g)	165/185	175/215
Displacement volume (ml)	91	121
Diameter (mm)	87.5	87.5
Material	Titanium and silicone rubber	Titanium and silicone rubber
Pump:		
Capacity (ml)	20.0	40.0
Residual volume (ml)	1.4 max	1.4 max
Pump tubing volume (ml)	0.199–0.289	0.199–0.289
Reservoir fill port:		
Septum puncture life (nr. of punctures)	500	500
Catheter access port:		
Residual volume (ml)	0.14 max	0.14 max
Septum puncture life (nr. of punctures)	500	500
Flow rate:		
Programmable rate (ml/day)	24 max, 0.048 min	24 max, 0.048 min
Minimum (nontherapeutic) rate (ml/day)	0.006	0.006
Leakage rate (stopped pump) (ml/day)	0.030 max	0.030 max

regulated by pulses from a battery-powered hybrid electrical control. The electrical circuitry adjusts the fluid delivery rate by altering the frequency of control pulses.

This pump will provide chronic infusion for about 4 years at typical dosage regimens. The pump utilizes a bacterial retention filter (pore size, 0.22 μm) in the fluid pathway to prevent the transmission of contaminants.

The pump functions properly at reservoir volumes as low as 3.5 ml. The pump output drops significantly below 2 ml. Therefore, a patient may experience a diminished efficacy of the baclofen treatment when the pump reservoir volume is less than 3.5 ml, but this is not necessarily observed in all patients unless the volume is less than 2 ml. The minimum infusion rate of the device is 0.096 ml/day (0.004 ml/h). When the pump is in its "stop" mode, the rotor is still functioning at its mechanical and electrical minimum. The reason for the pump's continuous function is to minimize leak rate, which under these conditions is never above a maximum of 5 μl/h (it is usually less than 1 μl/h). In order to ensure that absolutely no drug is being delivered, the pump reservoir must be emptied and eventually rinsed with saline solution.

The programming options allow the physician to achieve optimal spasticity relief and minimal side effects without readjusting the drug concentration or changing the reservoir contents (Fig. 6.5).

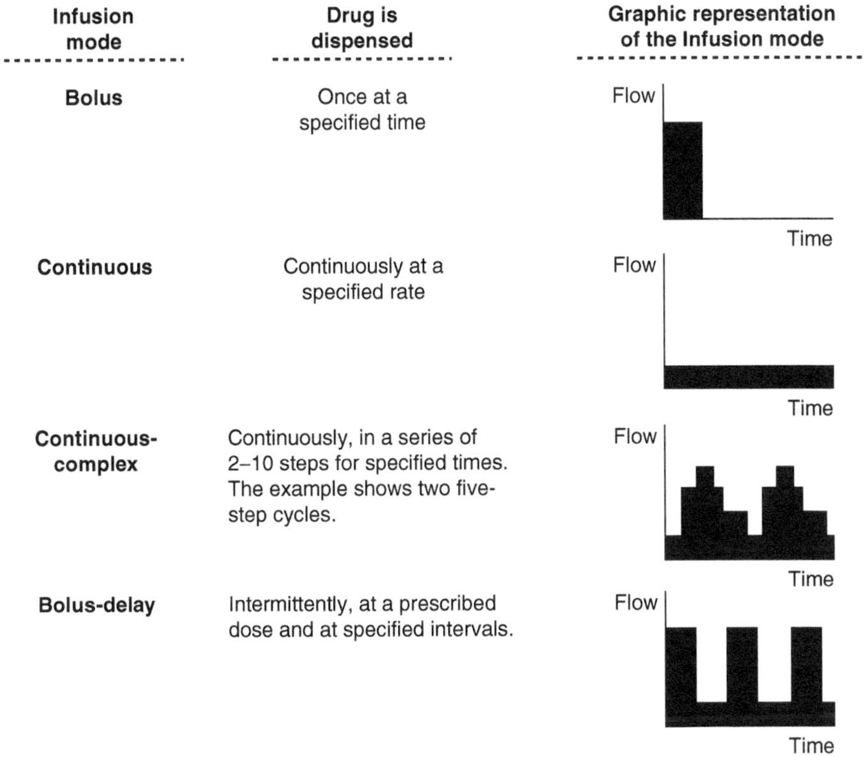

Fig. 6.5 Infusion modes possible with the implanted Synchromed II pump

6.3 Side-Effects and Complications of Baclofen

Adverse effects under continuous-infusion mode are infrequent and most often transient. If present, they may include drowsiness, dizziness, mental confusion, light-headedness, constipation, urinary retention. These side effects are reversed by decreasing the doses. Muscular hypotonia may also occur, leading to loss of muscular power and capacity to stand or walk in ambulatory patients. Adjusting the doses generally reverses hypotonia to the desirable level. Patients with multiple sclerosis or cerebral lesions are more inclined to present those adverse effects, especially fatigue and confusion. It is of practical importance to distinguish the symptoms associated with the disease that mimic overdose from those occurring as result of the ITB treatment.

Overdosing is infrequent and when it occurs it is rarely due to pump malfunctioning. It may rather be the consequence of inappropriate bolus dose, changes in drug concentration, or misprogramming the pump after reprogramming. Symptoms include weakness with rostral progression, blood pressure changes, respiratory depression, and alteration of consciousness: from somnolence to coma. There is no real antagonizing substance (antidote) of baclofen. However, physostigmine administered intravenously at a dose of 2 mg can reverse respiratory depression and lethargy. In the exceptional situation of respiratory distress, assisted ventilation should be performed on emergency.

An aspect of intrathecal baclofen that should not be underestimated is the **potential impairment of sexual function**. Administration of intrathecal baclofen may have deleterious effects on erectile function especially in men with spinal cord injury [13]. The inhibitory effect of intrathecal baclofen on erection and ejaculation is attributed to its agonist effect on GABA-B receptors in the lumbosacral spinal cord [14, 15]. Intrathecal baclofen impacts existing sexual function particularly at higher doses. However, the extent to which sexual function is impaired seems to be minimal and the effects are reversible with withdrawal or reduction of intrathecal baclofen administration. Clinicians should be aware of this risk and discuss it during routine clinic follow-up. Dosing adjustments need to be considered for these patients.

Baclofen withdrawal syndrome may happen if the pump is not refilled properly or at the scheduled intervals or in a case of pump or catheter malfunction. Symptoms include rebound motor spasticity and spasms, dysesthetic or itching sensations, headaches, drowsiness, confusion or even hallucinations, seizures, tachycardia, labile blood pressure, and fever. Treatment is readministration of intrathecal baclofen. In life-threatening situations baclofen should be given by lumbar puncture or external catheter. To avoid a withdrawal syndrome even in a mild form, after intrathecal baclofen has been initiated, oral baclofen should be withdrawn gradually over a period of several weeks.

Baclofen may also change the **convulsing threshold**, making seizure conditions difficult to control.

Tolerance to baclofen rarely develops. Most patients who are thought to have tolerance have in fact system malfunctions; responsiveness resumes once the system is revised. However, for around 5 % of the patients, especially those with some degree of dystonia, increase in doses is required. Such tolerance phenomenon occurs mainly over the first year, and doses have to be approximately doubled before clinical effect stabilizes.

6.4 Surgical Indications and Patient Selection

6.4.1 Spasticity of Spinal Origin

ITB is indicated for severe spasticity of spinal origin that is unresponsive to oral antispasticity agents at normal doses or patients experiencing intolerable side effects at effective doses. Patients may be ambulant, wheelchair-dependent, or bedridden.

Spasticity from spinal origin is encountered after multiple sclerosis, spinal cord injury or a variety of spinal cord diseases. Mechanisms include loss of supraspinal inhibition, damages in segmental inhibiting neurons, sprouting of collateral fibers, and changes in muscle fibers. Spasms can be triggered by physical or psychological noxious stimuli.

Criteria for selecting a patient as candidate for ITB are known chronic, stable spinal cord pathology as the etiology and severe, disabling spasticity and/or spasms, with an Asworth score of more than 3, interfering with activities of daily life, mobility, transfers, and nursing cares. Also ITB is the treatment of choice for familial spastic paraparesis.

Because of the constraints of the method, patient, family, and caregivers should agree to accept and follow all necessary steps to correctly maintain pump functioning and refilling. All the above should be included in the informed-consent form.

6.4.2 Spasticity of Brain Origin

Patients who survive after severe traumatic, hypoxic, or vascular injuries, especially those with midbrain damages responsible for unilateral or bilateral decorticated or decerebrated states, inevitably develop hypertonia or spasticity. Rapidly, as musculotendinous retractions and capsulitis appear, abnormal flexion/extension postures become permanent and contractures and ankyloses fixed, which makes mobilization and nursing care difficult and in addition increases pain and spasms.

Importantly, hypertonia after acute insult frequently develops within about a few weeks. In such eventuality, ITB should be started soon, before abnormal postures evolve toward irreversibility and the patient becomes bedridden with sores and infections. ITB can be delivered either through an implanted pump or by default through an access port connected with an external injector. The doses required for spasticity of supraspinal origin have been reported to be twice as high as those required for spasticity from spinal origin [16, 17]. Anticonvulsive protection is recommended, as some cases of seizure decompensation have been reported [17, 18].

6.4.3 Spasticity and/or Dystonia Due to Cerebral Palsy

Initially introduced for the treatment of patients with spasticity of spinal origin, indications of ITB were then extended to patients with spasticity of cerebral origin including cerebral palsy (CP), not only at the stage of young adult but also of childhood.

ITB may be an alternative to dorsal rhizotomy (DR) for spastic diplegia. In CP children (see Chap. 13), dystonia is frequently associated with spasticity under the clinical presentation of so-called mixed spasticity and dystonia. For these mixed syndromes, ITB is the treatment of choice as DR is less effective on the dystonia component than on the spastic component. In CP patients, dystonia may be the predominant or even the sole handicapping disorder. ITB can be considered when dystonia causes abnormal posturing and contributes to deformities. Preliminary ITB trials may help decision making, preferably using a percutaneous continuous infusion through a subcutaneous implanted access port. According to Albright [19], who screened more than 200 dystonic patients with ITB, the recommended protocol is the following. Infusion rate is 200 μg/day and increased by 75 μg every 12 h until a clinical response is achieved, namely, a 25 % decrease in Barry–Albright Dystonia scale (see Table 11.4) [20]. Infusion is stopped if and when unacceptable adverse side effects, i.e., lethargy, are observed, or if no significant response is obtained at 900 μg/day. If the patient is "responder" and no excessive weakness is manifested, permanent implantation of a pump is decided.

6.4.4 Alternative Methods for Patients with Brain Lesion or Cerebral Palsy Harboring Focalized and Severe Spasticity and/or Dystonia

For patients with brain lesion or CP harboring focalized and severe spasticity and/or dystonia, additional botulinum toxin injections can be indicated, and if they are not sustainably effective in spite of their repetitive administrations, peripheral neurotomy(ies) may then be considered.

In hemiplegic patients when spasticity and/or dystonia severely affect the upper limb, a cervical microsurgical DREZotomy, from C5–T1 segments, can be a remedy. Lesioning should be performed through the dorsal horn down to the ventral horn, in the order of 5 mm in depth so as to reach the grey matter of the base of ventral horn.

6.5 Patient Selection and Screening

Careful selection and screening of patients prior to decision for ITB is crucial to achieve successful outcome. The complex relationship between spasticity and daily functioning makes it necessary to evaluate each patient from his practical point of view and in a multidisciplinary manner. It is not sufficient to determine that spasticity and/or spasms will be diminished by treatment. It should be ascertained that no significant loss of function would occur due to reduction of spasticity. As a matter of fact, some degree of hypertonia is useful because it aids, e.g., in ambulation, standing, and transfers and also provides a feeling of "body control". It has been observed that some patients perceive the acute reduction in tone that results from ITB initiation as excessive weakness, thus triggering a sensation of anxiety.

For paraplegic or paraparetic patients with clinically typical hyperspasticity or those with handicapping mixed hypertonia in whom the spastic component is predominant, ITB will be effective on tone regulation. A preliminary bolus test of ITB would not be necessary to prove that such a patient will be a "responder". The patient can undergo implantation directly and doses should be adjusted thereafter.

In contrast to that situation, if the indication is not clear, that is, the diagnosis of spasticity is uncertain or involvement of the spastic component in the patient's handicap is not established, a primary test of ITB should be considered. A single (or a few) bolus of 50–100 μg through lumbar puncture will allow the caregivers to know whether the patient will be a "responder" or not. The problem is that the bolus method may be insufficient if performed at low dose(s) or conversely can reduce tone so much that weakness may occur leading the patient to consider the method not useful, if not harmful.

For patients for whom it is important to evaluate whether a reduction in spasticity will improve function, and to what degree, or on the contrary will weaken functionally useful hypertonia, a preliminary test prior to decision is mandatory. For such an evaluation a continuous infusion test for about 1 week is much preferable to the bolus method.

For performing a continuous-infusion test, an access port of the Ommaya reservoir, connected to the intrathecal catheter, is surgically implanted. The reservoir is then connected to an external pump. The system provides steady-state pharmaceutical levels with more prolonged effects of baclofen during hospitalization. With this technique the discomfort due to repeated lumbar punctures, the risk of infections, and the occurrence of side effects caused by overdosage are avoided as compared with the bolus mode.

Note that whatever the techniques used, lumbar puncture(s) or continuous infusions, and CSF depletion or leak may provoke headaches, nausea, and vomiting that confound interpretation until those symptoms disappear.

For **adult patients**, a bolus dose of 50–100 μg given by lumbar puncture is usually adequate. Effect often appears with 1–2 h delay and lasts for 8–12 h. In the absence of a positive response, which would be indicated by a two-point reduction in the Ashworth score, the bolus can be repeated with increments of 25–50 μg, up to 100 μg. No more than one bolus should be administered within a 24 h period. Once a positive response is observed without unacceptable loss of function, the patient is considered eligible for pump implantation. When a continuous infusion test is chosen to simulate the patient's ordinary life, different dosing regimens can be tried, with daily doses as high as twice or three times the baseline. In this way, the efficacy and adverse side effects of ITB can be evaluated in conditions resembling the mode of delivery of the implanted pump.

There are a few **pediatric specificities**. In small children, e.g., at an age of less than 8 years or with a body weight of less than 50 lb, bolus dose should start at 25 μg; doses of 50–100 μg may be secondarily used in those who do not respond. Spasticity decreases after approximately 2 h with a maximum at 4–6 h and returns to baseline after 12 h. In ambulant CP children, if gait worsens because of abrupt and excessive hypotonia in lower limbs, a percutaneous catheter may be inserted to perform repeated injections or, even better, a subcutaneous access port should be implanted to deliver a continuous baclofen infusion.

6.6 Surgical Technique

Implantation of the pump and the catheter is a simple procedure but should be performed meticulously. Patients must be free of infection prior to implantation. The site of the pump placement should be planned prior to surgery taking into consideration the patient's physical characteristics and conditions. The majority of teams use

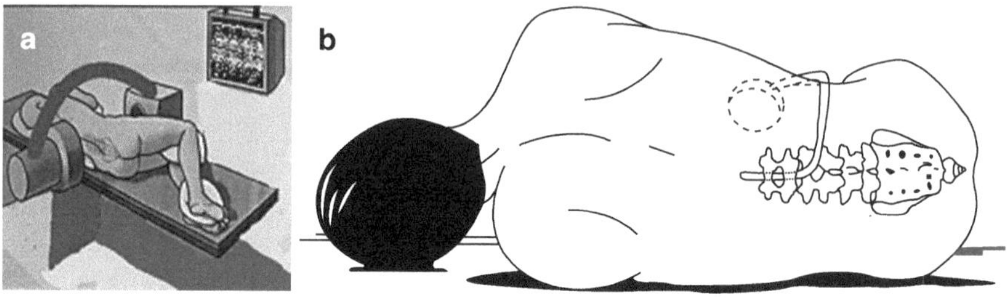

Fig. 6.6 (**a**) Positioning of the patient for implantation of the intrathecal catheter. (**b**) Schematic representation of pump implantation and catheter insertion in the lumbar region

Fig. 6.7 X-ray control of the implantation of the intrathecal catheter. *Arrowheads* show the traject of the catheter and *arrow* shows the catheter tip at the level of the thoracic vertebra T12

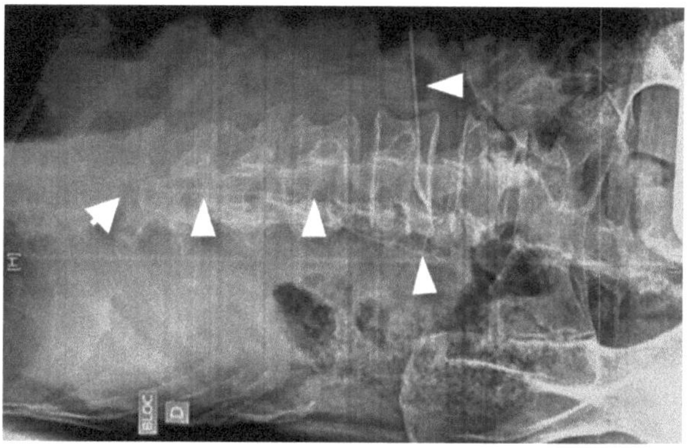

intravenous prophylactic antibiotics. Surgery is performed under either local or, more often, general anesthesia. The patient is placed in the lateral decubitus position to expose the abdominal wall and the lumbar spine at the same time. Lumbar lordosis should be reduced by positioning knees and hips in flexed postures, and the spinous processes aligned parallel to the table to make insertion of the catheter easier (Fig. 6.6). A C-arm fluoroscopy imaging is positioned so that the lumbar spine is visualized in an anterior-posterior view.

The catheter is inserted into the dural sac at the L3-4 or L4-5 interspace under radiographic control (Fig. 6.6). The trocar (a Tuohy needle) has the advantage to penetrate the dural sac obliquely in order to allow the catheter to be passed without sharp angulation. The catheter should ascend smoothly to the conus; otherwise it might be in the epidural or subdural space. For lower limb spasticity the catheter tip is placed at the conus level, i.e., between T10 and T12 vertebrae (Fig. 6.7). For upper limb spasticity, a higher position, i.e., at the mid- to high-thoracic levels is appropriate. The best test to confirm the placement in the subarachnoid space is to inject contrast medium, and not only to aspirate or reinject CSF. To secure the catheter, a purse string suture is placed around the catheter and anchors to the lumbar fascia as the catheter goes through it. If the catheter is not properly anchored, it will be pulled out due to patient's moves.

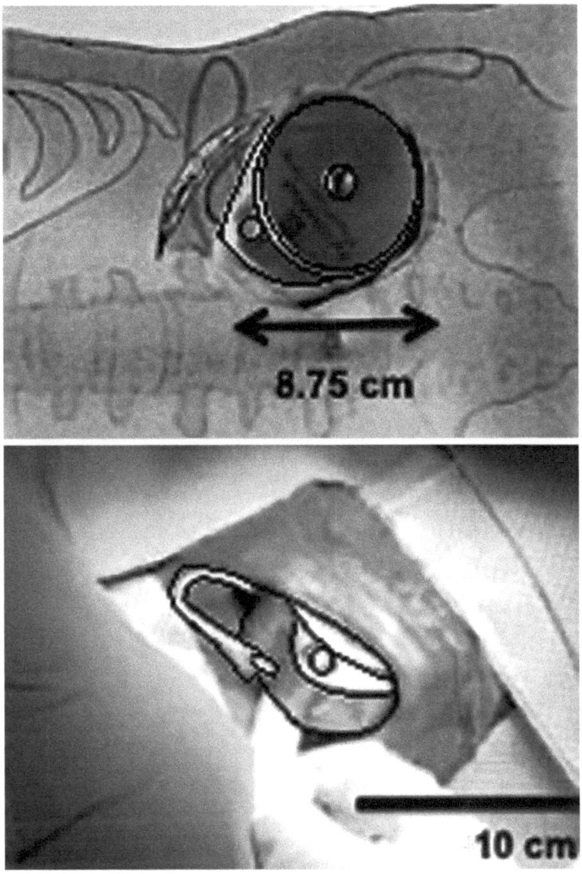

Fig. 6.8 Incision site and subcutaneous placement of the pump into the abdominal wall in the subcostal region

The pump mostly used for adults is the one with a 40 ml reservoir. Care must be taken to check if the abdominal wall has enough subcutaneous fat to support the bulky pump. Else, a 20 ml reservoir pump may be preferred.

The incision for placing the pump into the abdominal pocket is made just below the ribs (Fig. 6.8). The pocket should be medial enough to avoid the pump hitting the superior iliac crest. The pocket should be large enough so that the pump is not in front of the incision to prevent infection or erosion of the site. The outport of the pump should not press against the skin laterally and be best placed medially with the catheter underneath. The pump could move if not secured to the fascia; the loops at the pump edge are used to suture it to the fascia in two places. If the patient is obese, fat over the pump may need to be reduced, otherwise the pump will be difficult to fill or program.

Tunneling the larger catheter from the pump pocket to the lumbar incision is performed with a shuntlike tube passer, which is bent appropriately and advanced from the lumbar area to the abdomen. The intrathecal catheter and the larger catheter are then connected, after CSF is seen to drip out, assuring unobstructed flow

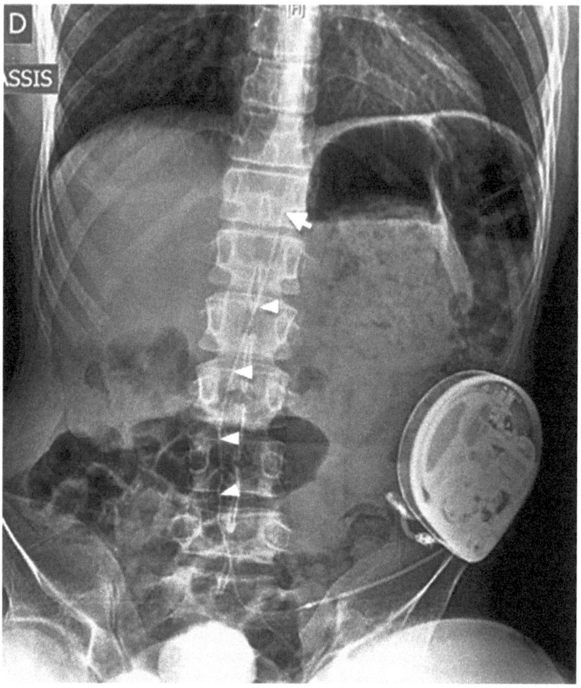

Fig. 6.9 Postoperative radiographic control of the implantation of the intrathecal catheter and its connection with the pump. *Arrowheads* show the trajectory of the catheter and *arrow* shows the catheter tip at the level of the thoracic vertebrae T11-T12

from the subarachnoid space. The excess catheter is looped under the pump to avoid stretching in case that the pump moves.

Before leaving the operating theater, a radiographic control of the whole implanted system is advisable to verify the accuracy of the procedure (Fig. 6.9).

Main pitfalls would be catheter being misplaced in the epidural or subdural spaces, catheter being damaged during maneuvers of the Tuohy needle because of its sharp cutting edges, catheter being pulled out due to akward moves or lack of anchorage, catheter being kinked.

For **pediatric patients** (or thin adult patients), a subfascial pocket provides better cosmesis and exposes less to a risk of skin erosion. However, it must be taken into account that the plan of dissection is more difficult to achieve and entails risk of blood loss.

In patients who have had a **midline spine fusion**, it may be necessary to drill through the fusion mass, but this has to be done minimally, just enough to insert the Tuohy needle. Any larger opening would create space for CSF leakage. In case of a difficult opening, it may be necessary to perform an interlaminar approach or laminectomy if a percutaneous insertion of the catheter seems impossible. In that case, care must be taken not to excessively open the dura and to perform tight suturing to avoid CSF leakage, pseudomeningocele, or fistula.

Traditionally, the catheter tip for baclofen delivery is placed in a low thoracic location. When hypertonia predominates in upper limbs, a **more rostral placement**, i.e., **cervical**, may be advisable. Because delivery of baclofen at an upper spinal cord level is potentially dangerous due to the risk of respiratory depression, effects of catheter placement in the cervical region were specially investigated [21]. That study with a group of 23 patients showed that cervical placement resulted in equal control of spasticity in the upper and lower extremities and did not increase complications, compared with the control group of 25 patients in whom the catheter was in the thoracic position.

6.7 Postoperative Management and Dosing After Implantation

During the postoperative period the site of implantation has to be kept protected from external pressure. To reduce the occurrence of CSF leakage, it is advantageous to position the patient in recumbent position for a few days. On the other hand, mobilization and physical therapy should be better started soon to lower the risk of venous thrombosis and pulmonary embolism. Low-dose heparin and stockings are also recommended.

Beginning on day 2, the initial infusion dose starts in between the effective screening dose and its double, usually between 100 and 200 μg/day. Doses are typically increased by 10–20 % for the first days to achieve the desired effect. The most useful criterion for dose adjustment in spastic patients is the suppression of reflexes – tendon jerk, clonus, and spasms, etc. – and "excessive" tone. Doses should be then titrated to optimize tone and function, especially in ambulatory patients. Response to dose adjustment is apparent with a delay of around 4–6 h. Infusion mode should be continuous, at least initially. In some patients the degree of harmful spasticity varies along the day. Because the programmable pump allows cyclical dose adjustments, it is possible for those patients to deliver baclofen levels that correlate with the variability of the spastic symptoms and their disabling effects. The mode most commonly used is the alternation of daytime rate and nighttime rate for bed rest.

Importantly, for patients who are still on oral baclofen or other antispastic drugs, the medications should not be stopped abruptly, but rather withdrawn progressively over the 2–4 weeks following implantation.

Approximately three-fourths of the patients require an increase in doses to maintain the desired effects, especially within the first year of the postimplantation period [22]. A sudden lack of efficacy would suggest a delivery system malfunction, necessitating its description and revision.

Doses required to reach efficacy may differ significantly according to etiologies, and from patient to patient [23]. For spasticity of spinal cord origin, daily doses ranged from 50 to 900 μg/day, with a mean of 350 μg/day. Mean maintenance dose was found higher for spinal cord injury than for multiple sclerosis patients, 462 and 320 μg/day, respectively.

For CP patients at 1 year after pump implantation, Albright [19] reported that the mean ITB effective dose was ±300 μg/day for treating spasticity, whilst for treating dystonia mean ITB dose was higher, ±600 μg/day; but doses of 600–1000 μg/day were not unusual for adequate relief of the most sever dystonic components to be achieved. For patients not completely relieved, increasing daily doses beyond 1500 μg/day is unlikely to produce any significant additional benefit, whether treating spasticity or dystonia [19].

Long-term management requires regular pump refilling and dose adjustments, usually three to five times a year.

It is to be noted that baclofen remains stable in the pump for at least 3 months, likely up to 6 months, according to data on file at Medtronic, Inc., 1999, available at www.medtronic.com. Baclofen for ITB therapy is not available in concentrations higher than 2000 μg/ml, because higher concentrations might result in precipitation and make delivery through pump unreliable.

When a refill is required, the programmable Medtronic pumps emit an alarm sound, usually at a preset level of 2 ml of their 20 or 40 ml capacity. At this level a decrease in efficacy on spasticity is often noticeable. Refilling pumps with dose adjustments is commonly performed in an outpatient clinic environment. Dedicated personnel is necessary as the procedure is always potentially dangerous due to the risk of infection and/or misprogamming.

The pump is refilled by puncturing the port. Prior to refilling, the reservoir must be emptied by aspiration with a syringe connected to an isolating tap so as to prevent air entrance when changing syringes. Meticulous asepsis is mandatory to avoid the inoculation of bacteria into the subcutaneous abdominal pocket of the pump or within the reservoir: Therefore a bactericidal filter should be mounted on the filling system [24].

Because the incorporated battery is not rechargeable, a new pump should be implanted when battery life expired, which is on average after 4–6 years of use.

6.8 Outcome

6.8.1 Effect on Spasticity and Dystonia

Successful use of ITB for the control of spasticity was first reported by Penn and Kroin for patients with **spasticity of spinal cord origin** [6]. Later, the same team published positive results of a double-blind study of effects of ITB infusions for a group of 20 adults affected with multiple sclerosis or spinal cord injury; Ashworth score decreased from 4 to 1.2 and muscle spasms from 3.3 to 0.4 after treatment [25]. A further study from the same team after 7 years of experience [26] and other studies demonstrated that ITB provided safe, titratable, and reversible control of spasticity in most (80–97 %) of the cases presenting with severe spasticity of spinal origin according to series [27, 28]. Also, our group found that the Ashworth score for lower extremities dropped from a mean of 3.8 ± 0.7 at baseline to 1.6 ± 0.8 after ITB ($p < 0.001$) and that the frequency and intensity of spasms both decreased from 2.8 ± 0.7 at baseline to 1.0 ± 0.7 ($p < 0.001$) (Fig. 6.10) [29].

Besides its major indication for the treatment of spasticity from spinal cord origin, applications of ITB were extended to other types of spasticity. ITB proved useful in the spastic and hypertonic states observed after **severe cerebral**, **midbrain**,

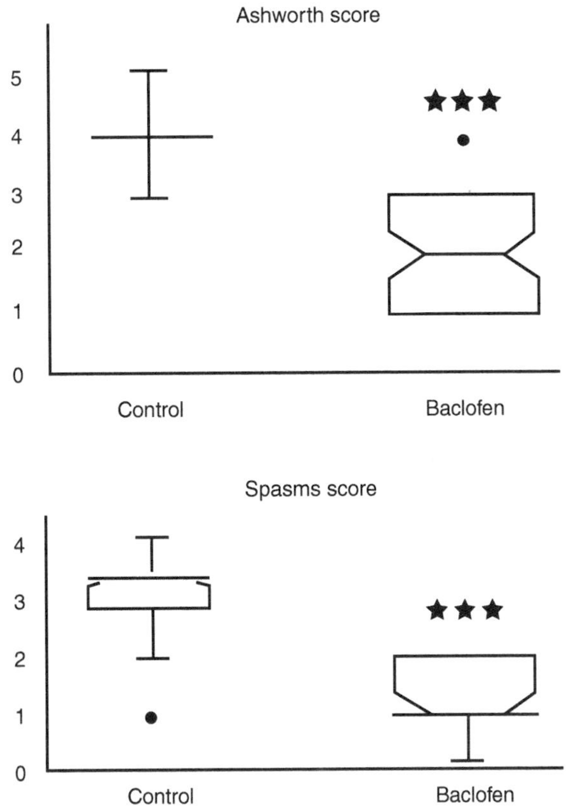

Fig. 6.10 Clinical scores before and during ITB therapy for patients affected with spastic paraplegia. Box plot graph of Ashworth scores and spasm scores obtained at control conditions and after ITB. Wilcoxon signed-rank test showed a significant reduction in both rigidity of lower limbs and frequency of spasms (***$p<0.001$) [29]. The *lower and upper borders* of the box represent the 25 and 75 % quartiles of the distribution, respectively, while the line inside the box corresponds to the median value. The upper and lower whiskers stand for the 10th and 90th percentile, the dot outside the whisker-range being the observed values exceeding those percentiles

or brainstem damage, before irreducible contractures and fixed deformities appeared [16].

ITB also became a first-line treatment for spasticity in **CP patients** whether spasticity is pure or mixed with dystonia [30, 31]. The earliest successful use of ITB in children was by Armstrong [32]. Independently, Albright et al. [33] reported a double-blind study with children which showed that a bolus injection of baclofen significantly decreased spasticity a few hours after injection. In 2003, Albright et al. [34] published a study of long-term effects of ITB with a series of 68 children and young adults, mostly with CP; follow-up was up to 10 years with a mean of 6 years. Daily dosage for optimal effects had to be augmented over the first 2 years, but then remained stable with a mean dose of 300 µg/day. In a study with 24 patients able to ambulate and a mean follow-up of 52 months after continuous ITB, ambulation improved by one of four functional levels in 9 patients, did not change in 12, and was worse in 2 [35, 36]. Effects of ITB on gait control in hereditary spastic paraparesis were published as positive by Dan et al. [37].

An excellent review of literature data by Albright is available in a special issue of the journal "Child's Nervous System" [19]. All studies converged to estimate that ITB improves spasticity and function, not only in children less than 8 years of age but also in adolescents between 8 and 18 years. Overall, improvement was observed for positioning in 69 % of the patients, transfers in 58 %, dressing in 69 %, hygiene in 51 %, reduction in startle reactions in 54 %, quality of sleep in 43 %, comfort in 53 % [28, 38, 39]. Besides, speech was improved in 33 % of the patients, self-feeding in 30 %, swallowing in 33 %, stool frequency in 25 % [40]. Overall 88 % of the patients would consent to undergo the procedure again [39]. According to Caregiver Questionnaire by the care providers, ease of care was improved in 88 % of the assessed children (mean age of 11 years), none of the children had rapid worsening of deformity or scoliosis, and 95 % would agree to have an operation again [41, 42].

Narayan et al. [43] were the first to report the successful use of ITB in pediatric dystonia, namely, for intractable axial dystonia in an 18-year-old adolescent.

The main report on pediatric patients is by Albright et al. [31], who used ITB in a series of 89 children affected with severe generalized dystonia; 70 % of them had CP and the remainder a variety of dystonic disorders. Dystonia improved in 90 % of the patients, ease of care in 85 %, and speech and function in 33 %.

In spite of some inconstant effects, ITB has proven especially valuable to treat dystonia in CP children. The goal is to improve posturing and comfort, decrease pain caused by dystonic arching of trunk and neck or by lower limb dystonic spasms, or abrupt "dystonic storms". In CP patients with mixed spasticity and dystonia, which is a frequent clinical situation, ITB improves both spasticity and dystonia.

6.8.2 Effect on Urinary Function

For patients with spasticity and normal micturition, ITB generally does not alter urinary function, except transiently during the dose adjusting time. For spastic patients with additional neurogenic hyperactive bladder, ITB may improve the clinical situation, namely, urinary urgencies, urine leakage in between intermittent catheterizations, or leak around the catheter in patients with permanent catheterization.

Urologic investigations include examination of the type of voiding (voluntary, triggered by suprapubic tapping, indwelling or intermittent catheterization), detection of urinary infections, measurement of the residual bladder volume, and urodynamic quantitive status. A neurogenic hyperactive bladder is characterized by uninhibited contractions with high bladder pressure elicited at a low volume of urine.

The benefit of ITB on the urinary function in spastic patients has been often mentioned in literature but rarely precisely documented. A personal study with a group of 17 patients with spasticity of spinal origin and presenting with a neurogenic bladder showed interesting but inconsistent results [28]. Under chronic ITB, urinary urgencies or incontinence were improved in 4 of the 5 noncatheterized explored patients, whereas urine leakage was reduced in all the 5 intermittently or permanently catheterized patients studied. At urodynamic examination under ITB, detrusor contractions were found to be totally suppressed in 1, occurring at a higher volume in 5, and unchanged in 3 of the 9 patients studied. Bladder capacity was found increased in 5 of the 9 explored patients; for those not improved the most likely cause of ineffectiveness was a high degree of fibrosis of the bladder wall.

6.8.3 Effect on Spasms

Spasms, especially in flexion, significantly impair quality of life for spastic patients; they render posturing in wheelchair and bed unsafe, provoke bladder incontinence, and disturb sleep. Approximately 82 % of patients with spasticity resulting from incomplete spinal lesion, and 50 % of those with complete lesion, have sleep disturbances as a result of increased nocturnal spasm activity. ITB has been shown to diminish spasms in most cases [44].

In a personal study with 17 patients with severe spasticity of spinal origin, we recorded polysynaptic flexion reflexes in control conditions and then under intrathecal baclofen, in order to quantify the spinal excitability responsible for spontaneous or induced spasms [28]. The flexion reflexes of lower limbs were recorded by a surface electrode applied over the short head of biceps femoris after electrical stimulation of the ipsilateral sensory sural nerve at the ankle, according to a method discussed elsewhere. Assessments using clinical spasm scales were combined with polysynaptic flexion reflex recordings. Flexion reflex thresholds were found to be increased and amplitudes significantly reduced by ITB in all patients' series.

6.8.4 Effects on Pain

There is a general agreement to consider that ITB achieves remarkable relief of **spasm-related pain** [27, 45–51]. This is also our experience with patients affected by spasticity of spinal origin, which we documented by studies on the effects of ITB on pain manifestations, sensation threshold, and polysynaptic flexion reflexes, the so-called nociceptive RIII reflexes [46].

Efficacy of ITB on **central neurogenic pain** remains controversial. Ochs et al. [27] and Sahuquillo et al. [49] reported that neuropathic pain was not affected in their series. In contrast to this, Herman et al. [50] and Taira et al. [51] reported that ITB reduced central pain caused by spinal or cerebral lesions, respectively. In our experience three of six patients who had central neuropathic pain of spinal cord origin had their pain reduced after ITB [28].

Stimulus-induced pain, i.e., hyperalgesia or allodynia, was considered more susceptible to baclofen than spontaneous pain. Experimental studies indicate that loss of GABA-ergic interneurons produce allodynia or hyperalgesia [52]. Since a significant decrease of dorsal horn GABA-ergic interneurons develops after spinal cord injury, GABA-ergic agonists might help restore the normal encoding of (exteroceptive) inputs. However, since baclofen affects the spontaneous hyperactivity of dorsal horn neurons, it would not be significantly effective on spontaneous pain.

6.8.5 Effects on Orthopedic Deformities

Effects on orthopedic deformities were mainly assessed in CP patients. In a study on hip subluxation with 33 children, adolescents or young adults, no deterioration of the annual migration rate was observed during the year of ITB therapy in as many as 91 % of the patients [53]. Evenmore, it is generally admitted that children needed less orthopedic surgery after ITB therapy [36].

Effects of ITB on scoliosis are controversial. On the one hand, aggravation of scoliosis was reported for a group of four patients [54]. On the other hand, decrease in spasticity or dystonia under ITB helps prevent deterioration of scoliosis as it allows better physical therapy program.

The main published series of the use of ITB for treating spasticity or dystonia for which a minimum of information is available are summarized in Tables 6.2 and 6.3.

6.9 Complications

6.9.1 Device-Related Complications

Catheter problems and CSF leaks are the most common complications. Pump malfunction occurs rarely, the latter approximately at 1 % per year.

Interruption of baclofen delivery results first in itching and rebound spasticity, which represent warning symptoms; this should lead to rapid re-hospitalization to avoid a life-threatening baclofen withdrawal syndrome (see above). The effective treatment is fixing the mechanical problem rapidly. Meanwhile, the patients can be managed with oral baclofen and benzodiazepine (e.g., clonazepam, diazepam).

Catheter problems include catheters being kinked, disconnected at the pump or connector, or dislodged; also their outlet can be encased in arachnoid or migrate to subdural space or be obstructed by fibrosis, more rarely by granuloma. Migration of catheter is likely to occur more frequently in children, because they are more active than adults [68].

The first steps to diagnose the problem are to query the pump by its programmer, so as to verify the reservoir is not empty and the pump is not misprogrammed, and then to check the catheter continuity by plain X-ray (Fig. 6.9). If the catheter is disconnected or has migrated out of the dural sac, its repositioning is performed; repair must be on emergency basis. If the cause is not obvious, the reservoir is emptied through the pump port to determine whether the appropriate amount of baclofen is present and CSF is aspirated. If no CSF can be aspirated, the catheter needs to be surgically revised. A contrast study is rarely required. According to Penn and Corcos [7], indium-111 can be injected through the port and scanned at 24 and 48 h to check patency. An alternative is to inject a radiopaque dye such as iohexal through the catheter under fluoroscopy to look for blockage or leak.

Also microscopic cracks in the catheter can lead to leakage without apparent loss of catheter patency [90, 91].

For prevention, care should be taken during surgery to check that the catheter is not pinched or kinked, and also that it is firmly fixed to the paraspinal muscles with the anchor devices in order to prevent secondary dislodgement under lumbar movements.

Table 6.2 ITB for treating spasticity (literature data)

Author(s) date reference(s)	No. of patients (age, years)	Etiology	Daily dose (µg/day) after equilibrium, range (average)	Results: Follow-up (months, m, or years, y), range (average)	Spasticity (Ashworth scale) Pre	Spasticity (Ashworth scale) Post	Spasms score Pre	Spasms score Post	Complications
Penn et al. (1989) [25]	20	Multiple sclerosis, spinal cord injury		10–33 m (19.2)	4.0	1.2			Pump failed (1), catheter dislodged (1)
Ochs et al. (1989) [27]	28	Multiple sclerosis, spinal cord injury, spinal cord disease	(350)	2–28 m (10)	3.6	1.8	2.8	1.4	
Parke et al. (1989) [55]	21	Multiple sclerosis, spinal cord injury		(6 m)	Decreased tone and improved performance in most patients				
Broseta et al. (1990) [56]	14	Spinal cord lesion	25–260	(11 m)	3.6	1.9	2.6	0.1	
Lazorthes et al. (1990) [48]	38	Multiple sclerosis, posttraumatic spastic syndrome, cerebral palsy, ischemic cerebral lesion, spinal ischemia, transverse myelitis	21–500 (160)	4–43 m (18)	Better results in traumatic medullary lesion than demyelinating disease, functional improvement, improvement of hypertonia confirmed by Hoffman (H) reflex, disappearance of painful muscular spasms				
Loubser et al. (1991) [57]	9 (22–63)	Spinal cord injury	(535)		3.8	1.3	3.6	0.6	
Sahuquillo et al. 1991 [49]	10	Spinal cord lesions	(193)	5–35 m (15)	4.6	1.2	3.2	0.8	

(continued)

Table 6.2 (continued)

Author(s) date reference(s)	No. of patients (age, years)	Etiology	Daily dose (µg/day) after equilibrium, range (average)	Results: Follow-up (months, m, or years, y), range (average)	Spasticity (Ashworth scale) Pre	Spasticity (Ashworth scale) Post	Spasms score Pre	Spasms score Post	Complications
Stewart-Wynne et al. (1991) [58]	6	Spinal origin, supraspinal origin		(5 y)	Decreased tone and spasms in most, improved capacities in most				
Herman et al. (1992) [50]	9	Multiple sclerosis, spinal cord injury, transverse myelitis			Decreased spasms in most				
Hugenholtz et al. (1992) [59]	6	Intractable spinal spasticity							
Meythaler et al. (1992) [60]	10	Spinal spasticity	(291)	(1 y)		2.2 points decrease		1.7 points decrease	Pseudo-meningoceles, catheter disruptions
Penn (1992) [26]	62	Spinal cord spasticity		(30 m)					
Saltuari et al. (1992) [61, 62]	9	Supraspinal spasticity, spinal spasticity			Decreased tone and improved performance in most				
Steers et al. (1992) [63]	10	Spinal cord origin		6–12 m	Decreased in inhibited bladder contractions in most patients decreased tone spasms in 97 %				
Albright et al. (1993) [64]	37 (5–27)	Cerebral palsy		3–48 m					
Coffey et al. (1993) [65]	93	Spinal cord injury, multiple sclerosis, other spinal pathology	(400)	5–41 m (19)	3.9	1.7	Decreased spasms in most		Pump pocket infection (1), overdose misprogramming (1)
Rifici et al. (1994) [17]	8	Traumatic brain injury			3.9	1.6	4.0	1.4	

Nance et al. (1995) [66]	7	Multiple sclerosis, spinal cord injury			3.9	1.8	3.5	0.8	
Azouvi et al. (1996) [22]	18	Multiple sclerosis, spinal cord injury, others	(339)	(1 y)	4.0	2.1	3.0	1.8	
Ordia et al. (1996) [67]	59	Multiple sclerosis, spinal cord injury, spinal cord disease	(272)	(1 y)	4.3	1.4	3.6	0.5	
Armstrong et al. (1997) [68]	19 (4–19)	Brain injury, cerebral palsy		3–48 m (23)	4	2	2.2	0.9	Pump pocket effusion (5), CSF fistula (1), local infection (3), meningitis (2)
Becker et al. (1997) [16]	18 (25–70)	Traumatic brain injury (9), hypoxic brain injury (9) (GOS 2 [vegetative] or 3 [severely disabled])	100–600 (310)	3–54 m (16)	4.1	2.7	2.1	0.9	Pump pocket infection (1), dislodged catheter (1)
Middel et al. (1997) [69]	22	Spinal origin			2.9	0.4	2.2	0.6	
Rawicki (1999) [70]	18	Cerebral origin	(301)	(1 y)	5	3	2.5	1.0	
Gerszten et al. (1998) [36]	48 (5–43)	Cerebral palsy: diplegia (8), quadriplegia (40)	25–1350 (306)			Reduced needs of orthopedic surgery in 36 % of patients			
Gianino et al. (1998) [71]	25	Multiple sclerosis, spinal cord injury, spinal cord disease	23–775 (298)	(1 y)	3.7	1.4	2.6	0.5	
Meythaler et al. (1999) [72]	17 (29±11)	Spastic-dystonic hypertonia after traumatic brain injury	100–412 (183)	(1 y)	3.5	1.7	1.8	1.2	

(continued)

Table 6.2 (continued)

Author(s) date reference(s)	No. of patients (age, years)	Etiology	Daily dose (μg/day) after equilibrium, range (average)	Results: Follow-up (months, m, or years, y), range (average)	Spasticity (Ashworth scale) Pre	Spasticity (Ashworth scale) Post	Spasms score Pre	Spasms score Post	Complications
Gilmartin et al. (2000) [73]	44	Cerebral origin	(402)	(39 m)	3.6	2.2	3.6	0.5	
Burns and Meythaler (2001) [74]	14	Tetraplegia	(300)	(1 y)	3.7	1.8	3.3	1.8	
Dario et al. (2002) [75]	20	Cerebral origin		12–36 m (22)	4.4	1.8	2.5	0.5	
Albright et al. (2003) [34]	68	Cerebral origin	(300)	(70 m)					CSF leaks, seromas, catheter problems
Plassat et al. (2004) [76]	40	Spinal cord injury, brain damage		(4 y)		1.8			Catheter problems, CSF leakage, subcutaneous collection
Boviatsis et al. (2005) [77]	22	Multiple sclerosis, spinal cord injury				2 point decrease			
Krach et al. (2005) [53]	31 (4–29)	Cerebral palsy			3	1			
Hoving et al. (2007) [78]	17 (7–16)	Cerebral palsy							
Delhaas et al. (2008) [79]	115			(12 m)					Wound complications, catheter problems, CSF leakage

Saval and Chiodo (2008) [80]	57 (19–86)	Cerebral palsy, traumatic brain injury, stroke, multiple sclerosis, spinal cord injury	MS, (227); non-MS, (127)	(3 y)					Catheter problems (8), meningitis (1)
Rekand and Grønning (2011) [81]	14	Multiple sclerosis		19–137 m (62)		1 point decrease			
Ucar et al. (2011) [82]	30	Cerebral palsy, brain injury, spinal cord injury	(156)	(10 y)	3.8	1.7	1.7	0.8	Wound complications, CSF collection
Natale et al. (2011) [83]	112	Quadriparesis (74), paraparesis (34), hemiplegia (4)	23–500	(55 m)	4.5	1.2			Catheter problems (7)
Taira et al. (2012) [84] (multicenter study)	369 adults, 31 juvenile			1 y for 313 out of 400 of patients					Catheter problems (8.5 %): catheter migration (6.5 %), breakage (1.5 %), obstruction (0.5 %), kinking (0.3 %) Pump trouble (1.5 %): alarm abnormality (0.3 %), memory error (0.3 %), delayed recovery (0.3 %), rotation (0,3 %), malfunction (0.3 %)
Lyon University (unpublished series 2013)	113	Supraspinal origin, spinal origin, cerebral palsy[a]	13–800 (212)	1–26 y (7.5)	3.9	1.9[b]			Catheter problems (5 %), infections (7 %)

[a]Analytical etiology. Spinal origin (52 %): multiple sclerosis (26 %), spinal cord injury (12 %), postsurgical paraplegia (6 %), spinal cord diseases (8 %; amyotrophic lateral sclerosis, hereditary spastic paraplegia, miscellaneous). Supraspinal origin (10 %): traumatic brain injury (5 %), posthypoxic ischemia (5 %). Cerebral palsy (38 %)

[b]Significant improvement after ITB implantation ($p<0.0001$)

Table 6.3 ITB for treating dystonia

Author(s) date, reference	No. of patients (age, years)	Etiology	Daily dose (μg/day), range (average)	Results: Follow-up (months, m, or years, y), average	Results: Dystonia (BADS) Pre	Results: Dystonia (BADS) Post	Remarks	Complications
Ford et al. (1996) [85]	13	Severe segmental dystonia, generalized dystonia		21 m			More effective when dystonia is associated with spasticity	
Grande et al. (2000) [86]	1 (26)	Heredo-degenerative dystonia					Improvement of hemicorps, disappearance of painful spasms	
Walker et al. (2000) [87]	14	Dystonia		6 y			Only two had clear clinical benefit	
Albright et al. (2001) [31]	77 (3–42; average, 13)	Generalized dystonia, predominant dystonia with coexisting spasticity	200–2000 (485)	29 m	18	4	More effective when catheter tip higher than T4	CSF leaks, infections, catheter problems
Albright (2007) [19]	>200	Severe dystonia, dystonia secondary to cerebral palsy or traumatic brain injury, heredo-degenerative dystonia, hemidystonia	25–900 (400)	10 y	12	9		Infections, catheter problems, CSF leaks in 10 % of patients
Van Rijn et al. (2009) [88]	42	Dystonia of complex regional pain syndrome	150–1300 (450)	12 m		Significant decrease	Improvement in dystonia, pain, disability, and quality of life	Pump or catheter defects
Motta et al. (2009) [89]	11	Secondary dystonia in upper limbs due to cerebral palsy		12 m		15 % decrease		

BADS Barry–Albright Dystonia scale [20]

CSF leaks may happen; their appearance is more commonly observed in children than in adults, 12 % vs. 3 % [92]. CSF may collect in the lumbar region or around the pump. Escape of CSF leads to low-pressure, postural headaches or even fistulae with potential infectious complications. If occurring in the initial postoperative period, it may resorb after bed rest and compressive bandage and rarely requires blood patches, lumbar drainage, or surgical closure. If it persists or is of secondary appearance, the site of leakage has to be surgically repaired. A purse-string suture can be placed around the catheter where it enters the dura so as to decrease the risk of further CSF leakage.

To overcome catheter-related complications, a catheter of the *Ascenda type* was recently developed by Medtronic Inc. (Fig. 6.2). Stronger than the former catheter, it should decrease risk of cracks and therefore CSF leaks; less soft, it should diminish occurrence of looping and kinking; with a more reliable anchorage system, it should decrease migration rate.

6.9.2 Infections

With trained hands, implant infections are rare. The bacteria filter of the pump is able to block contamination from the reservoir to the CSF. However, infection of the pump pocket and/or of the CSF may develop, in the order of 3 % of the patients treated with ITB. Clinical manifestations of infection may not become obvious before weeks or months after implantation. If only the pump pocket is infected, the wound should be reopened, the pump removed, and the cavity cleaned and irrigated with an antiseptic solution, and then the pump should be reimplanted followed by antibiotics administered intravenously according to the bacterial antibiogram. Such a management may be successful in around half of the cases. If both the pump and the CSF are infected, the whole implant should better be removed and antibiotics should be administered intravenously for at least 14 days. The system is then reimplanted a few months later, no less than 2 months after CSF has normalized. Infections generally result from intraoperative contamination or on the occasion of pump refilling. Responsible agents are most often Staphylococcus aureus or Gram-negative bacteria.

As reported by Penn [26], despite an overall 30 % of complications – mainly catheter problems, rarely infections, all requiring surgical revision – only 10 % of the patients with ITB decided to discontinue treatment, which corresponds to a good index of satisfaction.

6.10 Intraventricular Baclofen

Recently several studies have reported the use of intraventricular baclofen (IVB) in refractory spasticity or dystonia [93]. IVB can be indicated as remedy in a subset of patients who had experienced multiple revisions while receiving ITB therapy for spasticity [94]. IVB may be also the first option in patients with **generalized dystonia**.

The rationale for the use of IVB therapy is that for the treatment of dystonia the site of baclofen activity may be at the cortical level. As a matter of fact, intraventricular infusion results in a baclofen concentration over the cortex greater than that resulting from intrathecal infusion [95]. When treating generalized dystonia, baclofen would act by inhibiting the stimulation of the premotor and supplementary motor cortex [96]. Albright [97] reasoned that IVB may be less efficacious for patients with spasticity because baclofen needs to reach the spinal cord level, whereas for dystonia it needs to reach the cerebral convexities.

Prior to decision, patients with a history of intraventricular hemorrhage or meningitis should undergo a flow study to assess the potential risks of IVB [97]. As regards the site of implantation, Turner and colleagues [94] use the lateral ventricles, whilst Albright [95, 97] and Bollo and colleagues [98] prefer the third ventricle because the infused baclofen egresses directly down the aqueduct and fourth ventricle, then enters the subarachnoid space and distributes over the cerebral convexities. For third-ventricle catheter placement, Albright uses an endoscope to introduce the catheter in the third ventricle [97]. The length of the catheter is measured from the dura over the frontal cortex to a point 2–3 mm above the floor of the third ventricle. A subcutaneous or subfascial pocket is created for pump insertion. For patients cachectic secondary to the caloric expenditure associated with nearly continual dystonic movements and thus having minimal subcutaneous fat, a subfascial location is preferred.

The most frequent complications are infections, followed by catheter misplacement or migration.

IVB is a cost-effective option for patients with mounting revisions during ITB therapy. IVB might be also the first option for patients with generalized dystonia.

Conclusion

ITB is a potent inhibitor of spinal cord synaptic activity. Implantation of an intrathecal delivery system is only a means to an end: delivery of baclofen directly to the spinal cord. Worldwide therapeutic studies demonstrated efficacy and safety on spasticity of spinal origin, especially after multiple sclerosis or spinal cord injury. Indications were thereafter extended to spasticity and hypertonia of brain or brainstem origin and spasticity and dystonia in CP patients. For children with CP, ITB is particularly indicated for the subset of patients with spastic quadriparesis or generalized dystonia, for whom the method is able to achieve improvement in quality of life and to make caring much easier.

In well-defined situations with clinically typical spasticity, decision for implantation can be made straightforward. However, if the clinical pattern is complex, if it is feared that a reduction in tone could decrease motor strength and consequently locomotor function, a test before any such decision is mandatory. When a patient, family, and caregivers express some reluctance to decide an implantation, a screening trial may also be useful. However, the "easy" and simple bolus test through a single lumbar puncture, capable to tell whether the patient will be responder or not, can be fundamentally misleading as the bolus may reduce tone to such an extent that motor strength may be lost and the method considered not beneficial if not harmful. Therefore a continuous-infusion test for several days is preferable.

As benefits may differ from patient to patient and goals should be realistic depending on the initial patient status, the patient, family, and caregivers need to receive appropriate information to make the right decision. Realistic goal setting is the key to satisfaction. Also the patient and caregivers should understand the role that they will have to play in the therapeutic process, especially to be alert for emerging signs of overdosage, malfunction, or complications.

In spite of a significant complication rate, especially due to catheter-related problems, the dropout rate is rather low: less than 10 % over time, with most patients wishing to continue on ITB at the end of pump battery life [7, 99].

The method offers the advantage of reversibility and of adaptability to the desired degree of tone reduction, but it requires frequent refilling and delivery adjustments according to each patient's needs. Despite its high cost, ITB has an acceptable cost–benefit ratio, at least for developed countries [99].

References

1. Faigle JW, Keberle H (1972) The chemistry and kinetics of lioresal. Postgrad Med J 48(Suppl 5):9–13
2. Wuis EW, Dirks RJ, Vree TB, van der Kleyn E (1985) High-performance liquid chromatographic analysis of baclofen in plasma and urine of man after precolumn extraction and derivatization with o-phthaldialdehyde. J Chromatogr 337:341–350
3. Ahuja S (1985) Baclofen. In: Florey K (ed) Analytical profiles of drug substances, vol 14. Academic, New York, pp 527–548
4. Davidoff RA, Sears ES (1974) The effects of lioresal on synaptic activity in the isolated spinal cord. Neurology 24:957–963
5. Kroin JS, Penn RD, Beissinger RL, Arzbaecher RC (1984) Reduced spinal reflexes following intrathecal baclofen in the rabbit. Exp Brain Res 54:191–194
6. Penn RD, Kroin JS (1984) Intrathecal baclofen alleviates spinal cord spasticity. Lancet 1:1078
7. Penn RD, Corcos DM (2011) Management of spasticity by central nervous system infusion techniques. In: Winn HR (ed) Youmans neurological surgery, 6th edn. Elsevier-Saunders, Philadelphia, pp 1038–1048
8. Kroin JS, Ali A, York M, Penn RD (1993) The distribution of medication along the spinal canal after chronic intrathecal administration. Neurosurgery 33:226–230
9. Sallerin-Caute B, Monsarrat B, Lazorthes Y, Cros J, Bastide R (1988) A sensitive method for the determination of baclofen in human CSF by high performance liquid chromatography. J Liquid Chromatogr 11:1753–1761
10. Sallerin-Caute B, Lazorthes Y, Bastide R (1991) CSF pharmacokinetic of intrathecal baclofen administration. In: Sindou M, Abbott R, Keravel Y (eds) Neurosurgerry for spasticity. Springer, Wien/New York, p 95
11. Müller H, Zierski J, Dralle D, Krauß D, Mutschler E (1988) Pharmacokinetics of intrathecal baclofen. In: Müller H, Zierski J, Penn RD (eds) Local-spinal therapy of spasticity. Springer, Berlin, pp 223–226
12. Albright AL, Shultz BL (1999) Plasma baclofen levels in children receiving continuous intrathecal baclofen infusion. J Child Neurol 14:408–409
13. Jones ML, Leslie DP, Bilsky G, Bowman B (2008) Effects of intrathecal baclofen on perceived sexual functioning in men with spinal cord injury. J Spinal Cord Med 31:97–102

14. Denys P, Mane M, Azouvi P, Chartier-Kastler E, Thiebaut JB, Bussel B (1998) Side effects of chronic intrathecal baclofen on erection and ejaculation in patients with spinal cord lesions. Arch Phys Med Rehabil 79:494–496
15. Bitran D, Miller SA, McQuade DB, Leipheimer RE, Sachs BD (1988) Inhibition of sexual reflexes by lumbosacral injection of a GABAB agonist in the male rat. Pharmacol Biochem Behav 31:657–666
16. Becker R, Alberti O, Bauer BL (1997) Continuous intrathecal baclofen infusion in severe spasticity after traumatic or hypoxic brain injury. J Neurol 244:160–166
17. Rifici C, Kofler M, Kronenberg M, Kofler A, Bramanti P, Saltuari L (1994) Intrathecal baclofen application in patients with supraspinal spasticity secondary to severe traumatic brain injury. Funct Neurol 9:29–34
18. Meythaler JM, McCary A, Hadley MN (1997) Prospective assessment of continuous intrathecal infusion of baclofen for spasticity caused by acquired brain injury: a preliminary report. J Neurosurg 87:415–419
19. Albright AL (2007) Intrathecal baclofen for childhood hypertonia. Childs Nerv Syst 23:971–979
20. Barry MJ, Van Swearingen JM, Albright AL (1999) Reliability and responsiveness of the Barry–Albright dystonia scale. Dev Med Child Neurol 41:404–411
21. McCall TD, MacDonald JD (2006) Cervical catheter tip placement for intrathecal baclofen administration. Neurosurgery 59:634–640
22. Azouvi P, Mane M, Thiebaut JB, Denys P, Rémy-Neris O, Bussel B (1996) Intrathecal baclofen administration for control of severe spinal spasticity: functional improvement and long-term follow-up. Arch Phys Med Rehabil 77:35–39
23. Ochs G, Naumann C, Dimitrijevic M, Sindou M (1999) Intrathecal baclofen therapy for spinal origin spasticity: spinal cord injury, spinal cord disease, and multiple sclerosis. Neuromodulation 2:108–119
24. Rushton DN (2008) Intrathecal baclofen for the control of spinal and supraspinal spasticity. In: Barnes MP, Johnson GR (eds) Upper motor neurone syndrome and spasticity. Clinical management and neurophysiology, 2nd edn. Cambridge University Press, Cambridge, pp 181–192
25. Penn RD, Savoy SM, Corcos D, Latash M, Gottlieb G, Parke B, Kroin JS (1989) Intrathecal baclofen for severe spinal spasticity. N Engl J Med 320:1517–1521
26. Penn RD (1992) Intrathecal baclofen for spasticity of spinal origin: seven years of experience. J Neurosurg 77:236–240
27. Ochs G, Struppler A, Meyerson BA, Linderoth B, Gybels J, Gardner BP, Teddy P, Jamous A, Weinmann P (1989) Intrathecal baclofen for long-term treatment of spasticity: a multi-centre study. J Neurol Neurosurg Psychiatry 52:933–939
28. Mertens P, Parise M, Garcia-Larrea L, Benneton C, Millet MF, Sindou M (1995) Long-term clinical, electrophysiological and urodynamic effects of chronic intrathecal baclofen infusion for treatment of spinal spasticity. Acta Neurochir Suppl 64:17–25
29. Parise M, García-Larrea L, Mertens P, Sindou M, Mauguière F (1997) Clinical use of polysynaptic flexion reflexes in the management of spasticity with intrathecal baclofen. Electroencephalogr Clin Neurophysiol 105:141–148
30. Butler C, Campbell S (2000) Evidence of the effects of intrathecal baclofen for spastic and dystonic cerebral palsy. AACPDM treatment outcomes committee review panel. Dev Med Child Neurol 42:634–645
31. Albright AL, Barry MJ, Shafton DH, Ferson SS (2001) Intrathecal baclofen for generalized dystonia. Dev Med Child Neurol 43:652–657
32. Armstrong RW (1992) Intrathecal baclofen and spasticity: what do we know and what do we need to know? Dev Med Child Neurol 34:739–745
33. Albright AL, Cervi A, Singletary J (1991) Intrathecal baclofen for spasticity in cerebral palsy. JAMA 265:1418–1422
34. Albright AL, Gilmartin R, Swift D, Krach LE, Ivanhoe CB, McLaughlin JF (2003) Long-term intrathecal baclofen therapy for severe spasticity of cerebral origin. J Neurosurg 98:291–295

35. Gerszten PC, Albright AL, Barry MJ (1997) Effect on ambulation of continuous intrathecal baclofen infusion. Pediatr Neurosurg 27:40–44
36. Gerszten PC, Albright AL, Johnstone GF (1998) Intrathecal baclofen infusion and subsequent orthopedic surgery in patients with spastic cerebral palsy. J Neurosurg 88:1009–1013
37. Dan B, Bouillot E, Bengoetxea A, Cheron G (2000) Effect of intrathecal baclofen on gait control in human hereditary spastic paraparesis. Neurosci Lett 280:175–178
38. Krach LE, Kriel RL, Gilmartin RC, Swift DM, Storrs BB, Abbott R, Ward JD, Bloom KK, Brooks WH, Madsen JR, McLaughlin JF, Nadell JM (2005) GMFM 1 year after continuous intrathecal baclofen infusion. Pediatr Rehabil 8:207–213
39. Krach LE, Nettleton A, Klempka B (2006) Satisfaction of individuals treated long-term with continuous infusion of intrathecal baclofen by implanted programmable pump. Pediatr Rehabil 9:210–218
40. Bjornson KF, McLaughlin JF, Loeser JD, Nowak-Cooperman KM, Russel M, Bader KA, Desmond SA (2003) Oral motor, communication, and nutritional status of children during intrathecal baclofen therapy: a descriptive pilot study. Arch Phys Med Rehabil 84:500–506
41. Gooch JL, Oberg WA, Grams B, Ward LA, Walker ML (2004) Care provider assessment of intrathecal baclofen in children. Dev Med Child Neurol 46:548–552
42. Gooch JL, Oberg WA, Grams B, Ward LA, Walker ML (2003) Complications of intrathecal baclofen pumps in children. Pediatr Neurosurg 39:1–6
43. Narayan RK, Loubser PG, Jankovic J, Donovan WH, Bontke CF (1991) Intrathecal baclofen for intractable axial dystonia. Neurology 41:1141–1142
44. Kravitz HM, Corcos DM, Hansen G, Penn RD, Cartwright RD, Gianino J (1992) Intrathecal baclofen: effects on nocturnal leg muscle spasticity. Am J Phys Med Rehabil 71:48–52
45. Campbell SK, Almeida GL, Penn RD, Corcos DM (1995) The effects of intrathecally administered baclofen on function in patients with spasticity. Phys Ther 75:352–362
46. García-Larrea L, Sindou M, Mauguière F (1989) Nociceptive flexion reflexes during analgesic neurostimulation in man. Pain 39:145–156
47. Penn RD (1988) Intrathecal baclofen for severe spasticity. Ann N Y Acad Sci 531:157–166
48. Lazorthes Y, Sallerin-Caute B, Verdie JC, Bastide R, Carillo JP (1990) Chronic intrathecal baclofen administration for control of severe spasticity. J Neurosurg 72:393–402
49. Sahuquillo J, Muxi T, Noguer M, Jodar R, Closa C, Rubio E, Garcia-Fernandez L, Guitart JM (1991) Intraspinal baclofen in the treatment of severe spasticity and spasms. Acta Neurochir (Wien) 110:166–173
50. Herman RM, D'Luzansky SC, Ippolito R (1992) Intrathecal baclofen suppresses central pain in patients with spinal lesions: a pilot study. Clin J Pain 8:338–345
51. Taira T, Tanikawa T, Kawamura H, Iseki H, Takakura K (1994) Spinal intrathecal baclofen suppresses central pain after stroke. J Neurol Neurosurg Psychiatry 57:381–382
52. Yaksh TL (1999) Central pharmacology of nociceptive transmission. In: Wall PD, Melzack R (eds) Textbook of pain, 4th edn. Churchill Livingstone, Edinburgh, pp 253–308
53. Krach LE, Kriel RL, Gilmartin RC, Swift DM, Storrs BB, Abbott R, Ward JD, Bloom KK, Brooks WH, Madsen JR, McLaughlin JF, Nadell JM (2004) Hip status in cerebral palsy after one year of continuous intrathecal baclofen infusion. Pediatr Neurol 30:163–168
54. Sansone JM, Mann D, Noonan K, Mcleish D, Ward M, Iskandar BJ (2006) Rapid progression of scoliosis following insertion of intrathecal baclofen pump. J Pediatr Orthop 26:125–128
55. Parke B, Penn RD, Savoy SM, Corcos D (1989) Functional outcome after delivery of intrathecal baclofen. Arch Phys Med Rehabil 70:30–32
56. Broseta J, García-March G, Sánchez-Ledesma MJ, Anaya J, Silva I (1990) Chronic intrathecal baclofen administration in severe spasticity. Stereotact Funct Neurosurg 54–55:147–153
57. Loubser PG, Narayan RK, Sandin KJ, Donovan WH, Russell KD (1991) Continuous infusion of intrathecal baclofen: long-term effects on spasticity in spinal cord injury. Paraplegia 29:48–64
58. Stewart-Wynne EG, Silbert PL, Buffery S, Perlman D, Tan E (1991) Intrathecal baclofen for severe spasticity: five years experience. Clin Exp Neurol 28:244–255
59. Hugenholtz H, Nelson RF, Dehoux E, Bickerton R (1992) Intrathecal baclofen for intractable spinal spasticity – a double-blind cross-over comparison with placebo in 6 patients. Can J Neurol Sci 19:188–195

60. Meythaler JM, Steers WD, Tuel SM, Cross LL, Haworth CS (1992) Continuous intrathecal baclofen in spinal cord spasticity: a prospective study. Am J Phys Med Rehabil 71:321–327
61. Saltuari L, Kronenberg M, Marosi MJ, Kofler M, Russegger L, Rifici C, Bramanti P, Gerstenbrand F (1992) Long-term intrathecal baclofen treatment in supraspinal spasticity. Acta Neurol (Napoli) 14:195–207
62. Saltuari L, Kronenberg M, Marosi MJ, Kofler M, Russegger L, Rifici C, Bramanti P, Gerstenbrand F (1992) Indication, efficiency and complications of intrathecal pump supported baclofen treatment in spinal spasticity. Acta Neurol (Napoli) 14:187–194
63. Steers WD, Meythaler JM, Haworth C, Herrell D, Park TS (1992) Effects of acute bolus and chronic continuous intrathecal baclofen on genitourinary dysfunction due to spinal cord pathology. J Urol 148:1849–1855
64. Albright AL, Barron WB, Fasick MP, Polinko P, Janosky J (1993) Continuous intrathecal baclofen infusion for spasticity of cerebral origin. JAMA 270:2475–2477
65. Coffey JR, Cahill D, Steers W, Park TS, Ordia J, Meythaler J, Herman R, Shetter AG, Levy R, Gill B et al (1993) Intrathecal baclofen for intractable spasticity of spinal origin: results of a long-term multicenter study. J Neurosurg 78:226–232
66. Nance P, Schryvers O, Schmidt B, Dubo H, Loveridge B, Fewer D (1995) Intrathecal baclofen therapy for adults with spinal spasticity: therapeutic efficacy and effect on hospital admissions. Can J Neurol Sci 22:22–29
67. Ordia JI, Fischer E, Adamski E, Spatz EL (1996) Chronic intrathecal delivery of baclofen by a programmable pump for the treatment of severe spasticity. J Neurosurg 85:452–457
68. Armstrong RW, Steinbok P, Cochrane DD, Kube SD, Fife SE, Farrell K (1997) Intrathecally administered baclofen for treatment of children with spasticity of cerebral origin. J Neurosurg 87:409–414
69. Middel B, Kuipers-Upmeijer H, Bouma J, Staal M, Oenema D, Postma T, Terpstra S, Stewart R (1997) Effect of intrathecal baclofen delivered by an implanted programmable pump on health related quality of life in patients with severe spasticity. J Neurol Neurosurg Psychiatry 63:204–209
70. Rawicki B (1999) Treatment of cerebral origin spasticity with continuous intrathecal baclofen delivered via an implantable pump: long-term follow-up review of 18 patients. J Neurosurg 91:733–736
71. Gianino JM, York MM, Paice JA, Shott S (1998) Quality of life: effect of reduced spasticity from intrathecal baclofen. J Neurosci Nurs 30:47–54
72. Meythaler JM, Guin-Renfroe S, Hadley MN (1999) Continuously infused intrathecal baclofen for spastic/dystonic hemiplegia: a preliminary report. Am J Phys Med Rehabil 78:247–254
73. Gilmartin R, Bruce D, Storrs BB, Abbott R, Krach L, Ward J, Bloom K, Brooks WH, Johnson DL, Madsen JR, McLaughlin JF, Nadell J (2000) Intrathecal baclofen for management of spastic cerebral palsy: multicenter trial. J Child Neurol 15:71–77
74. Burns AS, Meythaler JM (2001) Intrathecal baclofen in tetraplegia of spinal origin: efficacy for upper extremity hypertonia. Spinal Cord 39:413–419
75. Dario A, Di Stefano MG, Grossi A, Casagrande F, Bono G (2002) Long-term intrathecal baclofen infusion in supraspinal spasticity of adulthood. Acta Neurol Scand 105:83–87
76. Plassat R, Perrouin Verbe B, Menei P, Menegalli D, Mathé JF, Richard I (2004) Treatment of spasticity with intrathecal baclofen administration: long-term follow-up, review of 40 patients. Spinal Cord 42:686–693
77. Boviatsis EJ, Kouyialis AT, Korfias S, Sakas DE (2005) Functional outcome of intrathecal baclofen administration for severe spasticity. Clin Neurol Neurosurg 107:289–295
78. Hoving MA, van Raak EP, Spincemaille GH, Palmans LJ, Sleypen FA, Vles JS; Dutch Study Group on Child Spasticity (2007) Intrathecal baclofen in children with spastic cerebral palsy: a double-blind, randomized, placebo-controlled, dose-finding study. Dev Med Child Neurol 49:654–659
79. Delhaas EM, Beersen N, Redekop WK, Klazinga NS (2008) Long-term outcomes of continuous intrathecal baclofen infusion for treatment of spasticity: a prospective multicenter follow-up study. Neuromodulation 11:227–236

80. Saval A, Chiodo AE (2008) Effect of intrathecal baclofen concentration on spasticity control: case series. J Spinal Cord Med 31:394–397
81. Rekand T, Grønning M (2011) Treatment of spasticity related to multiple sclerosis with intrathecal baclofen: a long-term follow-up. J Rehabil Med 43:511–514
82. Ucar T, Kazan S, Turgut U, Samanci NK (2011) Outcomes of intrathecal baclofen (ITB) therapy in spacticity. Turk Neurosurg 21:59–65
83. Natale M, Mirone G, Rotondo M, Moraci A (2012) Intrathecal baclofen therapy for severe spasticity: analysis on a series of 112 consecutive patients and future prospectives. Clin Neurol Neurosurg 114:321–325
84. Taira T, Ueta T, Katayama Y, Kimizuka M, Nemoto A, Mizusawa H, Liu M, Koito M, Hiro Y, Tanabe H (2013) Rate of complications among the recipients of intrathecal baclofen pump in Japan: a multicenter study. Neuromodulation 16:266–272; discussion 272
85. Ford B, Greene P, Louis ED, Petzinger G, Bressman SB, Goodman R, Brin MF, Sadiq S, Fahn S (1996) Use of intrathecal baclofen in the treatment of patients with dystonia. Arch Neurol 53:1241–1246
86. Grande MA, Chac6n J, Trujillo A, García-Moreno JM, Bravo M (2000) Bomba de perfusi6n intratecal de baclofén en la distonia generalizada (intrathecal perfusion pump with baclofen in generalized dystonia). Rev Neurol (Barcelona) 30:138–140
87. Walker RH, Danisi FO, Swope DM, Goodman RR, Germano IM, Brin MF (2000) Intrathecal baclofen for dystonia: benefits and complications during six years of experience. Mov Disord 15:1242–1247
88. van Rijn MA, Munts AG, Marinus J, Voormolen JH, de Boer KS, Teepe-Twiss IM, van Dasselaar NT, Delhaas EM, van Hilten JJ (2009) Intrathecal baclofen for dystonia of complex regional pain syndrome. Pain 143:41–47
89. Motta F, Antonello CE, Stignani C (2009) Upper limbs function after intrathecal baclofen therapy in children with secondary dystonia. J Pediatr Orthop 29:817–821
90. Bardutzky J, Tronnier V, Schwab S, Meinck HM (2003) Intrathecal baclofen for stiff-person syndrome: life-threatening intermittent catheter leakage. Neurology 60:1976–1978
91. Gaffen A, Nesic M, Coleman G (2005) Intrathecal baclofen (lioresal): suspected adverse incidents associated with implantable drug pump system. Can Adv React Newsl 15(4):1–2
92. Albright AL, Turner M, Pattisapu JV (2006) Best-practice surgical techniques for intrathecal baclofen therapy. J Neurosurg 104(4 Suppl):233–239
93. Albright AL, Ferson SS (2009) Intraventricular baclofen for dystonia: techniques and outcomes. Clinical article. J Neurosurg Pediatr 3:11–14
94. Turner M, Nguyen HS, Cohen-Gadol AA (2012) Intraventricular baclofen as an alternative to intrathecal baclofen for intractable spasticity or dystonia: outcomes and technical considerations. J Neurosurg Pediatr 10:315–319
95. Albright AL (2007) Long-term intraventricular baclofen infusion in beagles. J Neurosurg 107(3 Suppl):225–227
96. Siebner HR, Dressnandt J, Auer C, Conrad B (1998) Continuous intrathecal baclofen infusions induced a marked increase of the transcranially evoked silent period in a patient with generalized dystonia. Muscle Nerve 21:1209–1212
97. Albright AL (2011) Technique for insertion of intraventricular baclofen catheters. J Neurosurg Pediatr 8:394–395
98. Bollo RJ, Gooch JL, Walker ML (2012) Stereotactic endoscopic placement of third ventricle catheter for long-term infusion of baclofen in patients with secondary generalized dystonia. J Neurosurg Pediatr 10:30–33
99. Sampson FC, Hayward A, Evans G, Morton R, Collett B (2002) Functional benefits and cost/benefit analysis of continuous intrathecal baclofen infusion for the management of severe spasticity. J Neurosurg 96:1052–1057

Botulinum Toxin Injections for Spasticity

7

Justinus Kerner first recognized the potential of botulinum toxin (BTX) injections for a therapeutic use in 1817. He found that the toxin paralyzed muscles and proposed that it could be used as a therapeutic agent [1]. In 1989 Das and Park first reported the use of BTX in the treatment of adults with spasticity [2]. Injections can be administered with relative ease to almost every muscle affected by spasticity. The effects of the injections are reversible. The dose can be adjusted according to the patient's clinical response. The BTX therapy can be used to treat spasticity independent of its etiology, depending rather on the presence and distribution of increased tone and the treatment goals. Patients with focal spasticity are ideal candidates for BTX therapy. Since the 1990s, considerable experience has been gained with BTX-A for spasticity through pragmatic clinical practice and open studies, supported by randomized controlled trials. The spastic disorders for which BTX therapy has been studied include multiple sclerosis, traumatic brain injury, cerebral palsy, spinal cord injury, and stroke.

7.1 Clinical Pharmacology

BTX is a potent neurotoxin produced by the gram-negative anaerobic bacterium *Clostridium botulinum.* The paralytic effect of the toxin results from a blockade of neuromuscular transmission [3]. The effect is produced at the neuromuscular junction, where BTX inhibits the release of acetylcholine from the presynaptic nerve terminals, causing local chemodenervation. This effect, which is reversible, has led to the development of the toxin as a versatile therapeutic tool. Most of our knowledge about the mechanism of action of BTX and its efficacy in spasticity comes from work with serotype BTX-A.

There are seven serologically distinct toxin types named A, B, C, D, E, F, and G. They all inhibit acetylcholine release into the synaptic cleft by binding one or more of the transport protein chains with high specificity [4, 5]. These target proteins, on which the light chains of the toxin bind, vary for the different serotypes. Two antigenically distinct serotypes of BTX are available on the market as

M. Sindou et al., *Neurosurgery for Spasticity*,
DOI 10.1007/978-3-7091-1771-2_7, © Springer-Verlag Wien 2014

type A and B. BTX-A cleaves synaptosome-associated protein 25, whereas BTX-B cleaves vesicle-associated membrane protein. The specific site of action and the cleaved protein influence the duration of action of various BTX serotypes [6]. BTX-A has been shown to have a longer duration of effect compared with that of BTX-B [7]. The two serotypes differ from each other in their adverse effects. The unwanted effects of their anticholinergic action such as dry mouth, dysphagia, and voiding difficulties were found to be more common after BTX-B injections [8, 9].

Type A BTX formulations are available as Botox® (Allergan, Inc., Irvine, CA, USA) and Dysport® (Ipsen Ltd., Berkshire, UK). Type B is available as Myobloc® in the United States and NeuroBloc® in Europe (Solstice Neurosciences, South San Francisco, CA, USA) [10]. Although no direct comparison of these products has been made, approximate equivalence obtained from clinical experience and general survey of the literature is reported [11].

7.2 Site and Dose Determination

Treating all the muscles involved is often unnecessary and unfeasible. The treating physician needs to identify the muscles that appear to be the most disabling. The pattern of muscles to be injected can change later, depending on the patient's response. Direct injection via palpation may be appropriate for superficial muscles. Guidance by electromyography, electrical stimulation, and ultrasonography is commonly used to identify deeper muscles.

The treating physician should determine the starting dose by considering the factors shown in Table 7.1 [12]. This dose is further modified on subsequent visits, depending on the impact of prior treatments and the evolving clinical profile as it changes with treatment. If a trend toward a decreased response becomes apparent, muscle selection, muscle localization, BTX dose, injection technique, and finally the possibility of immunoresistance should be reassessed. Botox® is supplied in 100 U vials, while a vial of Dysport® contains 500 U. The vials must be reconstituted with normal saline without preservative. There is no consensus on the dilution that should be used in spasticity treatment, which varies from

Table 7.1 Possible modifiers of TBX dose

	Property of characteristic for dose to be:	
Clinical characteristic	Small	Large
Patient weight	Low	High
Muscle bulk	Small	Large
Likely duration of therapy	Chronic	Acute
Number of simultaneously injected muscles	Many	Few
Results of previous therapy	Too much weakness	Inadequate response
Ashworth score	Low	High

center to center. Studies with animals and humans show that diluted BTX-A is more effective than high concentrations, although this raises concerns about diffusion of the toxin to the adjacent muscles [13, 14]. The most appropriate number of injections per muscle depends on the size of the muscle. It is preferable to inject more sites with smaller volumes than one site with a large volume [15]. An increased number of sites provides a more even distribution of the toxin for optimum results.

7.3 Procedure

BTX-A is injected with a 23–27 gauge needle. Larger and superficial muscles are easily identified by palpation. Electromyography or electrical stimulation can identify small or deep muscle groups. Local anesthetic spray or sedation may be necessary, particularly for children. Tables 7.2 and 7.3 enumerate the muscles that can be targeted.

Table 7.2 Muscles involved in characteristic deformities of patients with spasticity in lower limb

Region	Clinical pattern	Muscle(s) involved
Hip	Flexed hip	Psoas, iliacus, rectus femoris
Thigh	Adducted thigh	Adductor group (longus, brevis, magnus), gracilis, obturator externus, ectineus
Knee	Extended knee	Quadriceps group (rectus femoris, vastus intermedius, vastus medialis, vastus lateralis)
	Flexed knee	Hamstring (biceps femoris, semitendinosus, semimembranosus)
Ankle	Equinovarus	Equinus: gastrocnemius, soleus, popliteal
		Varus: tibalis posterior
Toes	Claw toes	Flexor digitorum longus and brevis, flexor hallucis longus
	Hitchhiker' great toe	Extensor hallucis longus

Table 7.3 Muscles involved in characteristic deformities of patients with spasticity in upper limb

Region	Clinical pattern	Muscle(s) involved
Shoulder	Adducted or internally rotated shoulder	Pectoralis major, teres major
Elbow	Flexed elbow	Coracobrachialis, biceps, brachialis
Forearm	Pronated forearm	Pronator quadratus, pronator teres
Thumb	Thumb in palm	Flexor pollicis longus, adductor pollicis, opponens pollicis
Fingers	Clenched fist	Flexor digitorum superficialis, flexor digitorum profundus
	Swan neck	First and second lumbrical plus interosseous, third and fourth lumbrical plus interosseous

7.4 Onset and Duration of Therapeutic Effects

Depending on the location and severity of spasticity, BTX-A injections usually are needed at 3- to 6-month intervals to maintain the therapeutic benefit. Reinjections should be administered no sooner than 3 months after the last injections to decrease the possibility of antibody formation. Most patients begin to feel a therapeutic effect within 48–72 h after the injection. The peak effect occurs 10–14 days after injection.

A follow-up visit is recommended 10–14 weeks after injection to review the situation and consider further injections as the effect of previous injections wears off. Feedback from the patient, physiotherapist and caregivers is crucial for determining the dose and sites of the next injections.

The rehabilitation team has an important role in the evaluation and management of patients receiving BTX injections for spasticity. After injection, therapeutic interventions have multiple aims, including strengthening and facilitation, increasing range of motion, retraining of ambulation and gait, improving the fit and tolerance of orthoses and improving the function of the affected structure [16].

BTX injections can be used as a "prolonged" test for several weeks or months to mimic the effect of a corresponding neurotomy. This strategy of using preoperative injection tests allows both the patient and the medical team to appreciate the benefit that would follow a neurotomy [17].

BTX-B appears less effective but is still an alternative for individuals who have become resistant to BTX-A.

Conclusions

BTX has become a significant treatment for the management of spasticity. It is not an isolated treatment but is a valuable part of the overall therapeutic armamentarium, being relatively safe and easy to administer. Its main disadvantage is the need of repeated injections, especially when large doses and/or extended injections are required, which is a frequent situation in spastic or dystonic patients. The possible development of side effects and resistance are also significant disadvantages. Furthermore, the overall cost of the treatment is significant.

References

1. Erbguth FJ, Naumannn M (1999) Historical aspects of botulinum toxin: Justinus Kerner (1786–1862) and the "sausage poison". Neurology 53:1850–1853
2. Das TK, Park DM (1989) Effect of treatment with botulinum toxin on spasticity. Postgrad Med J 65:208–210
3. Burgen ASV, Dickens F, Zatman LJ (1949) The action of botulinum toxin on the neuromuscular junction. J Physiol 109:10–24
4. Dressler D, Adib Saberi F (2005) Botulinum toxin: mechanisms of action. Eur Neurol 53:3–9

5. Thakker MM, Rubin PA (2004) Pharmacology and clinical applications of botulinum toxins A and B. Int Ophthalmol Clin 44:147–163
6. Aoki KR (2003) Pharmacology and immunology of botulinum toxin type A. Clin Dermatol 21:476–480
7. Comella CL, Jankovic J, Shannon KM, Tsui J, Swenson M, Leurgans S, Fan W, Dystonia Study Group (2005) Comparison of botulinum toxin serotypes A and B for the treatment of cervical dystonia. Neurology 65:1423–1429
8. Dressler D, Eleopra R (2006) Clinical use of non-A botulinum toxins: botulinum toxin type B. Neurotox Res 9:121–125
9. Tintner R, Gross R, Winzer UF, Smalky KA, Jankovic J (2005) Autonomic function after botulinum toxin type A or B: a double-blind, randomized trial. Neurology 65:765–767
10. O'Brien CF (2002) Treatment of spasticity with botulinum toxin. Clin J Pain 18(6 Suppl):S182–S190
11. Pathak MS, Nguyen HT, Graham HK, Moore AP (2006) Management of spasticity in adults: practical application of botulinum toxin. Eur J Neurol 13(Suppl 1):42–50
12. Brin MF, Spasticity Study Group (1997) Dosing, administration, and a treatment algorithm for use of botulinum toxin A for adult-onset spasticity. Muscle Nerve 20(Suppl 6):S208–S220
13. Shaari CM, Sanders I (1993) Quantifying how location and dose of botulinum toxin injections affect muscle paralysis. Muscle Nerve 16:964–969
14. Bigalke H, Wohlfarth K, Irmer A, Dengler R (2001) Botulinum A toxin: Dysport improvement of biological availability. Exp Neurol 168:162–170
15. Borodic GE, Ferrante R, Pearce LB, Smith K (1994) Histologic assessment of dose-related diffusion and muscle fiber response after therapeutic botulinum toxin A injections. Mov Disord 9:31–39
16. Albany K (1997) Physical and occupational therapy considerations in adult patients receiving botulinum toxin injections for spasticity. Muscle Nerve 20(Suppl 6):S221–S231
17. Sindou M, Mertens P (2012) Surgery for intractable spasticity. In: Quiñones-Hinojosa A (ed) Schmidek and Sweet operative neurosurgical techniques: indications, methods, and results, 6th edn. Elsevier Saunders, Philadelphia, pp 1377–1392

8 Peripheral Neurotomies

Peripheral neurotomies (PN) were introduced more than a century ago [1, 2] (see Chap. 2) and more recently reactivated thanks to microtechniques and electrophysiological mapping. PN are indicated for severe focal spasticity, when botulinum toxin injections become less effective and cannot delay surgery any longer.

8.1 Rationale for Selectivity

PN aim at rebalancing the tonicity of agonist and antagonist muscular groups by reducing excessive spasticity (Fig. 8.1). A decrease in spasticity is obtained by sectioning both afferent and efferent fibers of the stretch reflex at the level of a muscular nerve (Fig. 8.2).

Surgery should be performed so that excessive hypertonia is reduced without a suppression of the useful muscular tone or an impairment of the residual motor and sensory functions. PN can be made "selective" by fine microsurgical dissection of the fascicles and their mapping by intraoperative electrical nerve stimulation [3–8].

Neurotomy consists of the partial sectioning of one or several motor branches of the nerves innervating the muscle(s) to be targeted, i.e., that in which spasticity is considered excessive. Motor branches must be accessed where they are already clearly isolated from the nerve trunk or they must be dissected and identified as motor fascicles within the nerve trunk proximal to the formation of an identifiable branch.

Up to now there is no scientific basis for defining the extent of the partial section. However, empirically, most experienced surgeons agree that sectioning must include 50–80 % (usually 75 %) of the fibers to a targeted muscle.

Before any decision on PN, testing with nerve blocks of the motor nerves innervating the selected target muscles is recommended [7, 9]. Also, botulinum toxin injections can be used as a "prolonged" test for a few months. Both mimic the effect of the neurotomy. Muscles and nerves to be targeted are listed in Tables 8.1 and 8.2.

M. Sindou et al., *Neurosurgery for Spasticity*,
DOI 10.1007/978-3-7091-1771-2_8,

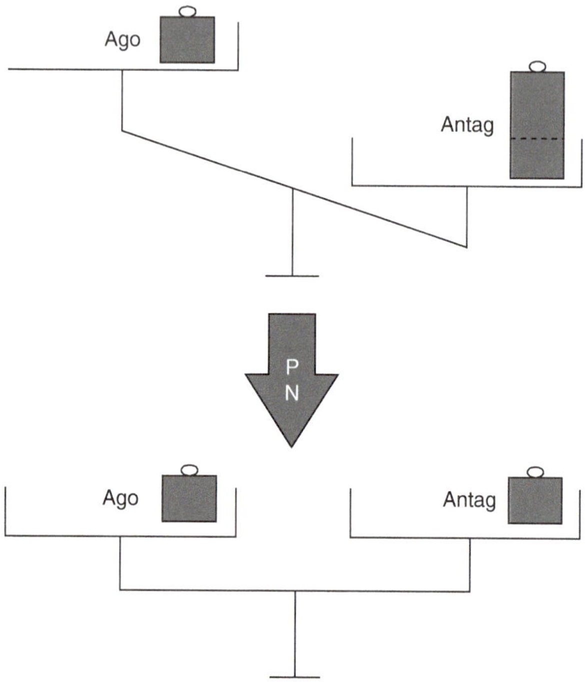

Fig. 8.1 Selective peripheral neurotomy (*PN*) improves motor function through reduction of excess tone by rebalancing agonist and antagonist muscular groups

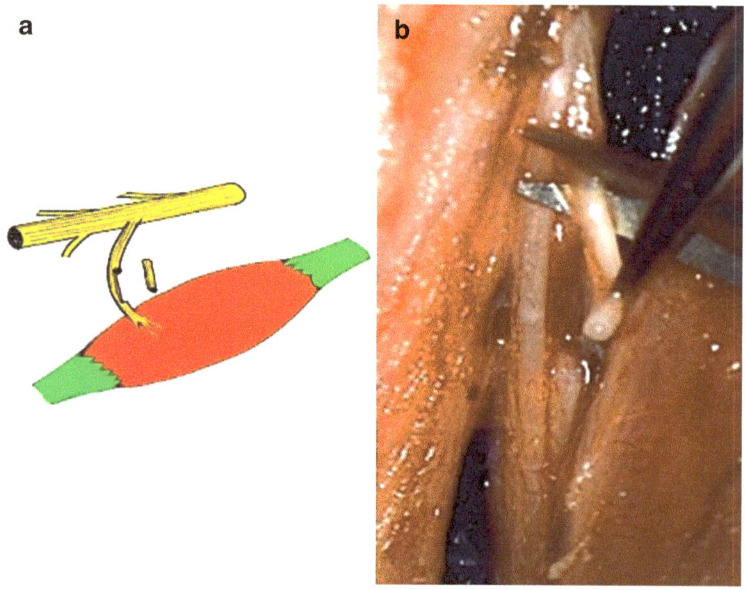

Fig. 8.2 (**a**) Sectioning of a muscular nerve, on principle including both afferent and efferent fibers of the stretch reflex. Commonly sectioning includes 50–80 % (usually 75 %) of the fibers to a targeted muscle. (**b**) Microsurgical view of the resection of one fascicle, one of the two constituting this motor nerve, for a length of 5 mm to avoid regrowing of fibers

Table 8.1 Muscles and nerves to be targeted according to clinical pattern for spasticity in lower limb

Region	Clinical pattern	Muscle(s) involved	Nerve
Hip	Flexed hip	Psoas, iliacus	Branch from lumbar plexus
		Rectus femoris	Femoral
Thigh	Adducted thigh	Adductor group (longus, brevis, magnus), gracilis, obturator externus, pectineus	Obturator
Knee	Extended knee	Quadriceps group (rectus femoris, vastus intermedius, vastus medialis, vastus lateralis)	Femoral
	Flexed knee	Hamstring (biceps femoris, semitendinosus, semimembranosus)	Sciatic
Ankle	Equinovarus	Equinus: gastrocnemius, soleus, popliteal Varus: tibalis posterior	Tibial
Toes	Claw toes	Flexor digitorum longus and brevis, flexor hallucis longus	Tibial
	Hitchhiker's great toe	Extensor hallucis longus	Peroneal

Table 8.2 Muscles and nerves to be targeted according to clinical pattern for spasticity in upper limb

Region	Clinical pattern	Muscle(s) involved	Nerve(s)
Shoulder	Adducted and internally rotated shoulder	Pectoralis major	Lateral, medial thoracic
		Teres major	Inferior subscapular
Elbow	Flexed elbow	Coracobrachialis, biceps, brachialis	Musculocutaneous
Forearm	Pronated forearm	Pronator quadratus, pronator teres	Median
Wrist	Flexed wrist	Flexor carpi radialis, palmaris longus	Median
		Flexor carpi ulnaris	Ulnar
Thumb	Thumb in palm	Flexor pollicis longus	Median
		Adductor pollicis, opponens pollicis	Ulnar
Fingers	Clenched fist	Flexor digitorum superficialis, flexor digitorum profundus	Median
	Swan neck	First and second lumbrical plus interosseous	Median
		Third and fourth lumbrical plus interosseous	Ulnar

8.2 Technical Bases for Neurotomy

8.2.1 Anesthesia

PN are performed under general anesthesia. It is useful to check the level of anesthesia by evaluating the stretch reflex (e.g., clonus); its presence implies that the anesthetic drugs do not depress reflex pathways. General anesthesia has to be performed without long-lasting muscle relaxants so that the motor responses elicited by electrical stimulation can be detected for identification of the nerve fascicles function. Nitrogen monoxide and propofol are contraindicated because they modify reflex excitability.

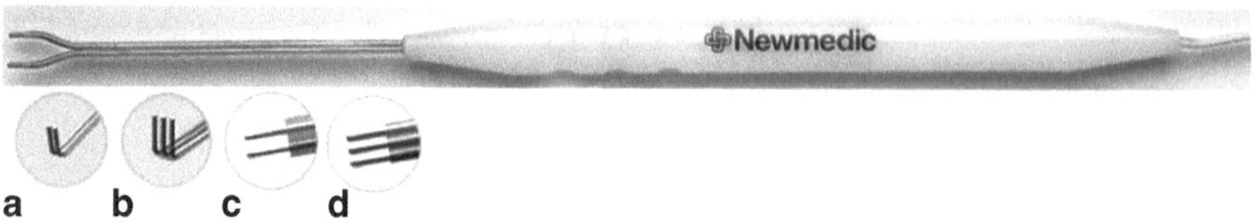

Fig. 8.3 *Angled* (**a**, **b**) and *straight* (**c**, **d**), *bipolar* (**a**, **c**) or *tripolar* (**b**, **d**) electrodes for mapping the muscular responses to electrical stimulation of nerve fascicles. The angled configuration allows moving away a fascicle from the surrounding ones, which increases stimulation selectivity. The tripolar electrode composed of a cathode positioned between two anodes produces less current diffusion, which provides better accuracy (Electrodes manufactured by Hemodia SAS, Labège, France, www.hemodia.com, www.newmedic.com)

8.2.2 Mapping

Mapping is an essential step to avoid cutting of sensory fascicles and to select the motor branches or fascicles to be interrupted. It requires the use of the operating microscope and intraoperative bipolar and/or tripolar stimulation. Frequent variations in the emergence of nerve branches and limited surgical access can make this a demanding step. The initial identification is based on descriptive anatomy, then on mapping of the muscular responses to electrical stimulation. For accuracy, a fine, flexible, angled or straight bipolar electrode or even a tripolar electrode (composed of a cathode between two anodes) for fascicle identification should be used (Figs. 8.3, 8.4 and 8.5). Stimulation is performed at low intensity, commonly 100 μA to 1 mA, to avoid "electrical diffusion" (Fig. 8.6). The response to stimulation shows in the form of a contraction in the corresponding muscle(s). Recordings of electromyography signals make identification more precise.

8.2.3 Sectioning

Once all motor branches or fascicles have been identified, those considered to be involved in harmful spasticity are marked separately with tiny differently colored tapes (Fig. 8.7). According to the preoperative evaluation and subsequent planning, variable proportions (50–80 %, depending on the degree of spasticity) of the selected motor branches or fascicles are resected. The section has to be done under the operating microscope and as close as possible to the muscle in order to ensure that only muscular branches are cut or, provided that fascicular identification is considered reliable, inside the nerve trunk itself. The resection should be approximately 5 mm long from the proximal stump, which is then coagulated with a fine bipolar forceps in order to prevent any regrowth of fibers.

The effect of each nerve resection is then evaluated by comparing the intensity of the muscular response to electrical stimulation, first distal (original maximal response) and then proximal to the resected portion of the nerve (Fig. 8.8). If the response after proximal stimulation is still intense, further resection is performed.

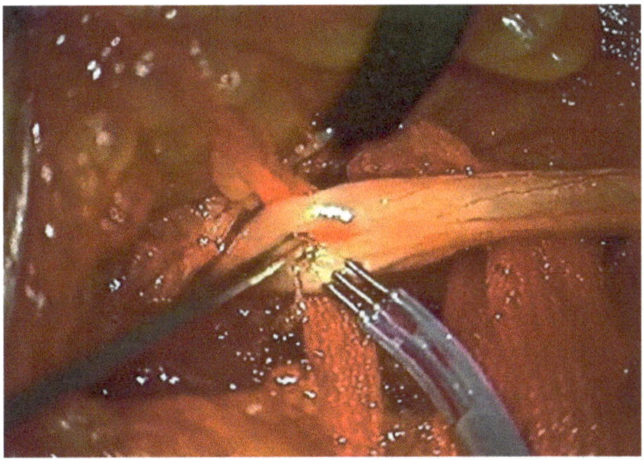

Fig. 8.4 Mapping by stimulation of a group of fascicles with a tripolar electrode before epineurium opening

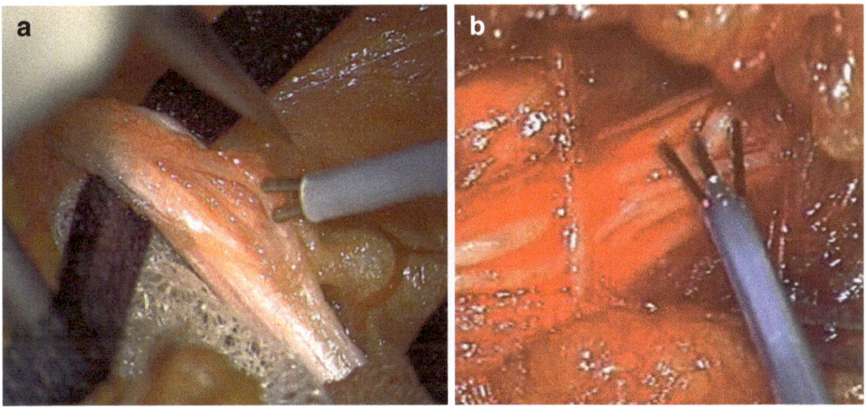

Fig. 8.5 Microsurgical dissection and exposure of the constituting fascicles of the targeted nerve after opening of the epineurium and fascicle mapping with electrostimulation. (**a**) Fascicle mapping by stimulation with a bipolar electrode. (**b**) Fascicle mapping by stimulation with a tripolar electrode

The goal is a decrease of motor innervation sufficient to avoid recurrence of spasticity by "takeover", that is, re-innervation or "adoption" of denervated muscular fibers by the surrounding intact motor fibers.

8.3 Operative Techniques for Lower Limb

8.3.1 Obturator Neurotomy

Obturator neurotomy (Fig. 8.9) aims at eliminating spasticity in the adductor muscles of the thigh and hip. It is recommended for patients with diplegia from

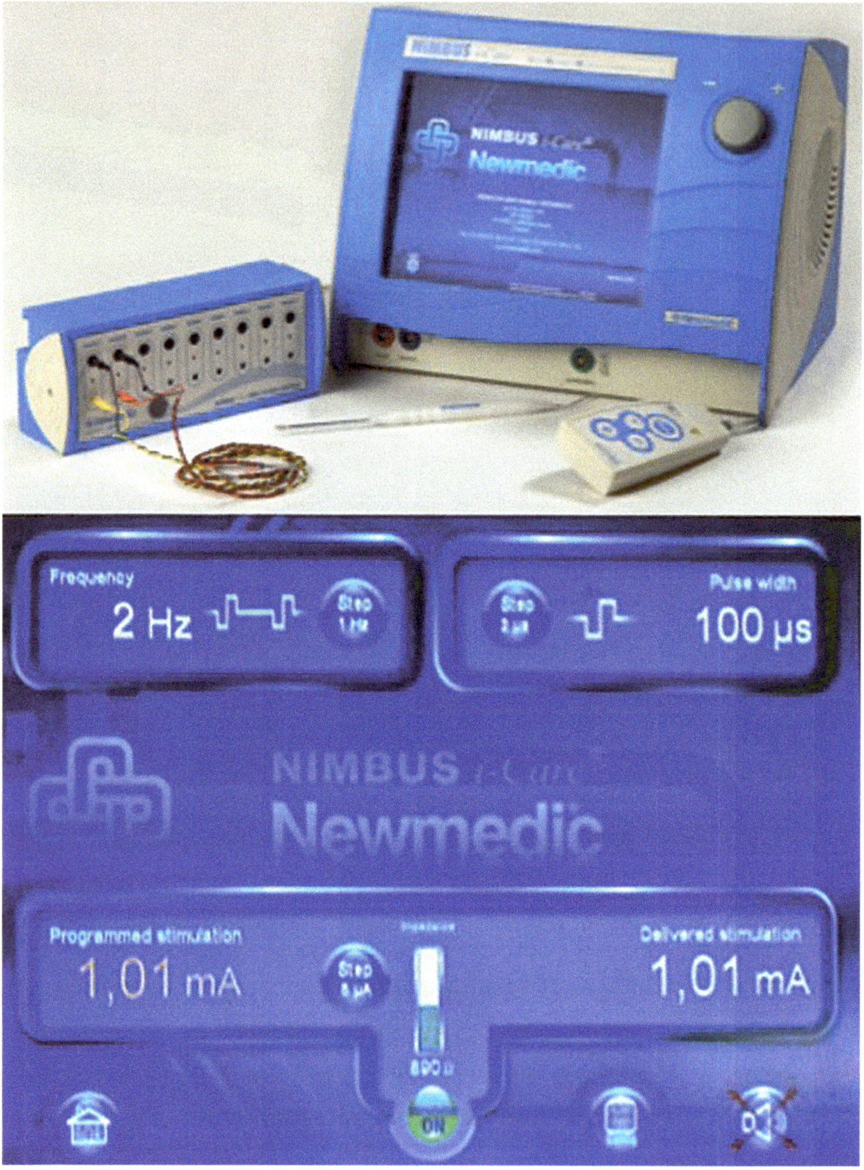

Fig. 8.6 Stimulation performed at low intensity, commonly 100 μA to 1 mA, to avoid "electrical diffusion" (Stimulator of the Nimbus i-Care model, manufactured by Hemodia SAS, Labège, France, www.hemodia.com, www.newmedic.com)

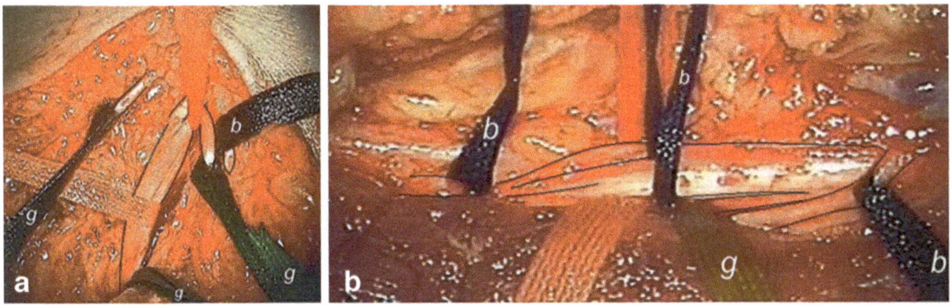

Fig. 8.7 (**a**) Operative view of the (*right*) popliteal region under operative microscope after dissection of the tibial nerve. (**b**) Operative view of the (*right*) median nerve under operative microscope. Tapes with different colors (usually three: *white*, *blue*, *green*) are used after identification of the several branches: *white tapes*, which change upon contact of blood tissue into *red*, indicate that keeping this branch totally intact is mandatory; *green tapes* (*g*) indicate that the branch is definitely a target for sectioning; *blue* ones (*b*) mean that the branch can be sectioned, but only after recheck the green-labelled branches having been cut

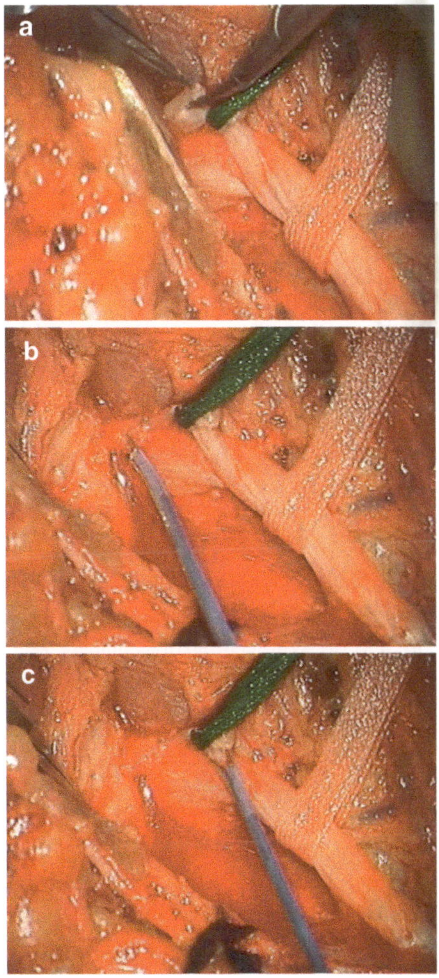

Fig. 8.8 Principle of stepwise checking the efficacy of fascicular resection with bipolar electrostimulation. (**a**) Resection of fascicle. (**b**) Stimulation distal to site of resection giving maximal muscular response. (**c**) Stimulation proximal to site of resection giving muscular response proportional to the quantity of resection

cerebral palsy if walking is hampered by a crossing of their legs. Obturator neurotomy may also be indicated in paraplegic patients to facilitate perineal toilet and self-catheterization.

The incision can be performed along the adductor longus at the proximal part of the thigh (Fig. 8.9a) or transversely at the hip flexion fold, centered on the prominence of the adductor longus tendon. In addition to its more aesthetic appearance, the latter incision facilitates adductor longus tenotomy when necessary (Fig. 8.9a). The anterior branch of the obturator nerve, which is the target of the neurotomy, is found after the dissection has been conducted laterally to the adductor longus muscle body. The posterior branch, which is situated more deeply, should be spared to preserve hip stability (Fig. 8.9b) [10, 11].

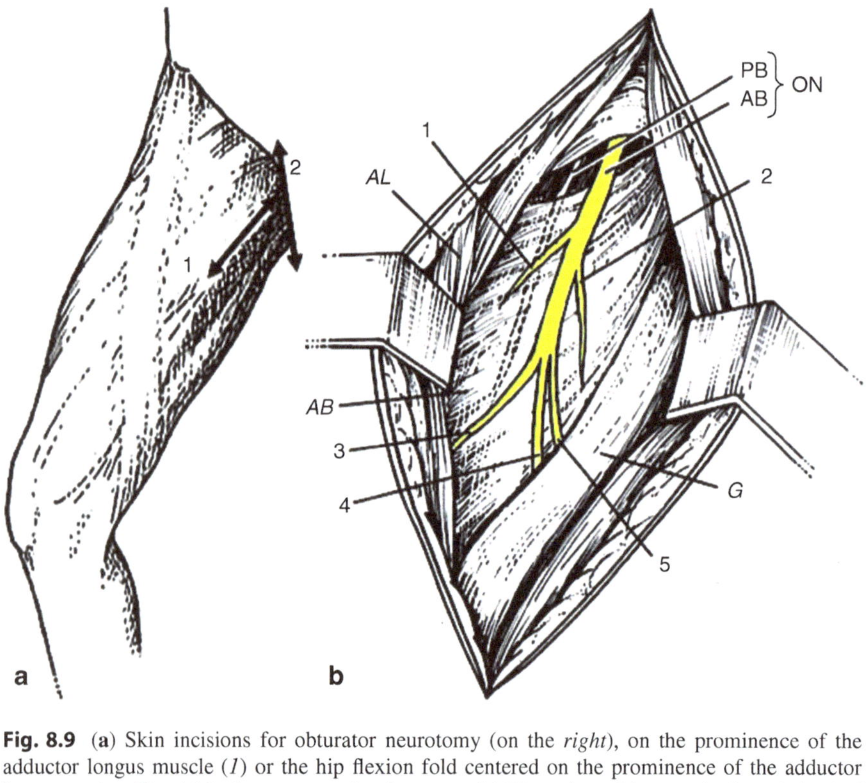

Fig. 8.9 (**a**) Skin incisions for obturator neurotomy (on the *right*), on the prominence of the adductor longus muscle (*1*) or the hip flexion fold centered on the prominence of the adductor longus tendon (*2*), which gives a cosmetic advantage. (**b**) Dissection of the anterior branch (*AB*) of the right obturator nerve (*ON*). The adductor longus (*AL*) is retracted laterally and the gracilis (*G*) medially. The nerve lies anterior to the adductor brevis (*AB*). Adductor brevis nerve (*1*, *2*), adductor longus nerve (*3*), gracilis nerve (*4*, *5*). The posterior branch (*PB*) of the obturator nerve lies under the adductor brevis and should spared

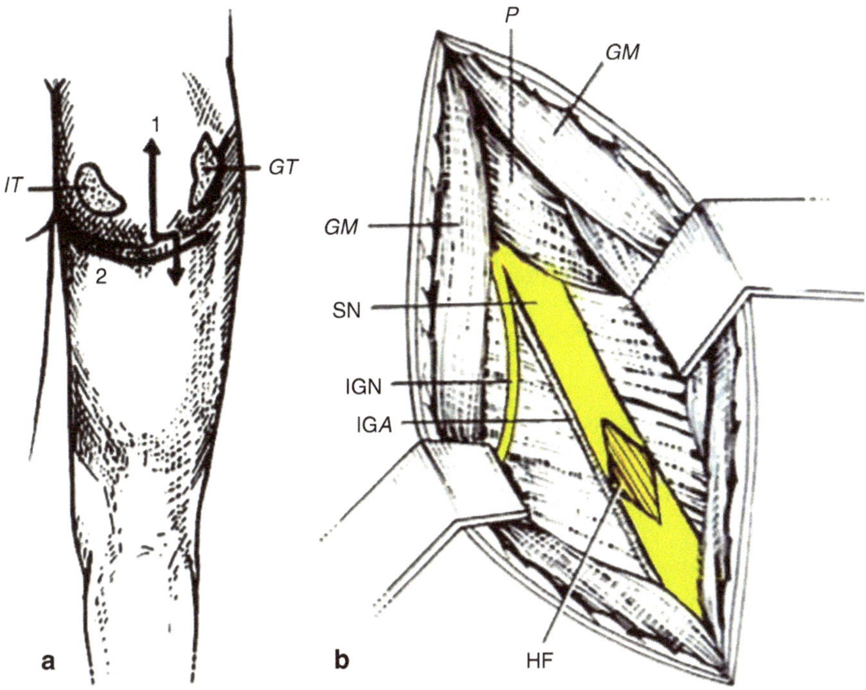

Fig. 8.10 (**a**) The skin incision for hamstring neurotomies (on the *right side*) is located on the midline (*1*) between the ischial tuberosity (*IT*) and the greater trochanter (*GT*). A transverse incision can also be performed in the gluteal fold (*2*) centered on the groove between the ischial tuberosity and the greater trochanter, for better cosmetic results. (**b**) Dissection of the right sciatic nerve (*SN*), under the piriformis (*P*), after passing through the gluteus maximus muscle (*GM*). The epineurium of the nerve is opened, and the fascicles for hamstring muscles (*HF*) are localized at the medial border of the sciatic trunk. *IGN* Inferior gluteal nerve, *IGA* inferior gluteal artery

8.3.2 Hamstring Neurotomy

Hamstring neurotomy (Fig. 8.10) is indicated for spasticity in the hamstrings with flexion deformity of the knee.

The target is the groove between the ischium and the greater trochanter (Fig. 8.10a). After crossing the gluteus muscles the sciatic nerve is identified in the depth of the incision. The branches to the hamstring muscles can be isolated at the side of the sciatic trunk, on the basis of responses of the biceps femoris, semimembranosus and semitendinosus muscles; the latter muscle being the major muscle responsible for spasticity [12] (Fig. 8.10b).

8.3.3 Tibial Neurotomy

Tibial neurotomy is indicated for the treatment of the so-called spastic foot, which is usually characterized by plantar flexion (equinus) and varus deformity, with or without claw toes [4, 7, 13–15]. Tibial neurotomy consists of exposing all motor branches of the tibial nerve at the popliteal fossa, i.e., the nerves to gastrocnemius and soleus, tibialis posterioris, popliteus, flexor hallucis longus and flexor digitorum longus (Fig. 8.11). The soleus has been demonstrated to be predominantly responsible for the spastic plantar flexion, which justifies for most patients to abstain from gastrocnemius nerve sectioning [16, 17], except when equinus is related to or significantly augmented by the maneuver of knee extension.

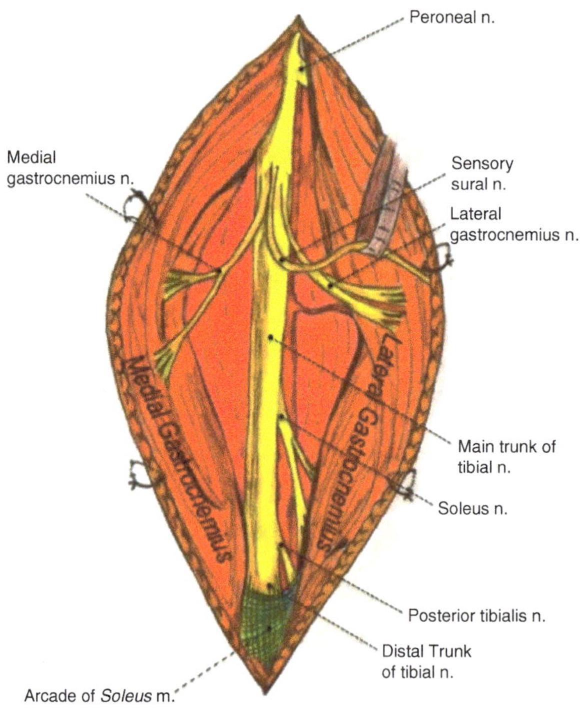

Fig. 8.11 Exposure of the tibial nerve in a dorsal view of the right popliteal region. The sensory cutaneous sural nerve lies superficially just beneath the subcutaneous aponeurosis and between the two gastrocnemius muscles. The medial and lateral gastrocnemius nerves may arise either separately from the both sides of the tibial trunk or posteriorly from a common origin, sometimes including the sensory cutaneous sural nerve. Each gastrocnemius nerve usually divides into two distal branches when approaching the muscle. The two soleus nerves may arise from a common origin, as shown, or quite separately from the tibial nerve. The posterior tibialis nerve, like the soleus nerve, originates from the ventro-lateral aspect of the tibial nerve but more distally at the level of the soleus arcade. Sometimes it may originate from a common trunk with the inferior branch of the soleus nerve. The distal trunk of the tibial nerve contains 5–8 fascicles averaging 1 mm in diameter each; two thirds of them are motor, most of them for the toes, and one third is sensory

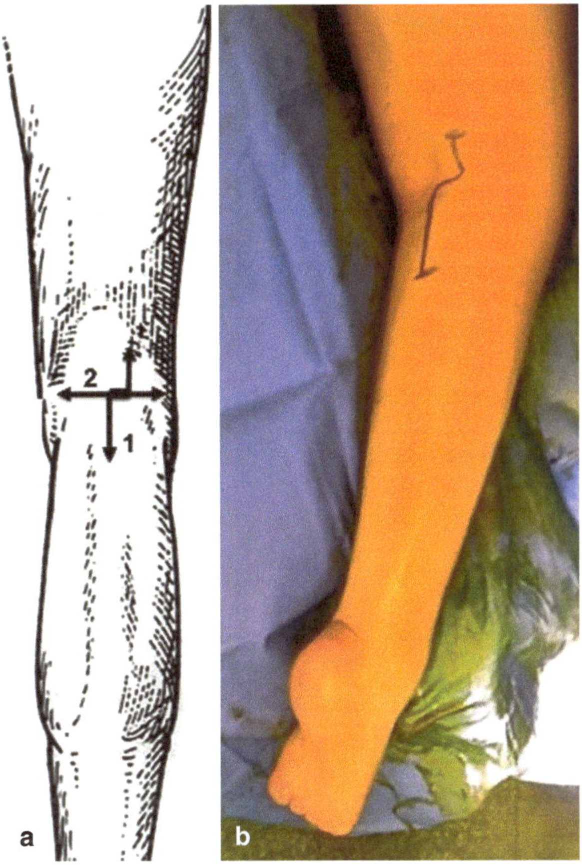

Fig. 8.12 (**a**) Skin incisions for the tibial neurotomy may be a vertical incision over the (*right*) popliteal fossa (*1*) or a transverse incision on the transverse popliteal fold (*2*) for a better cosmetic result. (**b**) Photograph of installation and bayonet-like skin vertical incision over the (*right*) popliteal fossa for tibial neurotomy. Note the equinovarus abnormal posture of the spastic foot

The incision can be vertical or transversal (Fig. 8.12), the latter providing a better aesthetic result. In addition, the transverse incision allows for a tenotomy of the insertion fascia of the gastrocnemius if necessary. The first nerve encountered is the medial cutaneous sural nerve, a sensory nerve innervating the lateral aspect of the foot; situated in a satellite position to the saphenous vein, it must be spared. More deeply lies the tibial nerve trunk. From top to bottom of the popliteal approach (Figs. 8.13 and 8.14), the first motor nerves to emerge are the nerves to the gastrocnemius muscles: one medial, the other lateral. The next is the superior soleus nerve. The effect of its sectioning is assessed by the immediate intraoperative disappearance of the ankle clonus. By retracting the tibial nerve trunk medially, the main other branches can be exposed and identified with electrical stimulation, as they emerge from the lateral edge of the tibial trunk. These are the inferior soleus nerve and, following it, the tibialis posterior nerve, responsible for equinus and varus, respectively. Before disappearing beneath the musculoaponeurotic arch derived from the soleus, the distal tibial trunk can be approached if treatment of toes in claw is needed. There the trunk may undergo a fascicular dissection after opening its epineural envelope in order to search for the flexor digitorum fascicles (Fig. 8.14c).

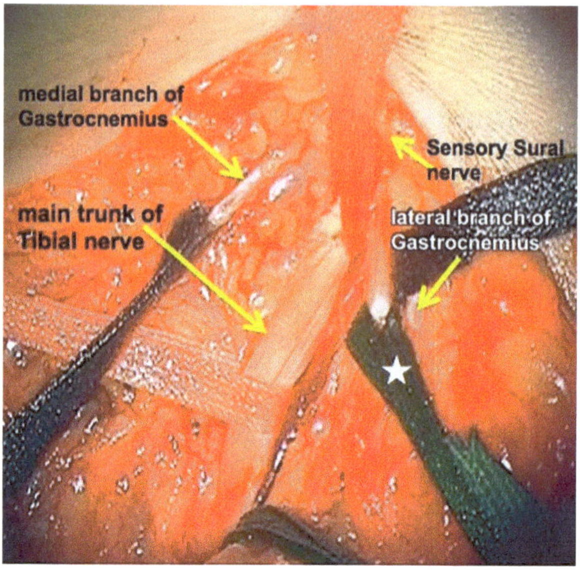

Fig. 8.13 View of the (*right*) popliteal region under operative microscope after dissection of the tibial nerve. *Arrows indicate* main trunk of the tibial nerve, the sensory cutaneous sural nerve and the medial and lateral branches for their respective gastrocnemius muscles. *Asterisk indicates* superior branch of soleus nerve

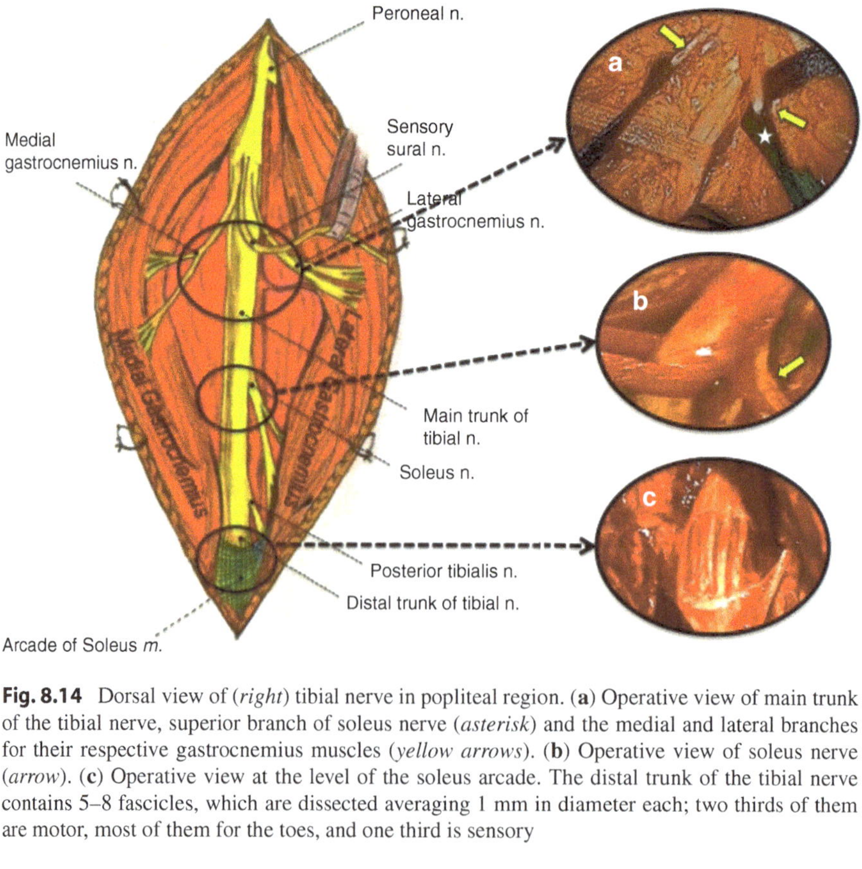

Fig. 8.14 Dorsal view of (*right*) tibial nerve in popliteal region. (**a**) Operative view of main trunk of the tibial nerve, superior branch of soleus nerve (*asterisk*) and the medial and lateral branches for their respective gastrocnemius muscles (*yellow arrows*). (**b**) Operative view of soleus nerve (*arrow*). (**c**) Operative view at the level of the soleus arcade. The distal trunk of the tibial nerve contains 5–8 fascicles, which are dissected averaging 1 mm in diameter each; two thirds of them are motor, most of them for the toes, and one third is sensory

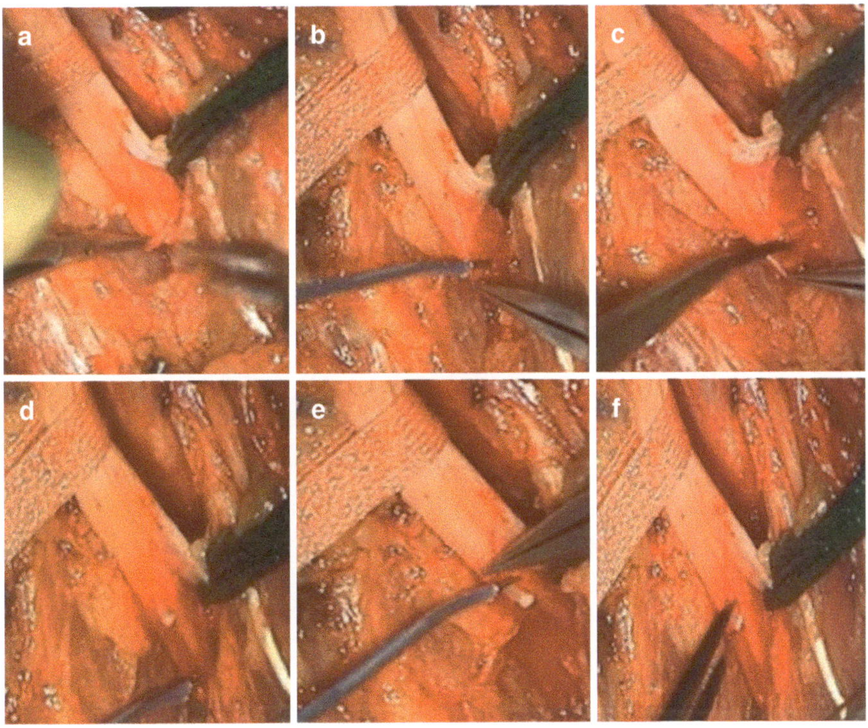

Fig. 8.15 Stepwise microsurgical technique for tibial neurotomy on the right side. (**a**) Fascicular dissection after opening of epineurium. (**b**) Mapping with bipolar electrode before fascicular resection. (**c**) Resection of targeted fascicle. (**d**) Stimulation distal to fascicular resection. (**e**) Stimulation proximal to fascicular resection. (**f**) Coagulation of the proximal fascicular stump to avoid postoperative neuroma formation

A very meticulous electrical mapping of every fascicle is important. The sectioning of fascicles might be dangerous if the motor fascicles cannot be clearly differentiated from the sensory ones, due to the risk of sensory disturbances (hypoesthesia, paraesthesias, dysesthesias) and trophic ulcers in the plantar sole [7].

Figure 8.15 illustrates the steps of the microsurgical procedure and mapping for tibial neurotomy.

8.3.4 Femoral Neurotomy

Femoral neurotomy (Fig. 8.16) is indicated for the treatment of excessive spasticity of the quadriceps muscle when it interferes with gait by limiting knee flexion during the swing phase [8, 18]. Given its "strategic" importance in the maintenance of an upright posture, a motor block test is an essential part of the preoperative evaluation. The neurotomy mainly concerns the motor branches to the rectus femoris and vastus intermedius muscles.

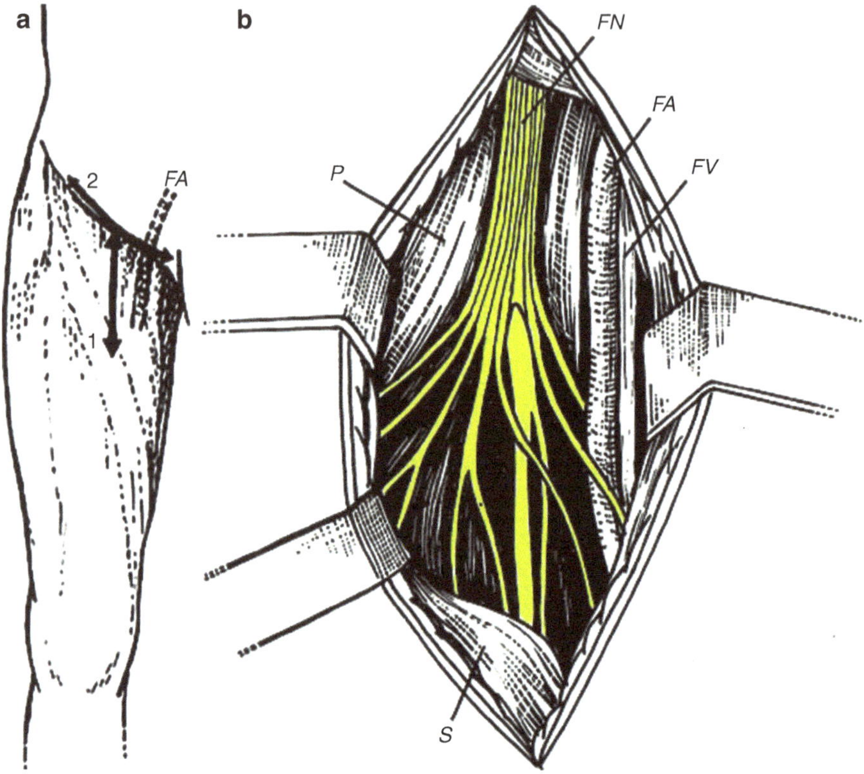

Fig. 8.16 (**a**) Skin incisions for femoral neurotomy, vertical below the inguinal ligament and lateral to the femoral artery (*1*) or horizontal in the hip flexion fold (*2*). (**b**) Dissection of the right femoral nerve (*FN*) and its branches after opening the anterior fascia of the psoas muscle (*P*). Bipolar stimulation allows identification of the two or three branches to the sartorius muscle (*S*) and of the three or four branches to the rectus femoris muscle. The nerve to the vastus intermedius can be found more deeply. *FA* femoral artery, *FV* femoral vein

The incision can be vertical or horizontal at the hip flexion fold (Fig. 8.16a). The dissection passes medial to the sartorius muscle and exposes the motor branches of the femoral nerve, first the nerve to the rectus femoris and then, more deeply, the nerve to the vastus intermedius (Fig. 8.16b). Identification of the respective function of the various exposed branches requires electrical mapping.

8.3.5 Anterior Tibial Neurotomy

Anterior tibial neurotomy, rarely performed, may be indicated for a permanent extension of the hallux, corresponding to a disabling Babinski sign, if it makes it difficult to wear shoes [8]. The vertical incision is centered on the junction between the tibialis anterioris and the extensor hallucis, at the middle third of the leg. The nerve is located between these two muscle heads, and the neurotomy is performed on the motor branch to the extensor hallucis.

8.4 Operative Techniques for Upper Limb

8.4.1 Pectoralis Major and Teres Major Neurotomies

Neurotomy of the collateral branches of the brachial plexus innervating the pectoralis major and the teres major muscle is indicated for spastic shoulder with internal rotation and adduction [19].

For pectoralis major neurotomy, the skin incision is made at the innermost part of the deltopectoral sulcus and curves along the clavicular axis. First the clavipectoralis fascia is opened and then the upper border of the pectoralis major muscle is reflected downwards. Close to the thoracoacromialis artery, the ansa of the pectoralis muscle is identified by stimulation.

For teres major neurotomy, the skin incision follows the inner border of the teres major, from the lower border of the posterior head of the deltoid muscle to the lower extremity of the scapula. The lower border of the long portion of brachii triceps constitutes the upper limit of the approach. The dissection continues deeply between the teres minor and major muscles. In the vicinity of the subscapularis artery, the nerve ending on the teres major is identified. The nerve is surrounded by thick fat when approaching the anterior facet of the muscle body.

8.4.2 Musculocutaneous Neurotomy

Neurotomy of the musculocutaneous nerve (Fig. 8.17) is indicated for spastic elbow with flexion depending on the biceps brachii and the brachialis muscles [8, 20, 21].

The skin incision is performed longitudinally; it reaches 5 cm down from the inferior edge of the pectoralis major, medial to the biceps brachii (Fig. 8.17a). The superficial fascia is opened between the biceps laterally and the coracobrachialis medially, which is crucial as in a more medial location the median nerve and vessels would be exposed. The dissection proceeds in this space; there the musculocutaneous nerve lies anterior to the brachialis muscle (Fig. 8.17b). Opening the epineurium allows the fascicles of the nerve to be dissected under the operating microscope (Fig. 8.18a). The function of the various fascicles is identified by electrical stimulation (Fig. 8.18b).

8.4.3 Median Neurotomy

Neurotomy of the median nerve (Fig. 8.19) is indicated for the so-called spastic hand [8, 22, 23]. The most frequent deformities are a forearm in pronation resulting from spasticity in the pronator teres and quadratus muscles, a wrist-with-flexion deformity because of spasticity in the flexor carpi radialis and palmaris longus muscles, two patterns of fingers in flexion, "swan neck" finger deformity, and thumb in adduction. For fingers in flexion, there may be either a flexion of the metacarpophalangeal joint and proximal interphalangeal joint due to spasticity in the flexor

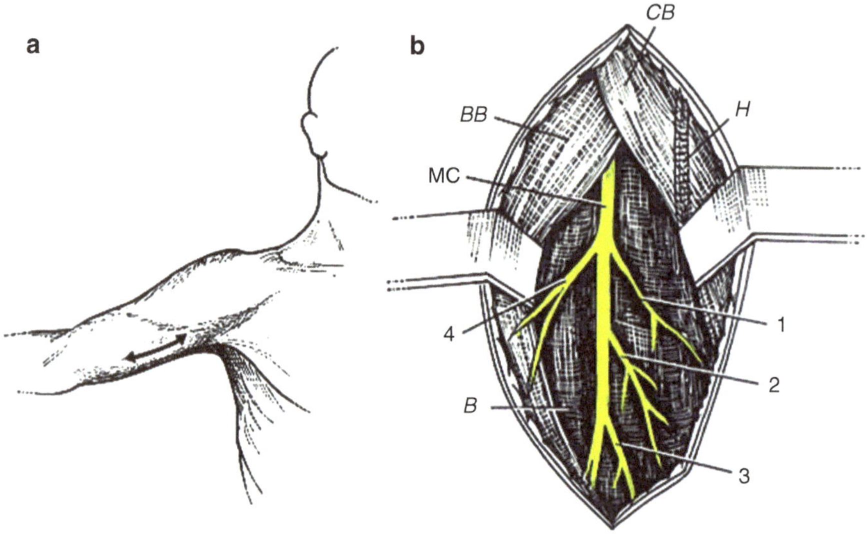

Fig. 8.17 (**a**) Skin incision for (*right*) musculocutaneous neurotomy, along the medial aspect of the biceps brachi, under the inferior edge of the pectoralis major muscle. (**b**) Dissection of the right musculocutaneous nerve (*MC*) in the space between the biceps brachii muscle (*BB*) laterally, the coracobrachialis muscle (*CB*) medially and the brachialis muscle (*B*) posteriorly. Branches to brachialis (*1*, *2*) and to biceps brachii (*3*, *4*) are recognized by stimulation provoking elbow flexion. The humeral artery (*H*) along with the median nerve is situated more medially and should not be exposed

digitorum superficialis or a flexion of the distal interphalangeal joint resulting from spasticity in the flexor digitorum profundus. The "swan neck" deformity consists of hyperextension of the proximal interphalangeal joint with flexion of the distal interphalangeal joint and depends on the lumbrical and interosseous muscles; these muscles are innervated by the median nerve for the first and second columns and predominantly by the ulnar nerve for the three other columns. A thumb in adduction is due to spasticity in the flexor pollicis longus muscle; the deep terminal branch of the ulnar nerve also supplies this muscle.

The skin incision begins 2–3 cm above the flexion line of the elbow, medial to the biceps brachii tendon, passes through the transverse elbow line and curves towards the junction of the upper and middle thirds of the anterior forearm (Fig. 8.19a). Thereafter, the median nerve is searched medially to the brachial artery and recognized at the elbow, deeply under the lacertus fibrosus, which is cut. Sharp dissection is used to separate the branches of the median nerve (Fig. 8.19b). The pronator teres belly with its two heads is retracted medially and distally so that its muscular branches can be identified. This muscle is then retracted upward and laterally while the flexor carpi radialis is pulled downward and medially. The muscular branches to the flexor carpi radialis and to the flexor digitorum superficialis can be seen then. Finally, the latter is retracted medially and thus the branches to the flexor digitorum profundus, the flexor pollicis longus and the pronator quadratus are uncovered.

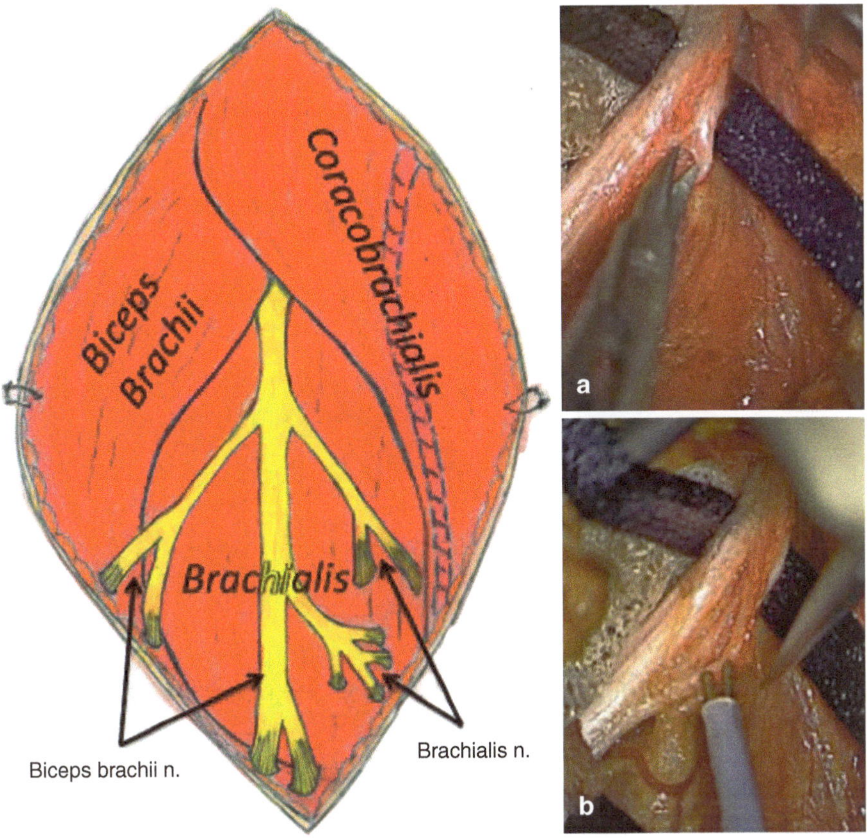

Fig. 8.18 View of the right musculocutaneous nerve in the space between the biceps brachii muscle laterally, the coracobrachialis muscle medially and the brachialis muscle posteriorly. (**a**) Epineurium opening of the trunk. (**b**) Fascicular stimulation with the bipolar electrode after interfascicular dissection

These muscular branches may appear as individual separate branches or remain together in the distal trunk of the anterior interosseous nerve. Sometimes, it may be useful to divide the fibrous arch of the flexor digitorum superficialis muscle to make the dissection easier (Fig. 8.20).

Besides this approach, which requires a long incision and extensive dissection, a "minimal" approach can be performed. The different fascicles in the trunk of the median nerve, just medial to the brachial artery, are dissected. This approach provides a better cosmetic outcome than the former. However, the exposure it provides is less favorable to the identification of the various motor branches in the form of fascicles which are supposed to contain fibers of the targeted muscle(s) only. At this level of the nerve, though, cutaneous sensory fibers are mixed with the muscle fibers. This entails the risk of sensory complications, especially the development of neuropathic pain together with a complex regional pain syndrome.

The microsurgical steps of this procedure are illustrated in Fig. 8.21.

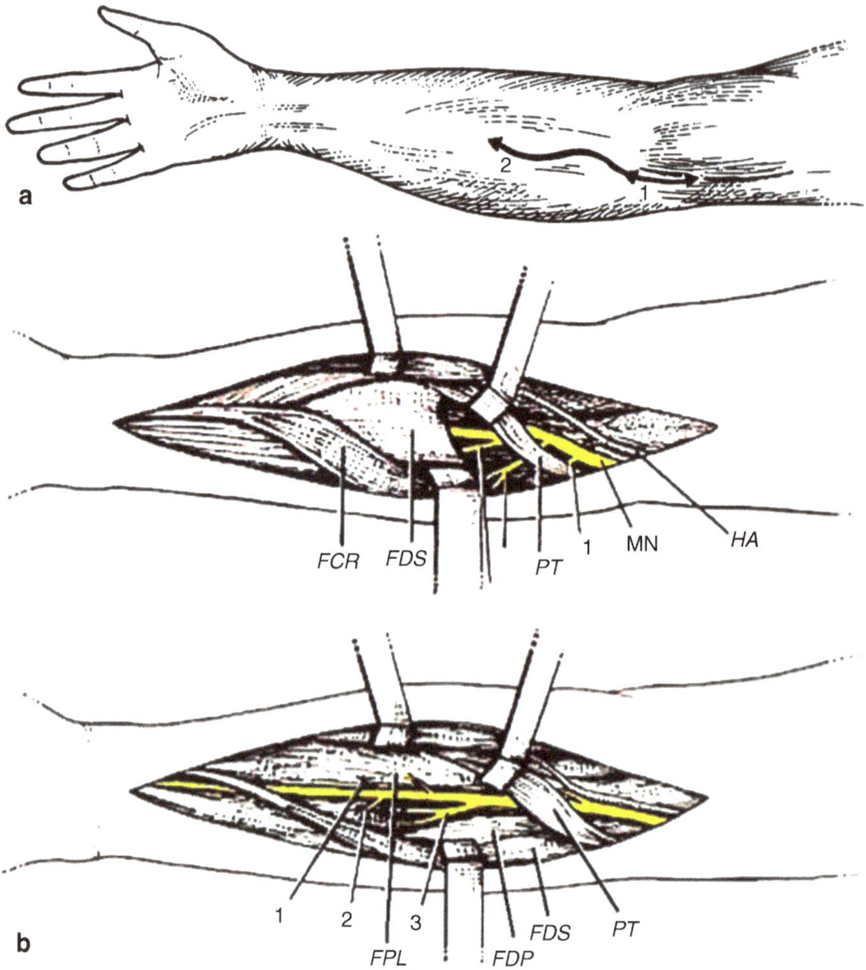

Fig. 8.19 (**a**) Skin incision for median neurotomy at the medial aspect of the biceps brachii, at the level of the elbow longitudinal along the bicipital crest (*1*). For more exposure, incision can be continued distally towards the midline above the wrist (*2*). (**b**) Dissection of the median nerve in two stages. In the first stage (*upper panel*), the pronator teres (*PT*) is retracted upward and laterally and the flexor carpi radialis (*FCR*) medially. Before median nerve (*MN*) passes under the fibrous arch of the flexor digitorum superficialis (*FDS*), branches to the pronator teres (*1*) and to nerve trunks to the flexor carpi radialis, palmaris longus and flexor digitorum superficialis (*2*, *3*) are dissected and identified. In the second stage of the dissection (*lower panel*), the fibrous arch of the flexor digitorum superficialis is sectioned to allow a more distal dissection of the median nerve. The flexor digitorum superficialis is retracted medially and identified are branches from the median nerve running to the flexor pollicis longus (*FLP*) (*1*) and to the flexor digitorum profundus (*FDP*) (*2*) and the interosseous nerve and its proper branches to these muscles (*3*)

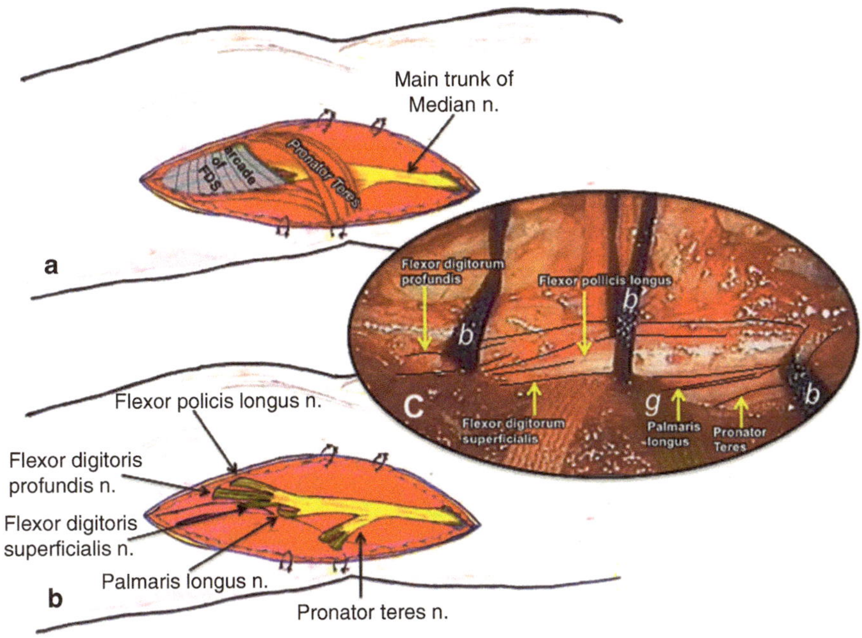

Fig. 8.20 Dissection of the (*right*) median nerve. (**a**) Pronator teres muscle and arcade of flexor digitorum superficialis (*FDS*) are almost covering the branches of the median nerve. (**b**) Pronator teres is retracted and arcade of flexor digitorum superficialis is divided to allow a more distal dissection of the median nerve branches to the pronator teres, palmaris longus, flexor digitorum superficialis, flexor digitorum profundis and flexor pollicis longus, as shown on the operative view (**c**) green tapes (*g*) indicate that the branch is definitely a target for sectioning; blue ones (*b*) mean that the branch can be sectioned, but only after recheck the green-labelled branches having been cut. Yellow arrows designate nerve branches with their corresponding muscle innervation

8.4.4 Ulnar Neurotomy

Neurotomy of the ulnar nerve at the elbow is indicated for a wrist-in-flexion deformity when related to spasticity in the flexor carpi ulnaris muscle [8, 22, 23]. Ulnar neurotomy can also be indicated for flexion deformity in the fingers when flexion predominates in the distal interphalangeal joints; as a matter of fact, such deformity results predominantly from spasticity of the portion of the flexor digitorum profundus muscle which is mainly innervated by the ulnar nerve.

Ulnar neurotomy may also be indicated for "thumb in adduction", which is due to spasticity in the flexor pollicis longus muscle. The deep terminal branch of the ulnar nerve supplies this muscle. Furthermore, ulnar neurotomy can be indicated for spasticity causing an adduction/flexion deformity of the thumb which shows as the so-called thumb in palm. This deformity is due to spasticity in the adductor pollicis and opponent muscles innervated by the ulnar nerve. These ulnar neurotomies can be used alone or in combination with median neurotomy.

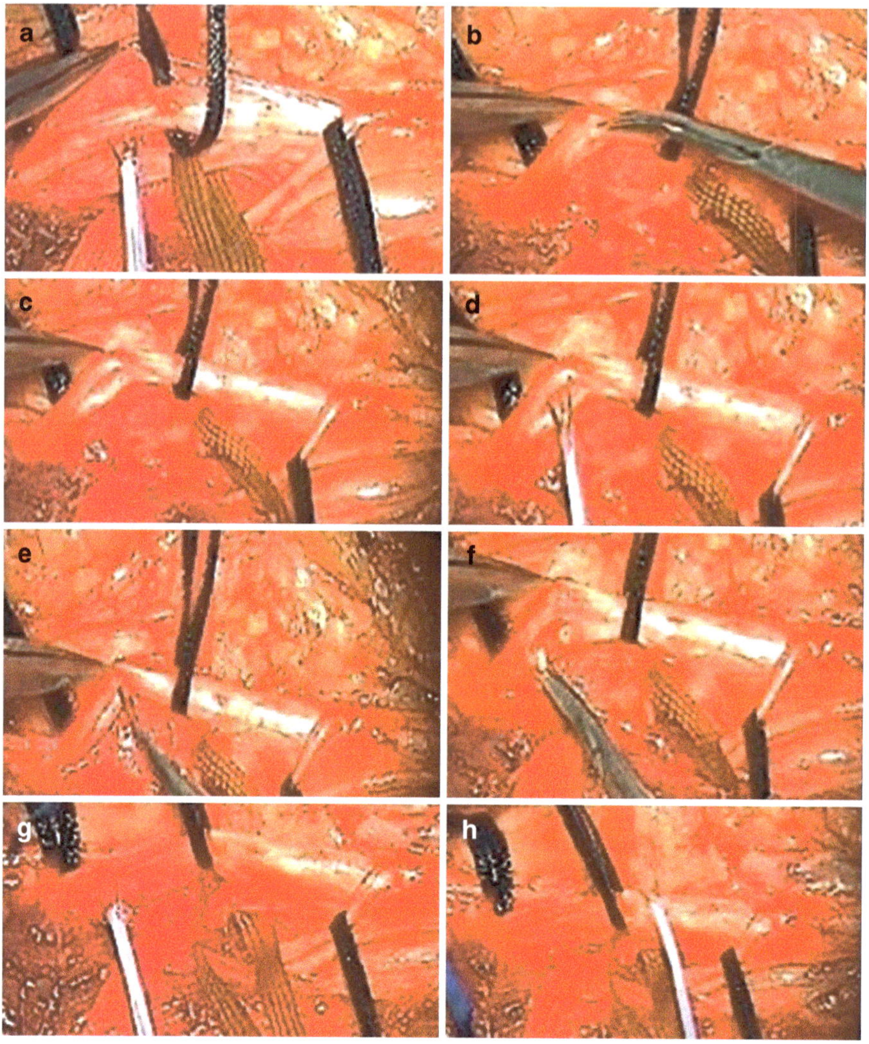

Fig. 8.21 Stepwise microsurgical technique for median neurotomy. (**a**) Mapping before fascicular dissection. (**b**) Interfascicular dissection in progress. (**c**) Exposure of dissected fascicles after opening of epineurium. (**d**) Fascicular mapping with tripolar electrode. (**e**) Proximal sectioning of fascicle. (**f**) Distal sectioning of fascicle. (**g**) Final distal stimulation. (**h**) Final proximal stimulation to check the quantitive effect of the neurotomy

Ulnar neurotomy can be performed at two different levels (Fig. 8.22). At the elbow, an arched skin incision is performed to expose the ulnar nerve at the medial part of the elbow. After subcutaneous dissection, the ulnar nerve is identified medially to the medial epicondyle, where it enters between the two heads of the flexor carpi ulnaris. There the motor branches to the flexor carpi ulnaris muscle are identified. More distally the branches to the medial half of the flexor digitorum

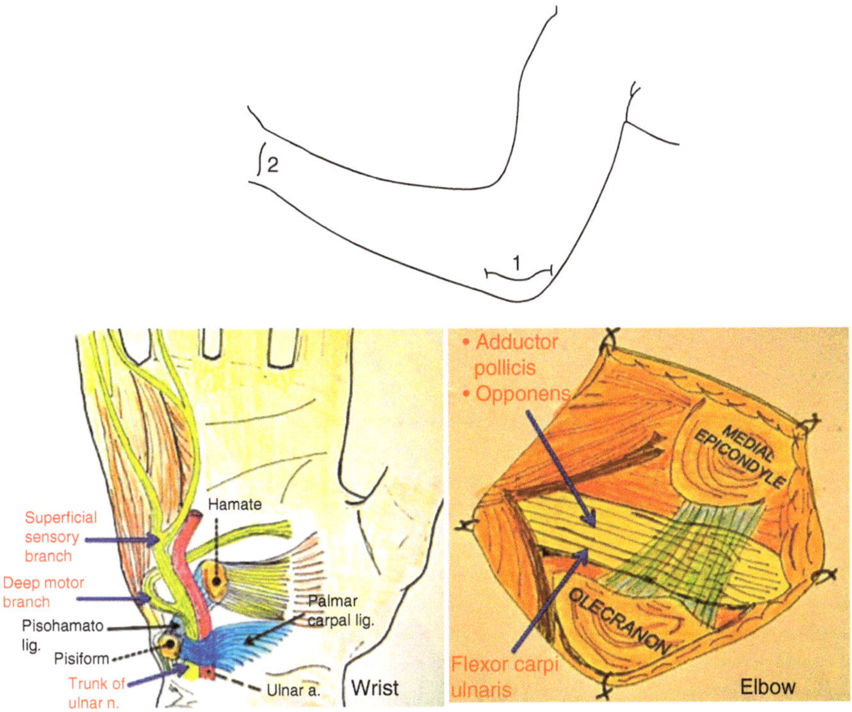

Fig. 8.22 (**a**) Skin incision(s) on the (*right*) forearm for ulnar neurotomy. Current approach is at elbow with a longitudinal incision posteriorly to the medial epicondyle and medially to the olecranon (*1*). An alternative is a transverse medial incision in the wrist fold (*2*), depending on the location of the spastic muscles (see text). (**b**) Schematic drawing of ulnar nerve at the level of wrist. Dissection of the trunk of ulnar nerve before entering Guyon's canal, which is opened by the section of the palmar carpal ligament. Identification of the deep motor branch. Dissection of fascicles for innervation of dorsal and palmar interossei muscles and adductor pollicis muscle. Section of approximately 75 % of fascicles for the innervation of the adduction and opposition of the thumb. (**c**) Schematic drawing of ulnar nerve after epitrochleo–olecranon approach. The epitrochleo–olecranon ligament is incised and then an incision is made along the two heads of the flexor carpi ulnaris aponeurotic arcade, to perform intrafascicular dissection distal to the arcade. This region is preferred because more proximally the ulnar nerve has still interfascicular anastomoses. *Arrows indicate* the fascicles innervating the flexor carpi ulnaris, the adductor pollicis and the opponens pollicis

profundus are found. For distal branch sectioning, the ulnar nerve can be approached at the wrist.

The microsurgical steps of this procedure are illustrated in Fig. 8.23.

8.4.5 Combined Neurotomies in Upper Limb

Combinations of several neurotomies, musculocutaneous and median/ulnar, in the same operative session are frequently accomplished (Fig. 8.24).

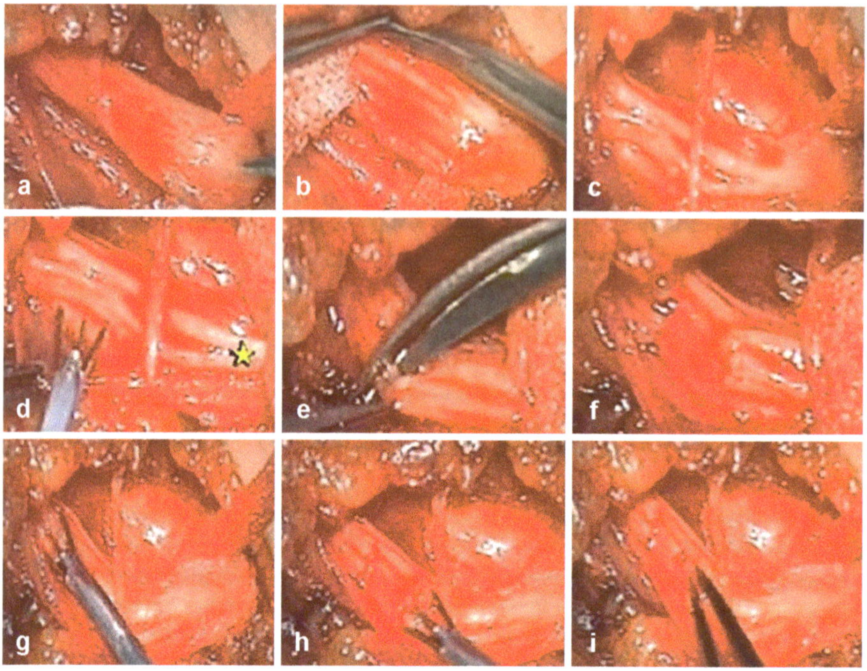

Fig. 8.23 Stepwise microsurgical technique for ulnar neurotomy at level of elbow on the right side. (**a**) Ulnar nerve before fascicular dissection. (**b**) Interfascicular dissection in progress. (**c**) Exposure of dissected fascicles after opening of the epineurium. (**d**) Fascicular mapping with tripolar electrode after interfascicular dissection. Note the interfascicular anastomoses at the proximal part of the nerve (*asterisk*). (**e**) Fascicular sectioning. (**f**) Exposure of proximal and distal extremities after sectioning. (**g**) Final distal stimulation. (**h**) Final proximal stimulation to check the quantitive effect of the neurotomy. (**i**) Coagulation of the proximal fascicular stump to avoid postoperative neuroma formation

8.5 Outcome

For a large majority of adult patients who underwent peripheral neurotomies – 80 to 85 % according to publications – surgery succeeded in the goals pursued [8, 24]:

- decrease the excess of spasticity
- reduce the abnormal postures and articular limitations
- unmask the eventual previously hidden voluntary movements
- relieve the pain and discomfort
- prevent the aggravation of the deformities

In our overall series of 475 cases followed over more than 1 year (5.4 years on average), 82 % of the patients benefited from a single or multiple neurotomies. For spasticity in the lower limb, the series includes neurotomies of the following nerves (in parentheses, the number of cases): obturator nerve (46), femoral nerve (7), hamstring branches (12), tibial nerve (317) and deep peroneal branch (22); a total of 404 cases. For upper-limb spasticity, neurotomies of the following nerves were

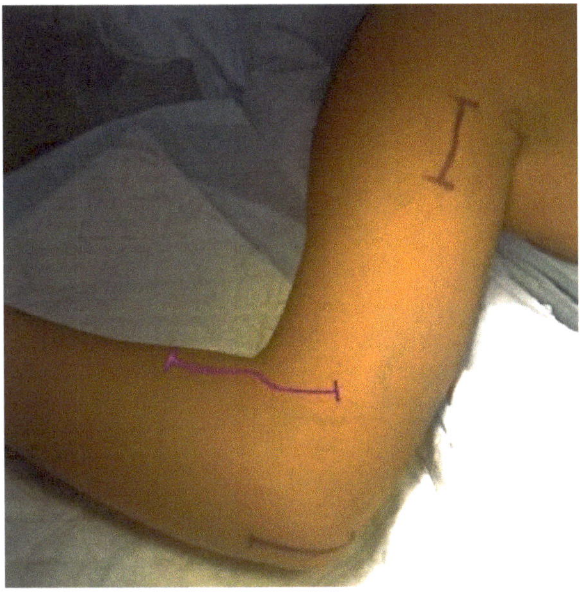

Fig. 8.24 Combination of several neurotomies: musculocutaneous and median/ulnar in the same operative session for (*right*) spastic upper limb in a hemiplegic patient

accomplished: brachial plexus branches (3), musculocutaneous nerve (15), median/ulnar nerve (53); a total of 71 cases.

In the group of patients who were treated by a tibial neurotomy for a *spastic, sometimes dystonic, foot*, assessment after 1 year of follow-up was the following [7, 8, 23].

With regard to **spasticity**, after surgery 92 % of patients were scored grade 1 or 2 on the Ashworth scale, whereas preoperatively all were in grade 3 or 4, the average score being decreased from 3.84 to 1.53.

Regarding **abnormal postures and articular limitations**, surgery eliminated equinus in 85.2 %, varus in 88.9 %, flexion of toes (when present) in 73.7 % and clonus of ankle (when present) in 66.7 %, and allowed return to normal passive dorsiflexion, 15° clinically, in 77.35 %.

Voluntary motility of dorsiflexion of the foot, quantified by Lovett's Motor scale from 0 to 5, was improved in 86.8 %. Motor power of the plantar flexion remained unchanged in most of the patients, but for 3.2 % it was significantly weakened, leading to a disabling talus foot.

Pain due to deformity of foot and/or cramping in triceps surae was significantly relieved in 85 %, with scores on the Visual Analog scale reduced from 8.5 to 1.8 on average, and any pressure sores in foot healed in 78 %. The orthopedic shoe or the splint could be dispensed with for 75 and 35 %, respectively. It is important to say, though, that those orthopedic shoes and splints have to be replaced by shoes high enough to maintain foot stability as surgery creates a relative "laxity" of the ankle.

Because of the return to a normal position of the foot on the ground on standing and a normalization of the alternance of stance and swing phases during walking, for 86.8 % of the series the dynamic and functional status of the entire lower limb including knee, hip and spine significantly improved. This can be verified and quantified by dynamic gait analysis (see Sect. 4.2.3).

At the **functional level** the preoperative goals were reached for 80 % of the patients. The walking distance was significantly increased for two thirds of the patients, from 65 to 750 m ($p<0.01$). The satisfactory index, ranging from 0 to 10, was 6.35 on average.

Failure to achieve long-term satisfactory reduction of spasticity was noted for 8.6 % of the hemiplegic adult group, likely as the result of an insufficient quantity of fascicles cut. Return of spasticity and of abnormal posture was rarely observed after the turn of the first year. This failure rate for adults was low, as opposed to that for children. As a matter of fact in two thirds of the 13 hemiplegic children with cerebral palsy who underwent a tibial neurotomy for a spastic or dystonic foot, the effect of neurotomy was transient with a recurrence of the same equinovarus deformity. Rather than a regrowth of fibers (as the fascicles were resected over a length of 5–10 mm), a reinnervation of the neurotomized muscles by collateral sprouting of the nearby healthy axons, i.e., a reinnervation into extensive motor units, was the likely cause of the recurrence. This could be demonstrated for 4 of the 13 children by a muscular biopsy of their denervated triceps surae, tibialis posterior and flexor hallucis longus on the occasion of a secondary tenotomy performed by the pediatric orthopedic surgeon [25].

For the group of hemiplegic adult patients who underwent peripheral neurotomies for *upper-limb spasticity, sometimes with dystonia*, surgery consisted of musculocutaneous, median and ulnar neurotomies performed individually or in various combinations according to patients' clinical patterns [8, 23]. The assessment after at least 1 year of follow-up was the following. Assessment with the Ashworth scale showed a significant decrease in spasticity in all muscular groups subjected to surgery ($p<0.001$). Resting position, range of motion, active joint amplitude, and antagonist motor strength were concomitantly improved ($p<0.01$). Antispastic medications could be withdrawn for 46 % of the patients.

With regard to their **hand function**, only one third of the patients were considered potential candidates for surgery to yield a functional improvement. Of them, 72.7 % could acquire the pressure paper function and 81.8 % an active hand opening after surgery. The remaining two thirds were operated only with the goal of a comfort and cosmetic gain. Most of them showed significant improvement in that respect. However, an increase in the degree of gross prehension was noted for 25 % and in that of fine prehension for 15 %. In the overall series, the average prehension score was 0.91 before and 2.45 after surgery [23] (Table 8.3 and Fig. 8.25). When present, permanent pain was reduced from 8.2 to 1.3 on average on the 1–10 Visual Analog scale. Improvement in daily activities was considerable [23] (Table 8.4).

Finally, at the latest examination, after 4.5 years of follow-up on average, the mean degree of satisfaction, evaluated with a scale ranging from 0 to 100, was on average 61.5 % for the patients and 64.1 % for the family and caregivers questioned.

Recurrence of spasticity occurred in 15.6 % of the patients. All of them had additional fascicle sectioning in the previously operated nerve and/or additional

Table 8.3 Evaluation of prehension of hand during everyday activities by patients with disturbances of muscle tone in upper limb

Definition	Score
Prehension impossible	0
Prehension possible with help and grasp	1
Prehension present but precautious or instable	2
Prehension functionally effective	3

Modified from Maarrawi et al. [23]

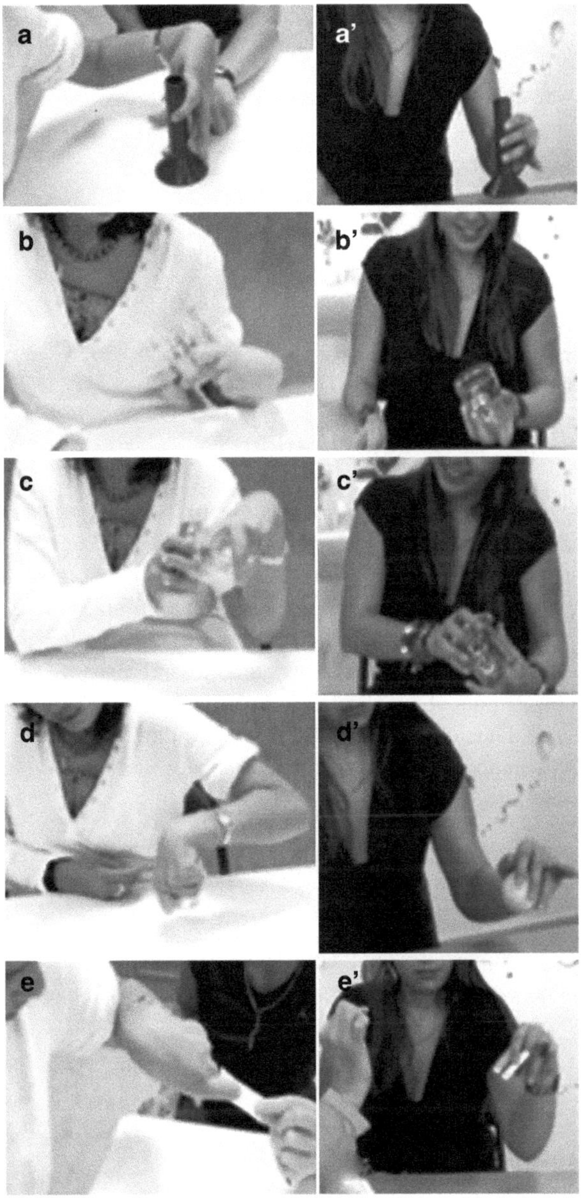

Fig. 8.25 Ability for prehension in left-hand of an hemiplegic adolescent presenting with both spasticity and dystonia after stroke due to thrombosis of right middle cerebral artery at the age of 2 years. Note improvement in capability for prehension after surgery (**a**′–**e**′) compared to the one before surgery (**a**–**e**). Surgery was combined (musculocutaneous, median, ulnar) neurotomies. Notice postoperative decrease in spasticity and dystonic flexion scheme during grip

Table 8.4 Improvement in everyday activities and aesthetic appearance of patients who underwent selective PN for upper-limb spasticity

Parameter	Total n. of patients (%)	Nr. of candidates (%) who were selected for and reached improvement in: Function	Comfort
N. of patients	31	11	20
Self-care	26 (84)	11 (100)	15 (75)
Hygiene	28 (90)	11 (100)	17 (85)
Dressing	23 (74)	9 (82)	14 (70)
Eating	15 (48)	8 (73)	7 (35)
Working	10 (32)	8 (73)	2 (10)
Leisure	21 (68)	10 (91)	11 (55)
Aesthetics	27 (87)	9 (82)	18 (90)

Modified from Maarrawi et al. [23]

neurotomy, namely, ulnar neurotomy as completion of a median neurotomy, with a beneficial effect in most cases.

8.6 Complications

8.6.1 Local Complications

In accord with literature as well as personal experience, hematomas and infections of the wound occurred only exceptionally. In contrast to this, delay in healing due to sweating and maceration at the folds was not infrequent, especially in bedridden patients. Repeated local care helps to minimize consequences. For lower-limb surgery, systematic administration of anticoagulation therapy, associated with early return to walking for patients able to ambulate, and intensive kinesitherapy for all despite pain at the operative site are effective to prevent thromboembolic complications. Dystrophic scarring, unesthetic at the skin level and responsible for local pain, may happen despite perfect hemostasis; there is little to do for its avoidance.

8.6.2 Neurological Complications

Postoperative hypoesthesia, paresthesias, dysesthesias are reported in most publications. Superficial cutaneous sensory nerves are at risk during approaches for tibial neurotomy, by excessive manipulation of the cutaneous sural branch, and for median neurotomy, by damaging the brachialis sensory nerves. In our series such disturbances occurred in 5 and 6.4 % of the patients, respectively; fortunately, they were transient in two-thirds of the affected patients [7, 23]. More severe are persistent dysesthesias, allodynia and some degree of anesthesia dolorosa in a hypoesthetic territory as the consequence of an inadvertent sectioning of sensory fascicles in mixed nerves. In our series such a complication appeared in the plantar sole in 2 % of the patients who underwent a tibial neurotomy including cut of the flexor fascicles for treating claw of toes. For half of these 2 %, the anesthesia dolorosa was accompanied by a plantar trophic ulcer that required surgical repair. Intraoperative mapping by meticulous fascicular electrostimulation is crucial to minimize the risk of such harmful side effects.

Loss of strength with increased disability may appear as the consequence of an excessive sectioning of the motor fascicles. In our series this occurred in 3.2 % of the patients who underwent a tibial neurotomy and it resulted in an abnormal talus posture of the foot, and in 3 % of the patients who were treated by a median/ulnar neurotomy and it resulted in the loss of the finger flexion-grip prehension.

Recurrence of spasticity may happen due to an insufficient extent of sectioning. If this can be confirmed by a motor block test, reoperation may be proposed with a significant chance of success.

Recurrence of preexisiting abnormal postures may also be observed after neurotomies even if performed with a theoretically appropriate sectioning of fibers attested by persistent suppression of the exaggerated stretch reflexes. Such situation can be attributed to rearrangements of the central nervous system in accordance with its plasticity or to a reinnervation of the denervated muscles.

Conclusion

PN are lesioning procedures with potential dangers. Provided that they are done prudently, they have few and minor side effects. When performed selectively, they not only reduce excessive spasticity and prevent increasing deformity but also improve motor function by rebalancing the tonicity between agonist and antagonist muscles (Figs. 8.26, 8.27, 8.28 and 8.29). In this way, PN are representative of the capability of sectioning procedures to improve function and be part of the armamentarium of functional neurosurgery.

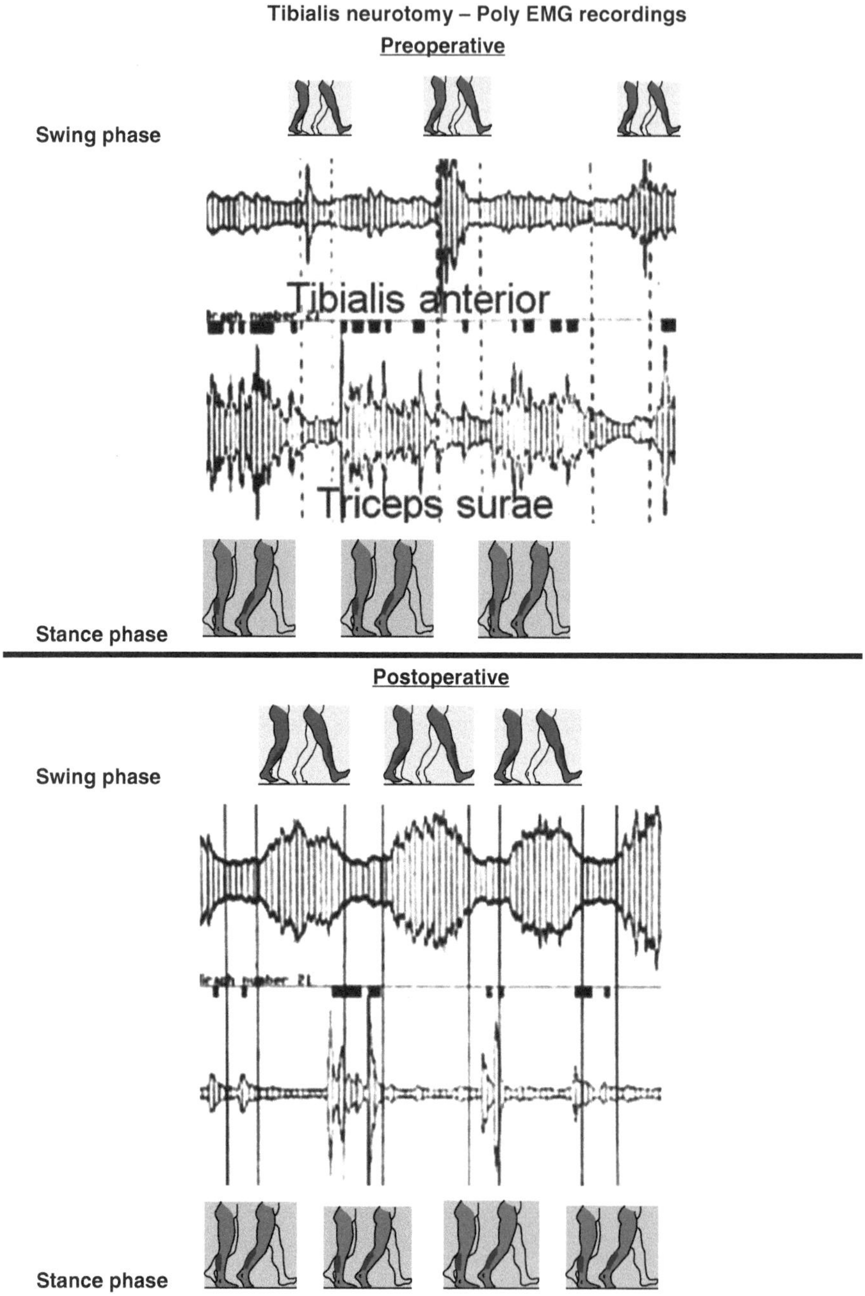

Fig. 8.26 Gait analysis in a hemiplegic patient with a spastic foot (equinovarus) before and after tibial neurotomy. Surface polyelectromyography of the tibialis anterior and triceps surae muscles on the spastic leg during walking, evaluating the change between pre- and postoperative state in stance and swing phase. Preoperative recordings show desynchronized activities of the triceps surae, with abnormal co-contractions of antagonist muscles: triceps surae and tibialis anterior. After tibial neurotomy, there is a reappearance of muscular activity in the tibialis anterior muscle, a clear decrease in triceps surae activity, and normal alternation of contractions of these muscles, i.e., the triceps surae at the end of the stance phase and the tibialis anterior during the swing phase

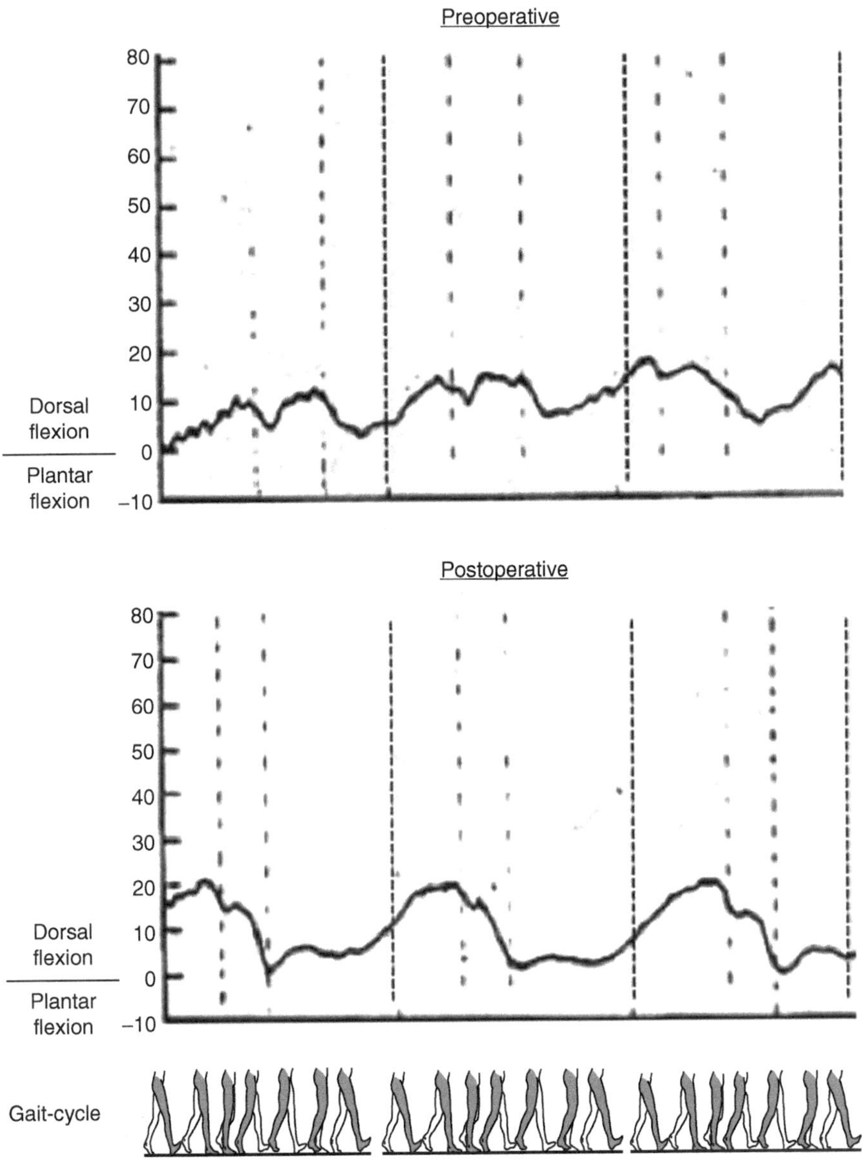

Fig. 8.27 Gait analysis in a hemiplegic patient with spastic foot (equinovarus) before and after tibial neurotomy. Three-dimensional movement analysis of the ankle flexion–extension amplitude during gait with the Vicon system. Preoperatively the amplitude of the spastic ankle was limited to 18° of dorsal flexion. After tibial neurotomy, dorsal flexion increased to 32°. Thus, the tonic balance at the ankle was established by the neurotomy; consequently motor function and gait improved

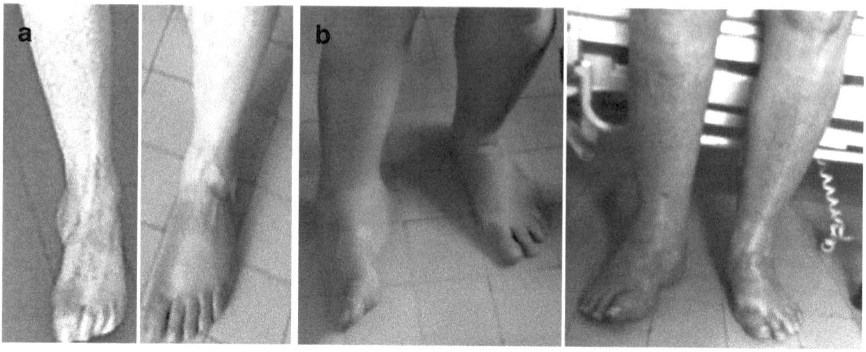

Fig. 8.28 (**a**) Hemiplegic patient with spastic left foot with severe equinus, slight varus, and moderate claw toes before and after tibial neurotomy. (**b**) Hemiplegic patient with right spastic foot with slight equinus and severe varus before and after tibial neurotomy

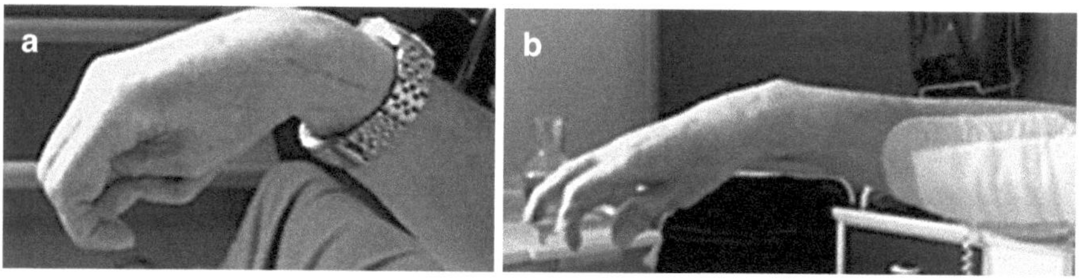

Fig. 8.29 Spastic hand with flexion of fingers and thumb in palm and impossibility of extension of wrist and fingers before (**a**) and after (**b**) median neurotomy

References

1. Lorenz F (1887) Über chirurgische Behandlung der angeborenen spastischen Gliedstarre. Wien Klin Rundsch 21:25–27
2. Stoffel A (1913) The treatment of spastic contractures. Am J Orthop Surg Ser 2(10):611–644
3. Gros C (1972) La chirurgie de la spasticité. Neurochirurgie 23:316–388
4. Gros C (1979) Spasticity: clinical examination and surgical treatment. In: Krayenbühl H, Brihaye J, Loew F, Logue V, Mingrino S, Pertuiset B, Symon L, Troupp H, Yaşargil MG (eds) Advances and technical standards in neurosurgery, vol 6. Springer, Wien/New York, pp 55–97
5. Sindou M, Abdennebi B, Boisson D, Eyssetie M, Goutelle A (1985) Traitement du pied spastique par la neurotomie selective du nerf tibial. Neurochirurgie 31:189–197
6. Mertens P (1987) Les neurotomies peripheriques dans le traitement des troubles spastiques des membres. Thèse de Médecine, Université de Lyon, Lyon
7. Sindou M, Mertens P (1988) Selective neurotomy of the tibial nerve for the treatment of the spastic foot. Neurosurgery 23:738–744
8. Mertens P, Sindou M (1991) Selective peripheral neurotomies for the treatment of spasticity. In: Sindou M, Abbott R, Keravel Y (eds) Neurosurgery for spasticity: a multidisciplinary approach. Springer, Wien/New York, pp 119–132
9. Mertens P, Sindou M (2001) Surgical management of spasticity. In: Barnes MP, Johnson GR (eds) Upper motor neurone syndrome and spasticity: clinical management of spasticity. Cambridge University Press, Cambridge, pp 239–265

10. Keats S (1957) Combined adductor-gracilis tenotomy and selective obturator-nerve resection for the correction of adduction deformity of the hip in children with cerebral palsy. J Bone Joint Surg Am 39:1087–1090
11. Banks HH, Green WT (1960) Adductor myotomy and obturator neurotomy for the correction of adductive contracture of the hip in cerebral palsy. J Bone Joint Surg Am 42:111–126
12. Decq P, Filipetti P, Feve A, Saraoui A (1996) Neurotomies périphériques sélectives des collaterals pour les muscles ischio-jambiers dans le traitement de la spasticité en flexion du genou: à propos d'une série de 11 patients. Neurochirurgie 42:275–280
13. Cahuzac M, Mansat C (1968) Le traitement chirurgical et ses résultats dans le pied spastique de l'enfant. Ann Podol 6:95–105
14. Fève A, Decq P, Filipetti P, Verroust J, Harf A, N'Guyen JP, Keravel Y (1997) Physiological effects of selective tibial neurotomy on lower limb spasticity. J Neurol Neurosurg Psychiatry 63:575–578
15. Deltombe T, Gustin T, Laloux P, De Cloedt P, De Wispelaere JF, Hanson P (2001) Selective fasicular neurotomy for spastic equinovarus foot deformity in cerebral palsy children. Acta Orthop Belg 67:1–5
16. Decq P, Cuny E, Filipetti P, Kéravel Y (1998) Role of soleus muscle in spastic equinus foot. Lancet 352:118
17. Roujeau T, Lefaucheur JP, Slavov V, Gherardi R, Decq P (2003) Long term course of the H reflex after selective tibial neurotomy. J Neurol Neurosurg Psychiatry 74:913–917
18. Decq P, Cuny E, Filipetti P, Fève A, Kéravel Y (1998) Peripheral neurotomy in the treatment of spasticity: indications, techniques and results in the lower limbs. Neurochirurgie 44:175–182
19. Decq P, Filipetti P, Fève A, Djindjian M, Saraoui A, Kéravel Y (1997) Peripheral selective neurotomies of the brachial plexus collateral branches for the treatment of the spastic shoulder: anatomical study and clinical results in five patients. J Neurosurg 86:648–653
20. Garland DE, Thompson R, Waters RL (1980) Musculocutaneous neurectomy for spastic elbow in flexion in non-functional upper extremities in adults. J Bone Joint Surg Am 62:108–112
21. Purohit AK, Raju BSV, Kumar KS, Mallikarjun KD (1998) Selective musculocutaneous fasciculotomy for spastic elbow in cerebral palsy: a preliminary study. Acta Neurochir (Wien) 140:473–478
22. Brunelli G, Brunelli F (1983) Selective microsurgical denervation in spastic paralysis. Ann Chir Main 2:277–280
23. Maarrawi J, Mertens P, Luaute J, Vial C, Chardonnet N, Cosson M, Sindou M (2006) Long-term functional results of selective peripheral neurotomy for the treatment of spastic upper limb: prospective study in 31 patients. J Neurosurg 104:215–225
24. Decq P (2003) Peripheral neurotomies for the treatment of focal spasticity of the limbs. Neurochirurgie 49:293–305
25. Berard C, Sindou M, Berard J, Carrier H (1998) Selective neurotomy of the tibial nerve in the spastic hemiplegic child: an explanation of the recurrence. J Pediatr Orthop B 7:66–70

9 Surgery in Dorsal Root Entry Zone

Surgery in the dorsal root entry zone (DREZ) was introduced in 1972 [1, 2] to treat some types of topographically limited pain. Because of its inhibitory side-effects on muscular tone, namely, the induction of marked hypotonia, the method was applied to patients with severe focalized hyperspasticity [3–6]. The technique was termed microsurgical DREZotomy (MDT) because it is performed by microsurgical techniques and with the bipolar coagulation microforceps as the lesion maker. The method attempts to selectively interrupt the small myelinated fibers (considered nociceptive) and the large myelinated myotatic fibers situated laterally and centrally, respectively, whilst partly sparing the large myelinated (considered sensory primary afferent) fibers located medially to reach and ascend through the dorsal columns (Fig. 9.1). Surgery in the DREZ requires strong knowledge of spinal cord anatomy [7, 8].

Basically, MDT consists of microsurgical lesioning, 3 mm in depth for pain, 5 mm for spasticity, at an angle of 35° at the cervical level and an angle of 45° at the lumbosacral level, according to the configuration of the dorsal horn (Fig. 9.2) [7]. After opening the dorsolateral sulcus ventrolaterally to the rootlets' entry, bipolar coagulations are performed ventrolaterally from the entrance of the rootlets into the opened dorsolateral sulcus down into the dorsal horn to the base of the ventral horn for spasticity, along all the selected target segments of the spinal cord.

9.1 Indications

MDT is indicated in severely disabled **paraplegic patients**, especially when they are bedridden (Fig. 9.3a, b) [9]; surgery is directed to the L2–S2 segments. Besides, MDT may be offered to patients harboring incontinent or retentive neurogenic bladder with uninhibited detrusor contractions resulting in voiding around the bladder catheter [10–12]. MDT is also indicated in **hemiplegic patients** especially for the treatment of the paralyzed upper limb when it is affected with severe, and sometimes also painful, hyperspasticity (Fig. 9.3c, d) [13]; surgery is directed to the C5–T1 segments.

M. Sindou et al., *Neurosurgery for Spasticity*,
DOI 10.1007/978-3-7091-1771-2_9, © Springer-Verlag Wien 2014

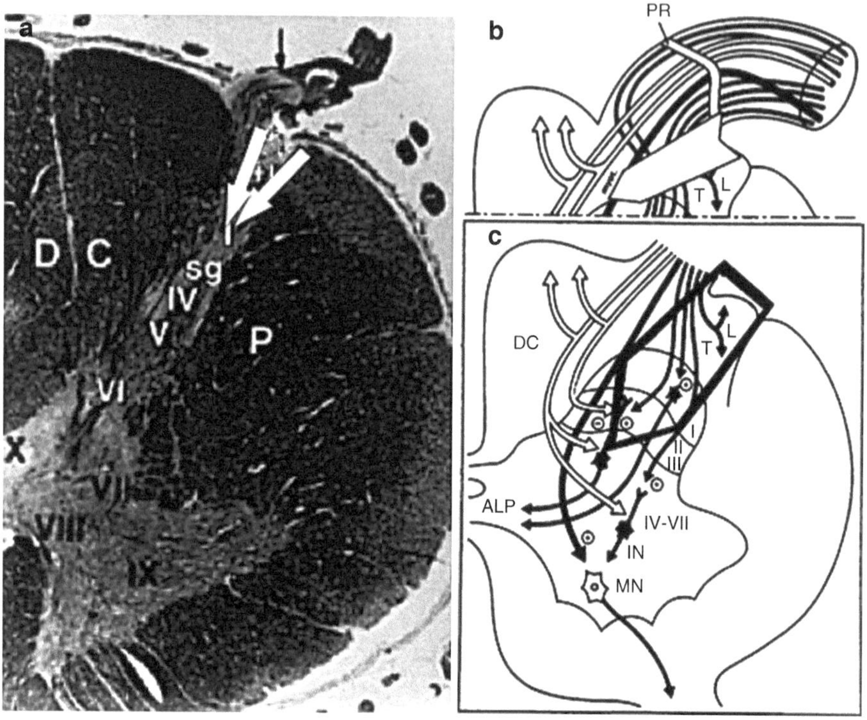

Fig. 9.1 (**a**) Rexed lamina of the dorsal horn (*I–VI*). Transverse hemisection of the spinal cord (at the lower cervical level) with myelin stained with luxol fast blue and fuchsin, showing the myelinated rootlet afferents that reach the dorsal column (*DC*). *P* pyramidal tract, *Sg* substantia gelatinosa, *tl* tract of Lissauer. *Small arrow* indicates the pial ring of the dorsal rootlet (diameter, 1 mm). *Large arrows* show the entry and axis of the MDT target. (**b**, **c**) Schematic representation of the DREZ area and the target of MDT. (**b**) Each rootlet can be divided, owing to the transition of its glial support; into a peripheral and a central segment. The transition between the two segments is at the pial ring (*PR*), which is located approximately 1 mm outside the penetration of the rootlet into the dorsolateral sulcus. Peripherally, the fibers are mixed together. As they approach the pial ring, the fine fibers (considered nociceptive) are located more toward the rootlet surfaces. In the central segment, they group in the ventrolateral portion of the DREZ and enter the dorsal horn (*DH*) through the tract of Lissauer (*TL*). The large myotatic fibers (*myot*) are situated in the middle of the DREZ, whereas the large myelinated sensory fibers are located dorsomedially to reach the dorsal column. (**c**) Schematic data on dorsal horn circuitry. Note the monosynaptic excitatory arc reflex of the myotatic fibers on ventral horn motoneurons (*MN*), the inhibitory influence of the recurrent collaterals of the large fibers to the dorsal column on dorsal horn cells and interneurons (*IN*), the fine fiber excitatory input onto the dorsal horn cells and the interneurons, the origin of the spino-reticulo-thalamic anterolateral pathways (*ALP*), and the projections of the interneurons onto the motoneuron (*MN*). The MDT (*arrowhead*) cuts most of the fine and the myotatic fibers, enters the medial (excitatory) portion of the tract of Lissauer, and penetrates more or less deep in the dorsal horn. MDT aims to preserve part of the large sensory fibers, and the lateral (inhibitory) portion of the tract of Lissauer

In severely affected patients harboring an intense spasticity and/or dystonia, MDT can be effective provided it is done deeply inside the spinal cord. Lesioning should be performed through the dorsal horn, down to the ventral horn, as deep as

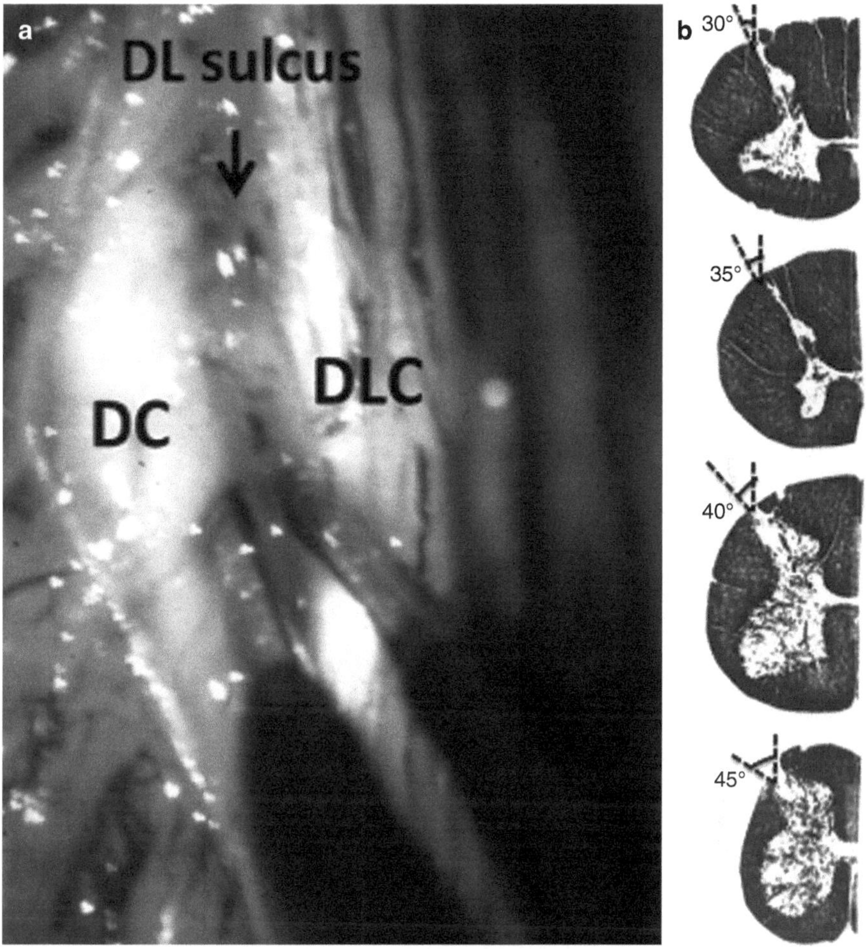

Fig. 9.2 (**a**) Microsurgical operative view of the dorsal horn (*DH*) after opening of the dorsolateral sulcus. Note the gelatinous aspect of the dorsal horn grey matter, in between the dorsal column (*DC*) and the dorsolateral column (*DLC*) white tracts, including the corticospinal pyramidal tract. (**b**) Variations of shape, width and depth of the DREZ area, according the spinal cord level. The axis of the dorsal horn is at an angle of 30–35° at the cervical and at an angle of 40–45° the lumbosacral level. Microsurgical incision of the dorsolateral sulcus and dorsal horn lesioning has to be done according to configuration of the dorsal horn to avoid damaging the dorsal column medially and the pyramid tract laterally. From *top* to *bottom*: cervical, C7; thoracic, T5; lumbar, L4; and sacral, S3. Note how the DREZ, the tract of Lissauer, and the dorsal horn are narrow and deep at the thoracic level

4–5 mm for spasticity and 5–6 mm for dystonia (which "pathway" is through the corticospinal tract and the descending tracts from basal ganglia and brainstem, to the ventral horn). This is particularly true for hemiplegic patients with severe spasticity associated with disabling focalized dystonia in the upper limb (Fig. 9.4).

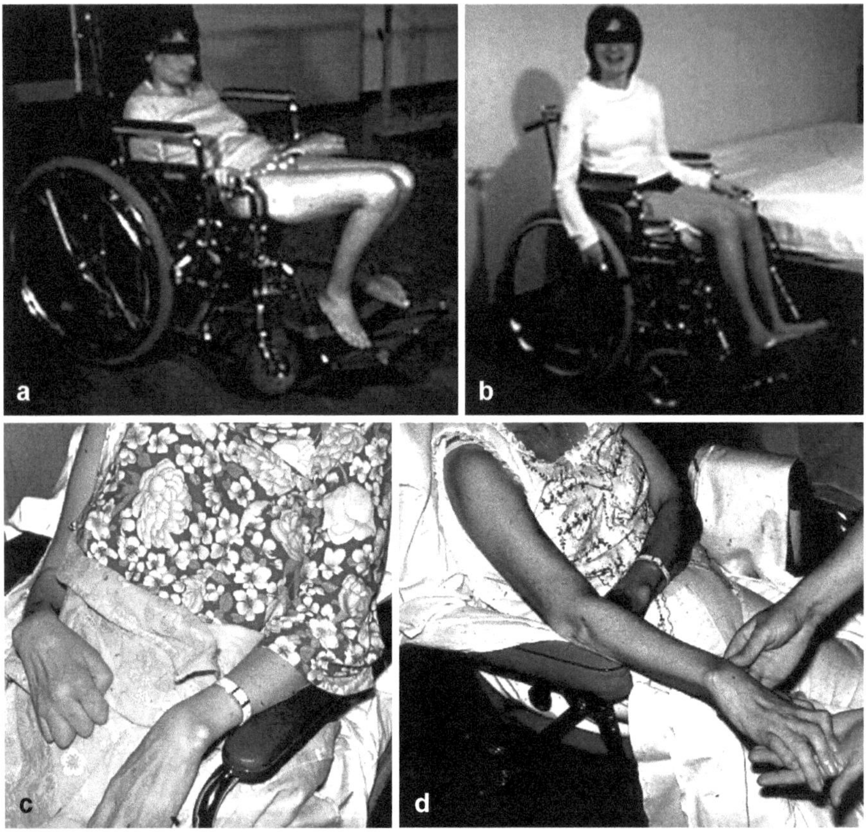

Fig. 9.3 (**a**, **b**) Hyperspastic paraplegic patient with advanced multiple sclerosis, before (**a**) and after (**b**) MDT directed to the L2–S2 segments. Note the improvement in comfort in wheelchair. (**c**, **d**) Severe right spastic hemiplegia in upper limb in a very disabled patient with paralyzed upper limb, posture in flexion and painful passive mobilization, before (**c**) and after (**d**) MDT directed to the C5–T1 segments. Note the relaxing effect on entire upper limb, allowing better comfort and easier and less painful passive mobilization

9.2 Surgical Technique

Surgery is performed with the patient under general anesthesia with endotracheal intubation. Curarization should be short-lasting to allow intraoperative identification of muscular responses to bipolar electrical stimulation of the exposed roots. Stimulation of the ventral and dorsal roots is most useful to determine the topographical level of the spinal cord segments to be targeted, as the anatomical landmarks are not identifiable reliably enough and innervation is subject to variation. Ventral roots have a motor threshold at least three times lower than that of the dorsal roots. Stimulation should preferably be bipolar to avoid diffusion of current. Frequency is commonly at 2 Hz. Intensity of stimulation should start between 0.1 and 1 mA. Microsurgery is performed at a magnification of ×10 to ×25. Specially designed microinstruments for MDT, microscissors and bipolar forceps, are available from Stryker Leibinger, Freiburg, Germany (Fig. 9.5a–c).

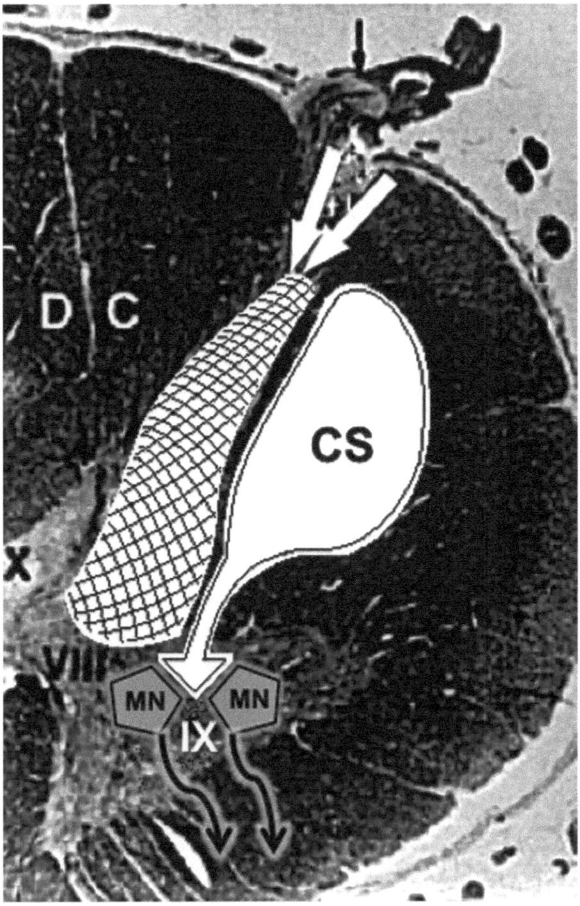

Fig. 9.4 Target of DREZ lesioning for severe spasticity and/or dystonia (at cervical level for upper limb). MDT is performed after incision of the dorsolateral sulcus (*double white arrows*), in the axis of the dorsal horn at an angle of 35° across the tract of Lissauer (*tl*) and the dorsal horn, down to the base of the ventral horn. Depth is 4–5 mm for (severe) spasticity or 5–6 mm for (severe) dystonia, as the "pathway" for the latter is through the corticospinal tract (*CS*) and descending extrapyramidal pathways, and projections to the motoneurons (*MN*). Target (*hatched area*) increases all layers of the dorsal horn and the base of the ventral horn and aims to spare the corticospinal fibers to the motoneurons. Microcoagulations of MDT are performed from C5 down to T1 for hemiplegic patients with upper limb entirely affected by severe disabling spasticity and/or dystonia. *DC* dorsal column, *VIII–X* rexed lamina

9.2.1 Operative Procedure at Cervical Level

The prone position with the head and neck flexed in the "Concorde" position has the advantage of avoiding brain collapse caused by depletion of cerebrospinal fluid. The head is fixed with a three-pin head holder. The level of laminectomy is determined after the prominent spinous process of C2 is identified by palpation. For unilateral DREZ surgery, a hemilaminectomy, usually from C4 to C7 included, with preservation of the spinous processes allows sufficient exposure of the posterolateral aspect

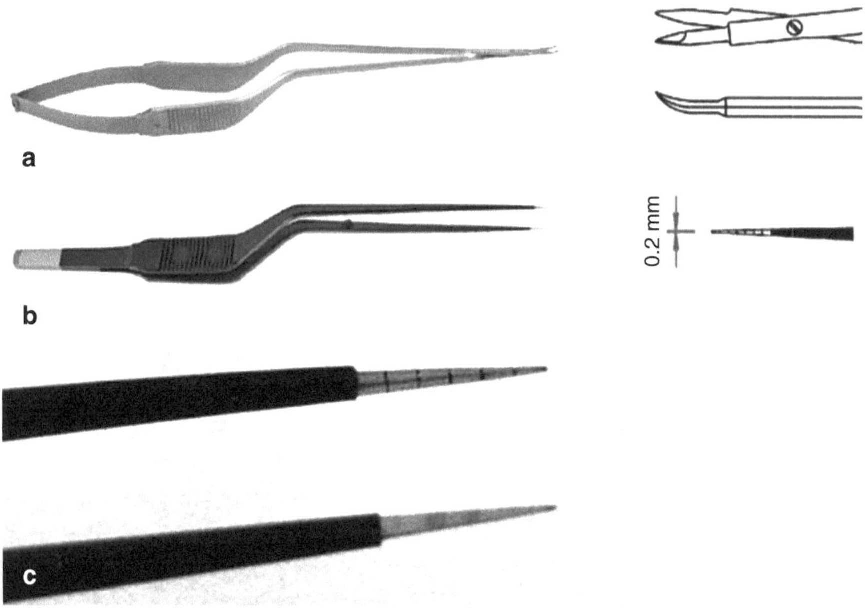

Fig. 9.5 Key microinstruments specially designed for MDT (Stryker Leibninger GmbH & Co. KG, Freiburg, Germany). (**a**) Microscissors bayonet shaped, fine, curved, 20 cm long. (**b**) Bipolar forceps, bayonet shaped, with graduated tip; width, 0.2 mm; working length, 8.5 cm; total length, 20 cm; graduation every millimeter over 6 mm. (**c**) Magnification of the uninsulated tip of the bipolar coagulation forceps. The insulated tip is incremented at 1 mm over 6 mm

of the cervical spinal cord segments that correspond to the upper limb innervation, i.e., the rootlets of C5 to T1 (Fig. 9.6).

Dura and arachnoid are opened longitudinally. The exposed roots are isolated by separating the tiny arachnoid filaments that bind them together to the arachnoid sheath and to the cord pia mater. The radicular vessels are preserved. Each ventral (and dorsal) root from C4 to T1 is electrically stimulated at the level of its corresponding foramen to identify its (their) muscular innervation and functional value. Responses are observed in the diaphragm for C4 (the response is palpable below the lower ribs), in the shoulder abductors for C5, in the elbow flexors for C6, in the elbow and wrist extensors for C7, and in the intrinsic muscles of the hand for C8 and T1.

Microsurgical lesioning is performed at the selected levels, which correspond to the upper-limb myotomes. Procedure is as follows (Fig. 9.7). The incision is made with a microknife; an ophthalmologic microscalpel is an appropriate instrument. Microcoagulations are performed in a "chain", i.e., a dotted manner. Each microcoagulation is performed in the axis of the dorsal horn, i.e., an angle of 35°, under direct magnification for a short duration (1–3 s) by low-intensity, bipolar electrocoagulation with an especially designed sharp graduated bipolar forceps (Fig. 9.5b, c). The depth and extent of the lesion depend on the desired therapeutic effect and preoperative neurological status; minimal depth into the dorsal horn should be 3–5 mm.

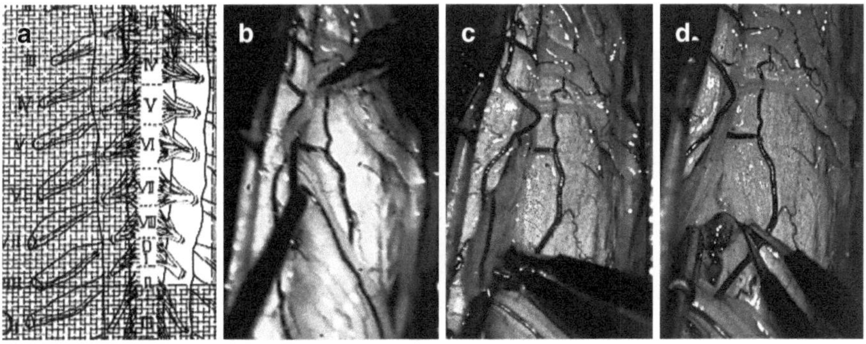

Fig. 9.6 Principles of MDT technique at cervical level. (**a**) Exposure of the right dorsolateral aspect of the cervical cord through right hemilaminectomy (in this example at the C6 level). The rootlets of the selected dorsal roots (in this example at C6 level), are displaced dorsally and medially with a hook (or a microsucker) for access to the ventrolateral aspect of the dorsolateral sulcus and dorsal rootlets. With microscissors the arachnoid adhesions between the spinal cord and the dorsal rootlets are cut. (**b**) After coagulation of the tiny pial vessels, a 2 mm deep incision at an angle of 35° ventrally and medially is made with a microknife at the lateral border of the dorsolateral sulcus. (**c**) Then microcoagulations for spasticity or dystonia are performed 3–6 mm down into the dorsal horn with a sharp graduated bipolar microforceps in a dotted manner every millimeter along the dorsolateral sulcotomy, as shown in (**d**)

If the root is loose enough, the incision is performed continuously in the dorsolateral sulcus, ventrolaterally along all the rootlets of the targeted root until the sulcomyelotomy is completed. Otherwise, a partial ventrolateral section is made successively on each rootlet after the surgeon has isolated each one by separating the tiny arachnoid membranes that hold the rootlets together.

9.2.2 Operative Procedure at Lumbosacral Level

The patient is positioned prone on thoracic and iliac supports. The head is placed 20 cm lower than the level of the surgical wound, in order to minimize the intraoperative loss of cerebrospinal fluid. The desired vertebral level is identified by a lateral X-ray study that includes the S1 vertebra as a reference. A laminectomy is performed from T10 to L2 (Fig. 9.8). The dura and arachnoid are opened longitudinally and the filum terminale is isolated. The root levels are identified by electrical stimulation (intensity, 0.1–1 mA; frequency, 2 Hz).

The L1 and L2 roots are easily identified at the site where they penetrate their respective dural sheaths. Stimulation of L2 produces a response of the iliopsoas and adductor muscles (Fig. 9.9).

Identification of L3 to L5 roots is difficult for several reasons. First, they exit through their respective dural sheaths, which are caudal to the exposure. Second, the dorsal rootlets enter the sulcus along an uninterrupted line. Third, the ventral roots are hidden in front of the dentate ligament. Finally, in the legs the motor responses to stimulation of the roots are difficult to observe intraoperatively because the

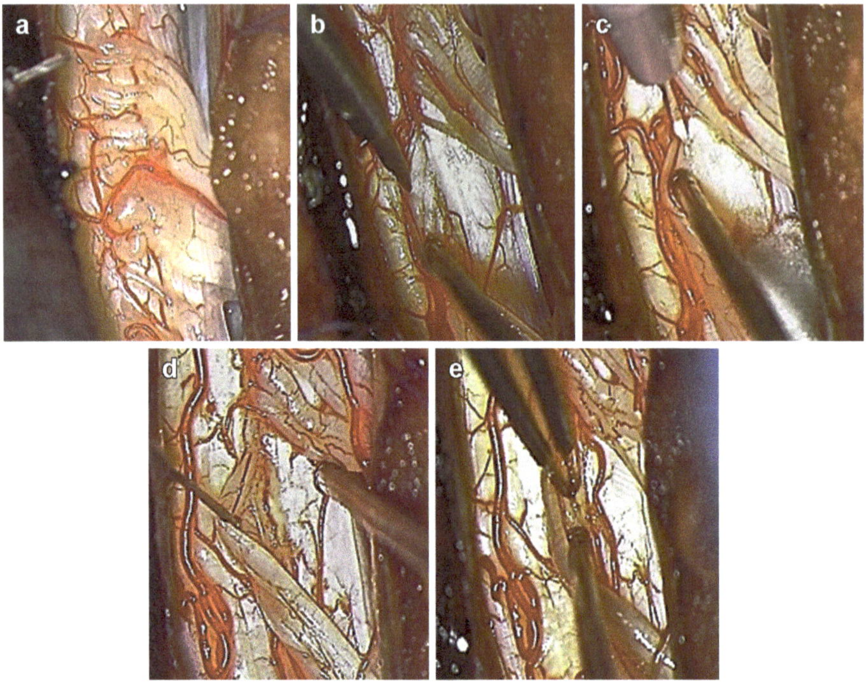

Fig. 9.7 Stepwise MDT technique at the cervical level (right side; rostral at top, caudal at bottom). (**a**) Exposure of the right dorsolateral aspect of the cervical cord at the C6 level through right hemilaminectomy. (**b**) The rootlets of the selected dorsal root(s) are displaced dorsally and medially with a microsucker for access to the ventrolateral aspect the dorsolateral sulcus. (**c**) A 2 mm deep incision at an angle of 35° ventrally and medially is made with a microknife in the ventral border of the dorsolateral sulcus. (**d**) Dorsolateral sulcus opened down to the dorsal horn apex. (**e**) Microcoagulations are performed 3–5 mm down into the dorsal horn with a sharp graduated bipolar microforceps in a dotted manner every millimeter along the dorsolateral sulcotomy

patient is in prone position. Stimulation of L3 produces a preferential response in the adductors and quadriceps; that of L4, in the quadriceps and the anterior tibialis; and that of L5, in the extensor of toes and the gluteal muscles (Fig. 9.10).

Stimulation of the S1 (dorsal) root produces a motor response in the gastrocnemius-soleus group. This response can be confirmed later by repeatedly checking the Achilles ankle reflex before, during, and after the DREZ lesioning.

Stimulation of the S2 to S4 (dorsal) roots (or better, of the corresponding spinal cord segments at the DREZ directly) can be assessed by recording the motor vesical or more easily the motor anal response by cystomanometry and rectomanometry, respectively, or much easier by electromyography of the anal sphincter or even simpler by inserting a gloved finger into the sphincter. Because neurophysiologic investigations are time-consuming, we found that measurements at the conus medullaris can be sufficient in patients who already have severe preoperative loss of their vesicoanal functions. These measurements, based on human postmortem anatomic studies, have shown that the landmark between S1 and S2 is situated approximately

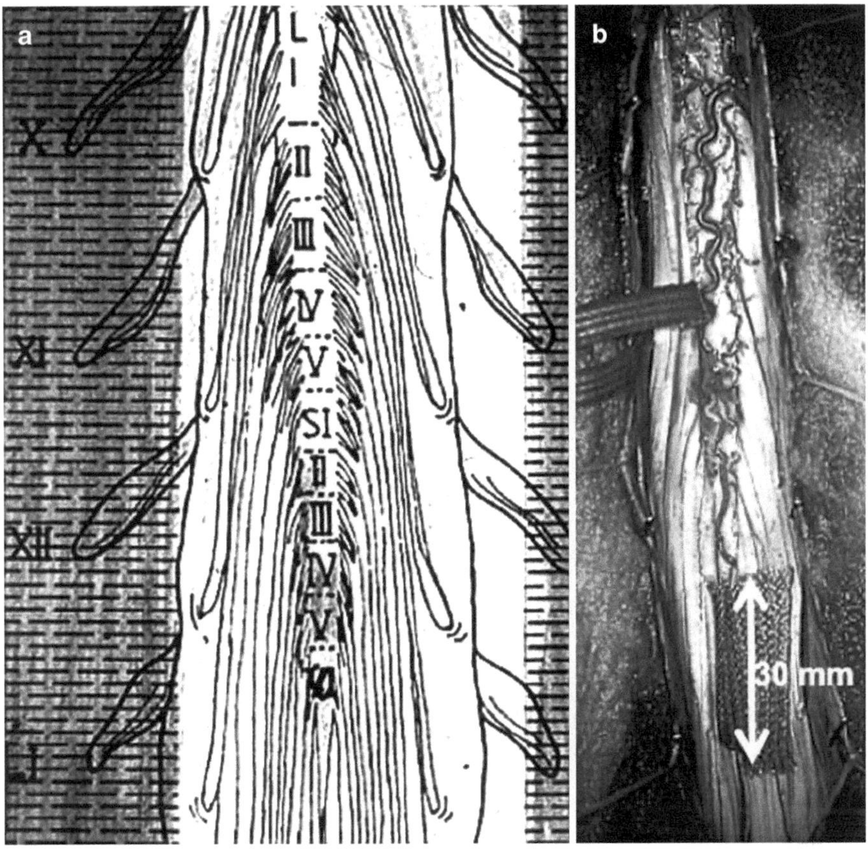

Fig. 9.8 Exposure of conus medullaris and identification of levels. (**a**) Schematic drawing of the conus medullaris approached through a laminectomy from T10 to L2. (**b**) Identification of S2-S5 spinal cord segments: the landmark between S1 and S2 spinal cord segments is situated approximately 30 mm above the exit of the (tiny) coccygeal root from the conus medullaris (operative view) [7, 8]

30 mm above the exit of the last (tiny) coccygeal root from the conus medullaris [7, 8], but this may vary (Figs. 9.8a and 9.9right).

MDT at the lumbosacral level follows the same principles as those at the cervical level (Fig. 9.11). But at the lumbosacral level, MDT is difficult and possibly dangerous because of the rich vasculature of the conus medullaris. The dorsolateral spinal artery courses along the dorsolateral sulcus; its diameter is 0.1–0.5 mm. It is fed by the posterior radicular arteries and joins caudally with the descending anterior branch of the artery of Adamkiewicz through the anastomotic loop of the conus medullaris. This artery must be freed from the sulcus and preserved, especially if the patient retains motor or sensory function (Fig. 9.12).

After opening the dorsolateral sulcus with a microknife, microcoagulations are performed under direct magnified vision, in a dotted manner, i.e., every millimeter, 3 mm in depth within the gray matter of the dorsal horn and with an angle of 45°,

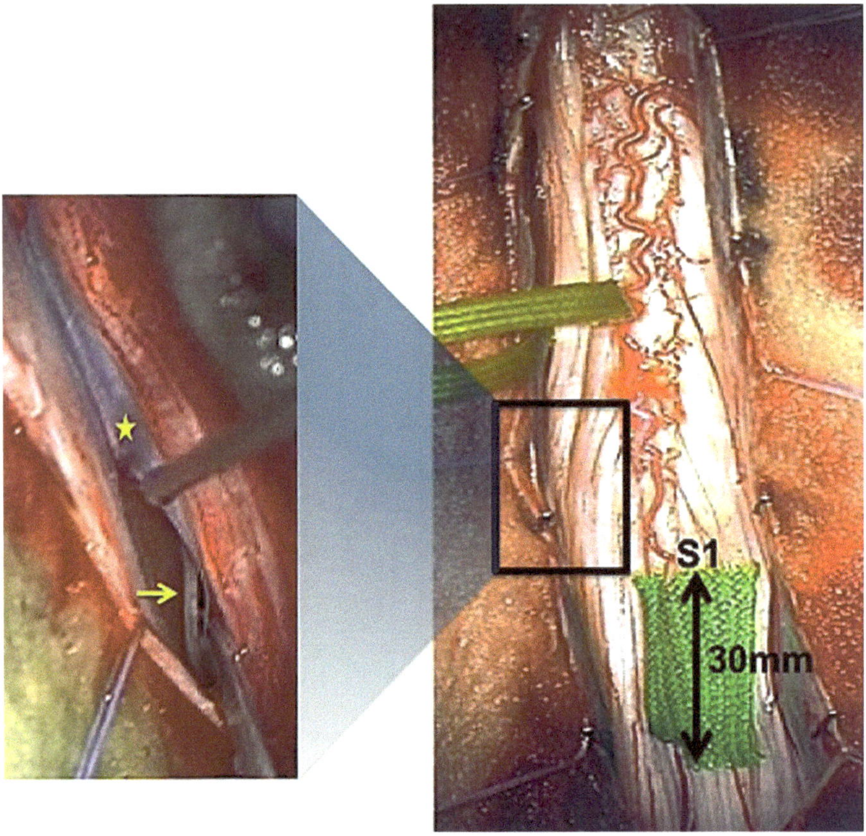

Fig. 9.9 Identification of L2 (*left image*): the boxed area on right inset is shown at greater magnification on left image. The left L2 ventral root (*arrow*) is visible anteriorly to the dentate ligament (*asterisk*). See projections of S2-S3 spinal cord segments *(double black arrow)*

which is the axis of the dorsal horn at the lumbar and sacral segmental levels (Fig. 9.12). Depth and extent of microcoagulation lesioning depends on the desired therapeutic effect and preoperative deficits.

9.3 Outcome, Side-effects, and Complications

For results of the operations we make recourse to our published reports. Our series consisted of three groups of patients.

94 hemiplegic patients underwent MDT at the cervical level for hyperspasticity in the paralyzed upper limb; MDT was performed from C5 to T1 through a C3–C7 hemilaminectomy.

175 patients underwent MDT at the lumbosacral level for excessive spasticity complicating severe paraplegic states such as those observed in advanced multiple

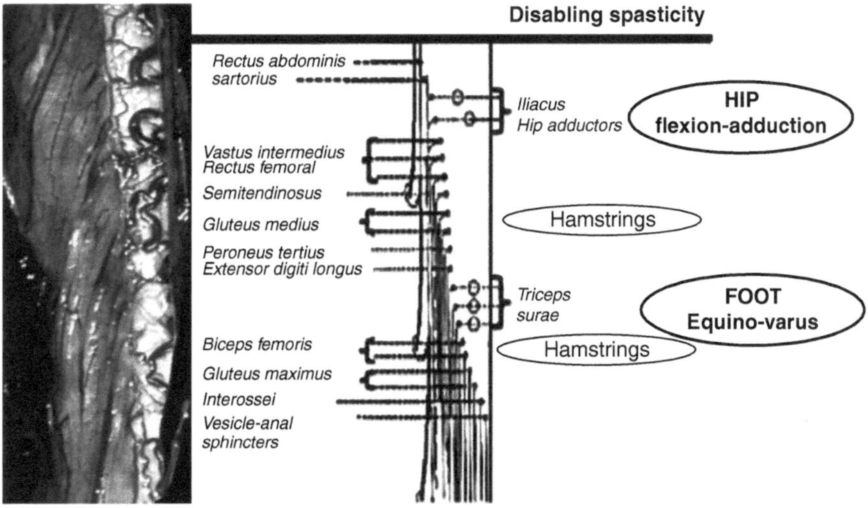

Fig. 9.10 Exposure of the conus medullaris for mapping. Stimulation of the ventral and dorsal roots is most useful to determine the topographical level of the root and spinal cord segments to be targeted, following the principle of lesioning the responsible segments for the disabling spasticity (*Right diagram*, modified from Gros [15])

sclerosis. MDT was performed bilaterally, through a T1–L2 laminectomy from L2 to S2, or to S5 in incontinent patients having a hyperactive neurogenic bladder with urine leakage around the catheter.

15 patients underwent MDT at the sacral (S2 to S3 or S4) level for an isolated hyperactive neurogenic bladder.

Outcomes have been detailed elsewhere [9–14] and will be only summarized here.

For **paraplegic patients**, spasticity and spasms, if any, were persistently suppressed or markedly decreased for 75 and 88.2 % of the patients, respectively. If patients suffered pain, as did 69.8 % of the group, it was relieved for 91.6 % of them. These benefits, combined with complementary orthopedic surgery (performed in approximately one third of the patients), resulted in a marked reduction in abnormal postures for 85.3 % and of articular limitations for 96.8 % of the patients. The Global Functional Disability score, using the 0–20° quantifying disability score of the Lyon University scale (Table 9.1), improved on average for the series from 15.6 of disability to 3.6 of disability (Fig. 9.13). Motor activity, preoperatively very poor if not absent in almost all the patients of the series, was unchanged for 79.6 %, improved for 11.2 %, and worsened for 10.2 % of the patients. Urinary function was unchanged for 81 %, improved for 7 %, and impaired for 12 % of the patients. If in the operated territories any sensation was felt preoperatively, it was impaired moderately for 38 % and severely for 20 % of the patients. Chronic cutaneous trophic lesions, with which 43.1 % of the patients presented, were transiently aggravated for one third of them, but in the long term ameliorated for all patients, care being easier after surgery.

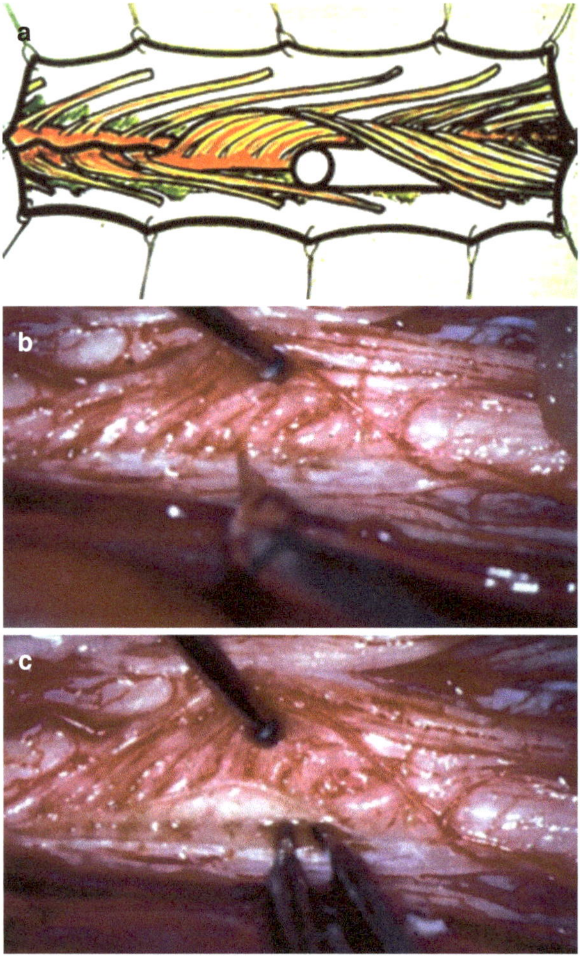

Fig. 9.11 Principles of the MDT technique at the lumbosacral level (in this example on the left side of the conus; rostral at left, caudal at right). Exposure of the conus medullaris through a T11 to L1 laminectomy. Approach of the dorsolateral sulcus. (**a**) Dorsal rootlets of the selected roots are displaced dorsally and medially to obtain proper access to ventrolateral aspect of the dorsolateral sulcus and held with a (specially designed) ball-tip microsucker used as a small hook. After division of the fine arachnoidal filaments binding the rootlets together and to the pia mater with curved sharp microscissors, the arteries running along the dorsolateral sulcus are dissected free. Smaller arteries are coagulated with a sharp bipolar microforceps, main arteries are preserved. (**b**) Then a continuous incision is made with a microknife at an angle of 45° and to a depth of 3 mm. (**c**) Once the dorsolateral sulcus is opened, the surgical lesion is completed by low-intensity microcoagulations performed under direct magnified vision inside the dorsolateral sulcomyelotomy, 3–5 mm down into the dorsal horn. These microcoagulations are made in a dotted manner, every millimeter, along all the segments of the spinal cord selected for lesioning with a special sharp bipolar forceps

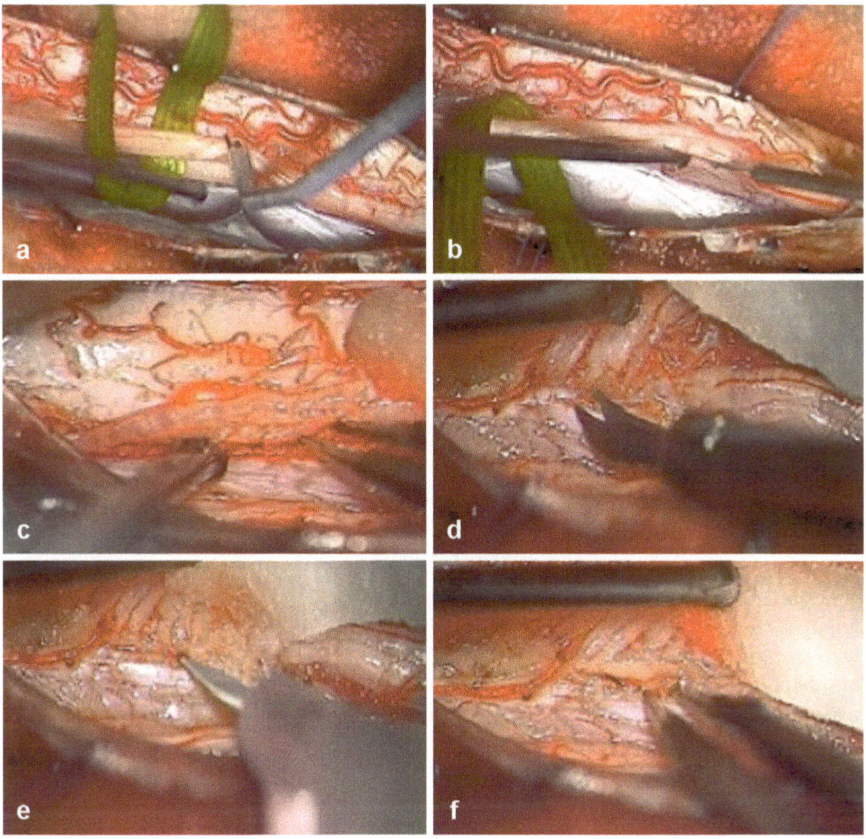

Fig. 9.12 Stepwise MDT technique at the lumbosacral level (left side of conus medullaris; rostral at left, caudal at right). (**a**) Identification of the segmental levels by electrical stimulation eliciting muscular responses. (**b**) Exposure of the dorsolateral sulcus by retracting the dorsal roots posteriorly and medially. (**c**) The ventral aspect of the dorsolateral sulcus is marked by the dorsolateral artery running along the sulcus. In this case, the artery could not be spared and was coagulated with the fine sharp bipolar microforceps. (**d**) Incision of the pia mater along the ventral border of the dorsolateral sulcus with sharp curved microcissors. (**e**) Incision of the sulcus with a microknife (of the ophthalmologic type), at an angle of 45°. (**f**) Microcoagulations inside the opened dorsolateral sulcus, 3–5 mm down into the dorsal horn, every millimeter in a dotted manner, with the bipolar microforceps

For **hemiplegic patients**, spasticity was abolished or markedly reduced for 87 %, pain relieved for 81 %, voluntary motility improved for 50 % of the group. Global functional status was ameliorated, with better passive mobilization for 87 % and gain in active motility for 56 % of the patients. As regards patients' satisfaction, surgery was considered very useful by 69 %, moderately useful by 12 %, and a failure by 19 % of them.

Table 9.1 Global Functional Disability scale of Lyon University for paraplegic patients with spasticity in lower limbs

Criterion	Score
Pain:	
Absent	0
Rare and mild; no disability	1
Frequent; minimal disability	2
Marked und frequent; marked disability	3
Permanent and severe	4
Spasms:	
Absent	0
Rare and mild spasms only during mobilization; no disability	1
Frequent, spontaneous but moderate spasms; some disability	2
Frequent, spontaneous and marked spasms; marked disability	3
Almost constant and severe spasms; severe disability, major problems for sitting and lying	4
Sitting position:	
Normal	0
Mild difficulty	1
Moderate difficulty	2
Severe difficulty, patient has to be tied down in position	3
Impossible	4
Body transfer:	
Normal	0
Mild difficulty	1
Moderate difficulty	2
Marked difficulty, needs one person helping	3
Severe difficulty, needs two persons helping	4
Washing and dressing:	
Normal	0
Mild difficulty	1
Moderate difficulty	2
Marked difficulty, needs one person helping	3
Severe difficulty, needs two persons helping	4

A score of 10 out of 20 corresponds to a functional disability indicating neurosurgery to be considered for spasticity

Briefly summarized, long-term outcome with a follow-up ranging from 2 to 25 years (mean, 9 years) was the following. For paraplegic patients, a useful effect for lower limbs, i.e., a lasting decrease in tone allowing easy passive mobilization, was achieved for 80 % of them. Bladder capacity was improved for 85 % of the patients whose detrusor muscle was hyperactive and not fibrotic. For hemiplegic patients with harmful spasticity in the upper limb, a useful effect was obtained for 83 % of them. The effect on the upper limb was more pronounced and lasting at the level of the shoulder and elbow than at the hand and fingers. Additional peripheral neurotomies together with orthopedic surgery were often required to complete the effect of the MDT.

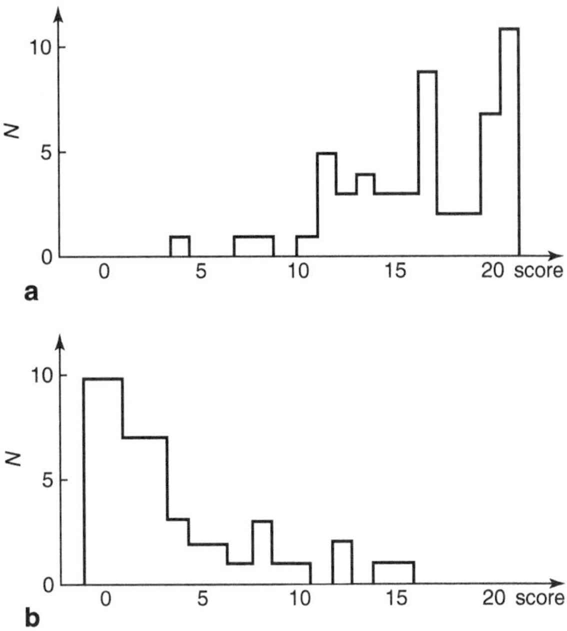

Fig. 9.13 Results of MDT in a group of paraplegic patients, evaluated using the Global functional disability scale of Lyon University (see Table 4.6, for scoring). Histogram for the authors' group of 53 patients before (**a**) and after (**b**) MDT. Note that most patients shifted from the range of 10–20 (average, 15.6) before surgery, to 0–10 (average, 3.6) after surgery. *N* number of patients

For both groups of patients (paraplegic and hemiplegic), MDT consistently decreased sensation in the operated territories; the decrease was mild for 40 %, marked for 40 %, and severe for 20 % of the patients. Any pain was relieved for 88 % of both groups. Permanent neurological disturbances due to adjacent long-tract impairment may be observed (ipsilaterally) after MDT. Ataxia due to arthrokinesthetic hypoesthesia and tactile hypoesthesia with some degree of paresthesias may happen if DREZ lesioning is performed too far medially and damages the dorsal column tract. Also, motor weakness may occur if lesioning is done too far laterally toward the pyramidal tract.

Hypotonia and reduction in reflex automatisms produced by MDT in the lumbosacral segments can exceed the desired effects, which would be a major concern for paraparetic patients who are able to walk or have genito-sphincterian function.

Lesioning surgery in the DREZ, because it entails risk of creating new or aggravating preexisting deficits, has to be performed with caution, especially in patients retaining significant neurological functions.

Conclusion

On the basis of our experience, the indications for severe disabling spastic states are as follows. The hyperspastic hemiplegic upper limb can benefit from MDT when spasticity predominates in the shoulder and elbow. Wrist and fingers are less favorably influenced, especially when there are irreducible contractures and deformities in flexion and poor motor function in the extensors. Peripheral neurotomies combined with tendon surgery may be preferred or associated to MDT for patients with poor extensor function. For hemiplegic patients with focalized dystonia associated to spasticity in upper limb, MDT can be effective on both components, provided it is performed deeply down to the base of ventral horn.

MDT has a dramatic effect on tone in lower limbs. Surgical indications must be restricted to paraplegic patients with severe disability who are unable to walk autonomously. MDT is indicated if patients cannot be installed comfortably in a wheelchair or are at risk of pressure sores in bed, especially if additional pain from spasms, contractures, or neurotrophic disturbances is present. Intrathecal baclofen therapy is an alternative to MDT and the first neurosurgical option.

MDT can be indicated to treat neurogenic bladder when there is no voluntary micturition and if uninhibited detrusor contractions result in voiding around the catheter or in between intermittent self-catheterization.

Indications for surgery in the DREZ must be considered and discussed within the context of the entire armamentarium available for the treatment of spasticity.

References

1. Sindou M (1972) Etude de la jonction radiculo-médullaire posterieure: la radicellotomie postérieure selective dans la chirurgie de la douleur. Thèse de Médecine, Université de Lyon, Lyon
2. Sindou M, Quoex C, Baleydier C (1974) Fiber organization at the posterior spinal cord-rootlet junction in man. J Comp Neurol 153:15–26
3. Sindou M, Fischer G, Goutelle A, Schott B, Mansuy L (1974) La radicellotomie postérieure selective dans le traitement de la spasticité. Rev Neurol (Paris) 130:201–216
4. Sindou M, Millet MF, Mortamais J, Eyssette M (1982) Results of selective posterior rhizotomy in the treatment of painful and spastic paraplegia secondary to multiple sclerosis. Appl Neurophysiol 45:335–340
5. Sindou M, Abdennebi B, Sharkey P (1985) Microsurgical selective procedures in the peripheral nerves and the posterior root-spinal cord junction for spasticity. Appl Neurophysiol 48:97–104
6. Sindou M, Pregelj R, Boisson D, Eyssette M, Goutelle A (1985) Surgical selective lesions of nerve fibers and myelotomies for the modification of muscle hypertonia. In: Eccles J, Dimitrijevic MR (eds) Upper motor neuron functions and dysfunctions, vol 1, Recent achievements in restorative neurology. Karger, Basel, pp 10–26
7. Sindou M, Fischer G, Mansuy L (1976) Posterior spinal rhizotomy and selective posterior rhizidiotomy. In: Krayenbühl H, Maspes PE, Sweet WH (eds) Pain: its neurosurgical management, vol 7, Progress in neurological surgery. Karger, Basel, pp 201–250
8. Sindou M, Goutelle A (1983) Surgical posterior rhizotomies for the treatment of pain. In: Krayenbühl H, Brihaye J, Loew F, Mingrino S, Pertuiset B, Symon L, Troupp H, Yaşargil MG (eds) Advances and technical standards in neurosurgery, vol 10. Springer, Wien/New York, pp 147–185
9. Sindou M, Jeanmonod D (1989) Microsurgical DREZ-otomy for the treatment of spasticity and pain in the lower limbs. Neurosurgery 24:655–670
10. Beneton C, Mertens P, Leriche A, Sindou M (1991) The spastic bladder and its treatment. In: Sindou M, Abbott R, Keravel Y (eds) Neurosurgery for spasticity: a multidisciplinary approach. Springer, Wien/New York, pp 193–199
11. Sindou M (1998) Spinal entry zone interruption for spasticity. In: Gildenberg P, Tasker RR (eds) Textbook of stereotactic and functional neurosurgery. McGraw-Hill, New York, pp 1257–1266

12. Sindou M (1995) Microsurgical DREZotomy (MDT) for pain, spasticity and hyperactive bladder: a 20-year experience. Acta Neurochir (Wien) 137:1–5
13. Sindou M, Mifsud JJ, Boisson D, Goutelle A (1986) Selective posterior rhizotomy in the dorsal root entry zone for treatment of hyperspasticity and pain in the hemiplegic upper limb. Neurosurgery 18:587–595
14. Decq P, Mertens P (eds) (2003) La neurochirurgie de la spasticité. Neurochirurgie 49:135–416
15. Gros C (1979) Spasticity: Clinical classification and surgical treatment. In Krayenbuehl H, Brihaye J, Loew F, Logue V, Mingrino S, Pertuiset B, Symon L, Troupp H, Yasargil MG (eds) Advances and Technical Standards in Neurosurgery, vol 6. Springer, Wien/New York, pp 55–97

Part III

Children

Spasticity in Cerebral Palsy

10

The most frequent cause of spasticity and hypertonia in childhood is by far cerebral palsy (CP). In 1861 Little was the first to draw the medical community's attention "on the influence of abnormal parturition, difficult labours, premature birth, and asphyxia neonatorum, on the mental and physical condition of the child, especially in relation to deformities" (Figs. 10.1, 10.2 and 10.3) [2, 3]. The term "cerebral palsies of children" was established in 1889 by Osler (Fig. 10.4) [4]. The presently adopted description of CP was given by Ingram [5]. CP is now worldwide used to designate nonprogressive disorders of the motor and related functions that result from an insult to the brain which occurs in the prenatal, perinatal, or approximately 2-year postnatal period, or due to excessive prematurity. There are different clinical patterns of hypertonia within the frame of CP disorders [6, 7].

Spasticity is defined as muscular resistance to stretching which is velocity-dependent, thus giving a "catch sensation" at high-velocity stretching. Features of spasticity are modified variably with time and under environmental conditions and emotional factors, so that examination should be repeated and performed by not only one examiner.

Spasticity is frequently accompanied by other motor and tone disturbances. Spasticity may be mixed to some degree with **rigidity**, which is a resistance to movement but not velocity-dependent, giving a "lead-pipe impression".

Spasticity is frequently associated with **dystonia**, which is a stereotype pattern of contorted and prolonged hypertonic state induced by attempts at voluntary motion. When examined, the limb resists to passive mobilization. Like spasticity, dystonia is very susceptible to anxiety and emotional factors.

Hypertonia and dystonia may also be affected by the coexistence of **choreoathetoid** "parasite" movements that will not be influenced by the treatment of hypertonia and spasticity.

Because of the complexity of clinical presentations of these children and the therapeutic implications of the various disturbances frequently mixed with spasticity, a rigorous analysis of all the components of motor and tone disorders is crucial to establish the appropriate and optimal surgical management and plan when needed.

M. Sindou et al., *Neurosurgery for Spasticity*,
DOI 10.1007/978-3-7091-1771-2_10, © Springer-Verlag Wien 2014

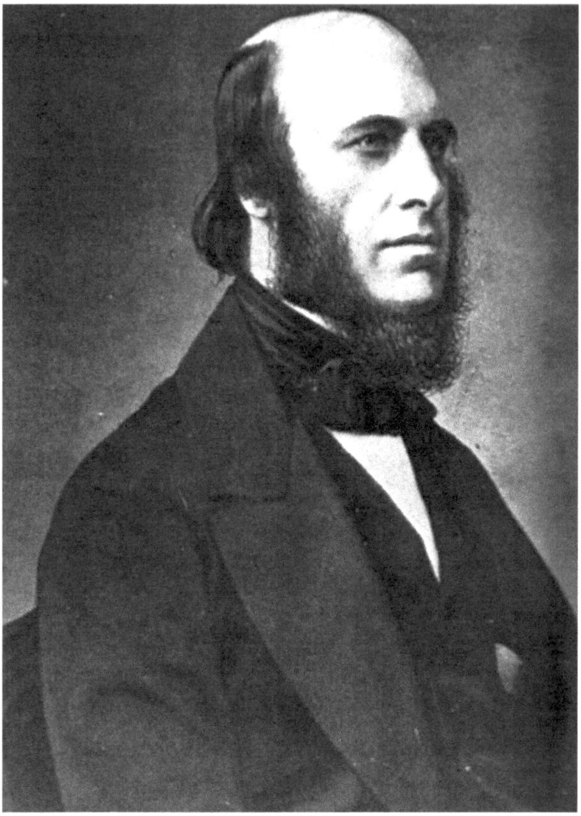

Fig. 10.1 William J Little (1810–1894), English surgeon who first described the medical identification of spastic diplegia in 1861. William John Little had in many respects a unique career. He suffered childhood poliomyelitis with residual left lower-extremity paraparesis, complicated by severe talipes. After medical studies at Medical School at the London Hospital, he was admitted to the Royal College of Surgeons in 1832. He later travelled to Germany to study the technique of subcutaneous tenotomy with its originator, Louis Stromeyer, who subsequently corrected Little's deformed foot by this method. His doctoral dissertation (1837) was the first monograph on tenotomy ever published, and he became the apostle of this operation for the correction of skeletal deformity secondary to neuromuscular disease. Little founded the Royal Orthopaedic Hospital of London. Among his many publications, major ones deal with cerebral spastic palsy (Little's Disease). The techniques introduced by Stromeyer and applied by Little are used today in the surgical management of muscular dystrophy. William Little was one of the first to bridge the gap between neurology and orthopedics and his important work continues to impact on both these fields [1]

Fig. 10.3 Illustration of children with representative patterns of spastic diplegia in the publication of Little [2]. (**a**) General spastic contraction of the lower extremities due to premature birth and asphyxia neonatorum of 36 h duration. (**b**) Contraction of adductors and flexors of lower extremities due to asphyxia neonatorum of 1 h duration

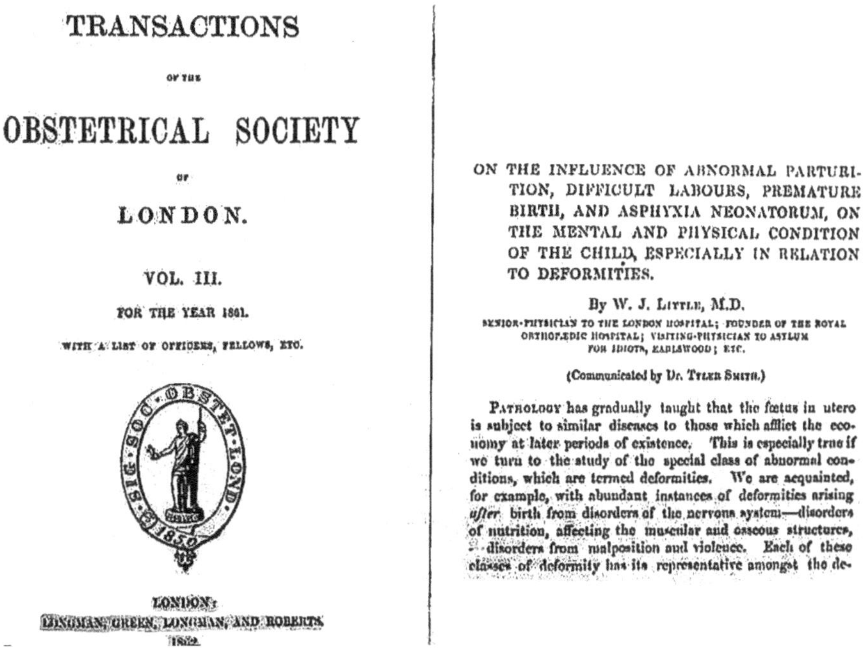

TRANSACTIONS

OF THE

OBSTETRICAL SOCIETY

OF

LONDON.

VOL. III.

FOR THE YEAR 1861.

WITH A LIST OF OFFICERS, FELLOWS, ETC.

LONDON:

LONGMAN, GREEN, LONGMAN, AND ROBERTS.

ON THE INFLUENCE OF ABNORMAL PARTURITION, DIFFICULT LABOURS, PREMATURE BIRTH, AND ASPHYXIA NEONATORUM, ON THE MENTAL AND PHYSICAL CONDITION OF THE CHILD, ESPECIALLY IN RELATION TO DEFORMITIES.

By W. J. Little, M.D.

SENIOR-PHYSICIAN TO THE LONDON HOSPITAL; FOUNDER OF THE ROYAL ORTHOPÆDIC HOSPITAL; VISITING-PHYSICIAN TO ASYLUM FOR IDIOTS, EARLSWOOD; ETC.

(Communicated by Dr. Tyler Smith.)

Pathology has gradually taught that the fœtus in utero is subject to similar diseases to those which afflict the economy at later periods of existence. This is especially true if we turn to the study of the special class of abnormal conditions, which are termed deformities. We are acquainted, for example, with abundant instances of deformities arising *after* birth from disorders of the nervous system—disorders of nutrition, affecting the muscular and osseous structures, —disorders from malposition and violence. Each of these classes of deformity has its representative amongst the de-

Fig. 10.2 Title page and first page from the classical description by Little

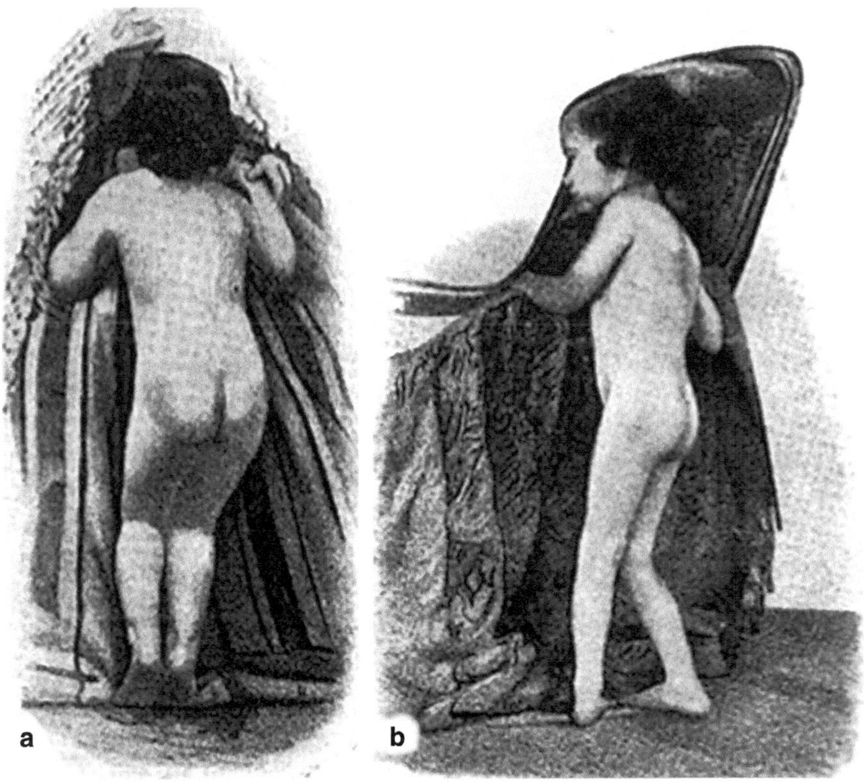

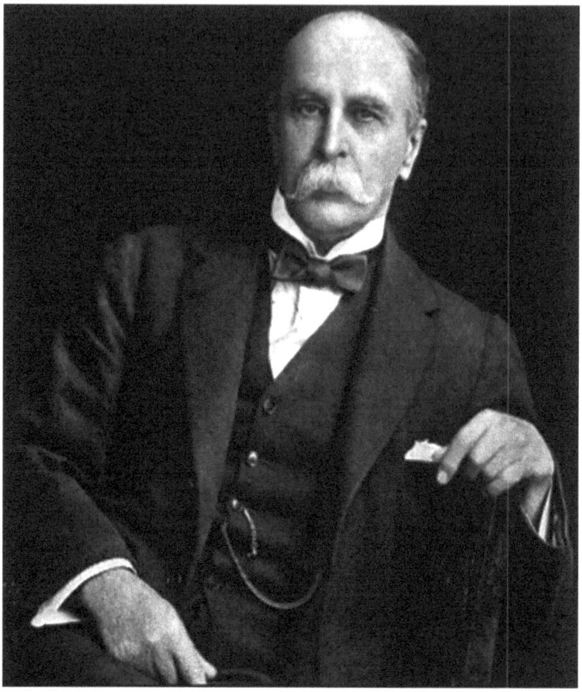

Fig. 10.4 Sir William Osler (1849–1919), Canadian physician who first introduced the term "cerebral palsy" in 1889

As pointed out by Little in his visionary publication, deformities are the consequences of the – primary – damage in the central nervous system [2]. Deficiency in selective motor control and dependence on primitive automatisms for ambulation and equilibrium, as well as imbalances in tone between agonist and antagonist muscular groups, are at the origin of bone deformities and muscle contractures.

Deformities develop as the child ages, because of imbalance in tone, postures, and gait. Axes and shapes of bones and joints become distorted due to abnormal remodeling under disturbed growth.

These – secondary – abnormalities, together with a deterioration in quality of muscular elasticity, result in evolving muscular contractures. They progressively aggravate disturbances in gait and deformities.

In ambulatory patients these abnormalities are at the origin of compensations used to circumvent disability in the locomotor function, which is a vicious circle that impairs gait and increases deformities. Whereas primary and secondary abnormalities become irreversible if the child is treated too late, the – tertiary – compensatory responses will disappear when no longer required [8].

When spasticity in children becomes harmful and threatens to induce irreversible contractures and deformities in spite of intensive physical therapy, an effective surgical armamentarium is available. Peripheral neurotomies for focal spastic muscles can be considered if botulinum toxin injections are not sufficient. Dorsal rhizotomies can be performed especially in spastic diplegic children able to ambulate, also intrathecal baclofen therapy especially in cases with strong associated dystonia.

Orthopedic surgery is of paramount interest, either on front row or as an adjuvant to neurosurgical treatment that aimed to decrease spasticity prior to orthopedic correction. The choice among the various therapeutic options is difficult at the pediatric age, because children are continuously developing and the evolution of spasticity and dystonia, which are frequently associated, has dynamic characteristics.

To analyze spasticity, scales are available; gait analysis is paramount to select the optimal therapeutic options. The developmental status of the child must be forecast. Fighting against disabling hypertonia must be carried out within the framework of a multidisciplinary team and global caring.

References

1. Siegel IM (1988) Historical vignette #9. Little big man: the life and genius of William John Little (1810–1894). Orthop Rev 17:1156, 1161–1166
2. Little WJ (1861) On the influence of abnormal parturition, difficult labours, premature birth and asphyxia neonatorum on the mental and physical condition of the child, especially in relation to deformities. Trans Obstet Soc Lond 3:293–344
3. Siegfried J, Lazorthes Y (1985) La neurochirurgie fonctionnelle de l'infirmité motrice d'origine cérébrale. Neurochirurgie 31(Suppl 1):1–118
4. Osler W (1989) The cerebral palsies of children: a clinical study from the Infirmary for Nervous Diseases. Blakiston, Philadelphia
5. Ingram TT (1955) A study of cerebral palsy in the childhood population of Edinburgh. Arch Dis Child 30:85–98
6. Abbott R (2007) The management of childhood hypertonia. Childs Nervous Syst 23:937–941
7. Sanger TD, Delgado MR, Gaebler-Spira D, Hallett M, Mink JW, Task Force on Childhood Motor Disorders (2003) Classification and definition of disorders causing hypertonia in childhood. Pediatrics 111:e89–e97
8. Novacheck TF, Gage JR (2007) Orthopedic management of spasticity in cerebral palsy. Childs Nerv Syst 23:1015–1031

Assessment of Spasticity in Pediatric Patients

11

Children are most often referred with the generic diagnosis of hypertonia. The first concern then is to determine the real nature of this hypertonia. Is it real spasticity? Is there an excess of spasticity which interferes with the capability of the child to ambulate, stand, and rest, as well as with the ability of the caregivers to provide optimal ease for caring and helping the child in daily living activities? Establishing the cause of the spasticity is an important prerequisite. Past factors supporting a diagnosis of cerebral palsy (CP) are to be searched: history of perinatal difficulties, premature birth, low weight at birth. A developmental profile of the child should be obtained, as well as all details on prior treatments.

Definitions of the various disorders that might be demonstrated by children with so-called hypertonic or spastic CP have been published by the Task Force on Childhood Motor Disorders [1].

Hypertonia is defined as "abnormally increased resistance to externally imposed movement about a joint" [2, p. 821]. Hypertonia may be caused by spasticity or dystonia individually or in combination.

Spasticity is defined as "hypertonia in which one or both of the following signs are present: (1) resistance to externally imposed movement that increases with increasing velocity and varies with the direction of joint movement. (2) rapid rise in resistance to externally imposed force movement above a threshold speed or joint angle" [2, p. 821]. After the rise, there may be a rapid decrease in resistance if the externally imposed force is maintained; this is the so-called clasp-knife response.

Dystonia – that may accompany hypertonia and spasticity – is defined as a movement disorder in which sustained muscle contractions cause twisting and repetitive movements or abnormal postures or both [1]. Dystonia may cause hypertonia, but dystonia may be present in the absence of hypertonia.

The motor disorders in children with CP are even more complex. Weakness and incoordination are common. There usually is co-contraction of agonists and antagonists if excessive reflex spreads to other muscle groups. Selective motor control is often reduced. This leads to an inability to achieve an isolated activation of muscles in a selected voluntary pattern of posture or movement [2].

M. Sindou et al., *Neurosurgery for Spasticity*,
DOI 10.1007/978-3-7091-1771-2_11, © Springer-Verlag Wien 2014

The diagnosis of spasticity must be established by the demonstration of an increase in velocity-dependent tone responses to stretching, hyperactive tendon reflexes, and clonus. Then the joint range of motion and functional abilities have to be graded for decision-making.

After having determined the specific nature of the hypertonia, the next concern is whether it is the hypertonia or the contractures and deformities that are impairing the child's function. As a matter of fact, as the child grows, contractures and deformities develop that become flexed and reduce the ease of care.

The assessment of children with CP consists of four successive fundamental stages. The first stage is the physical observation in order to assess the **child's global function.** The second stage is measurement of the **range of motion** to detect permanent and fixed contractures, which would be little accessible to neurosurgical treatment. The third stage is the **assessment of spasticity** with the Ashworth scale and/or the Tardieu scale. The fourth stage consists of grading the disability especially with the standardized **gross motor function measure (GMFM)** system and of evaluating its evolution by observing motor function in relation to time. This assessment of a child with CP is crucial for decision-making.

11.1 Physical Observation

Observation of the child in a **lying position** permits identification of abnormal postures in lower limbs, particularly their asymmetry. This is particularly important for nonambulatory children. They often exhibit left or right windswept posture, bilateral flexion and internal rotation and adduction, batracoid, crossed, or scissoring postures of lower limbs (Figs. 11.1 and 11.2) [3].

For the clinical examination of the gait of **ambulatory patients** there is a classification into five different groups: true equinus, jump gait, apparent equinus, crouch gait, and asymmetric gait (Fig. 11.3). These types of gait reflect pelvic tilt, hip extension or flexion, knee extension or flexion, and ankle dorsiflexion or plantar flexion (Table 11.1) [4]. Triceps surae is the dominant spastic muscular group for

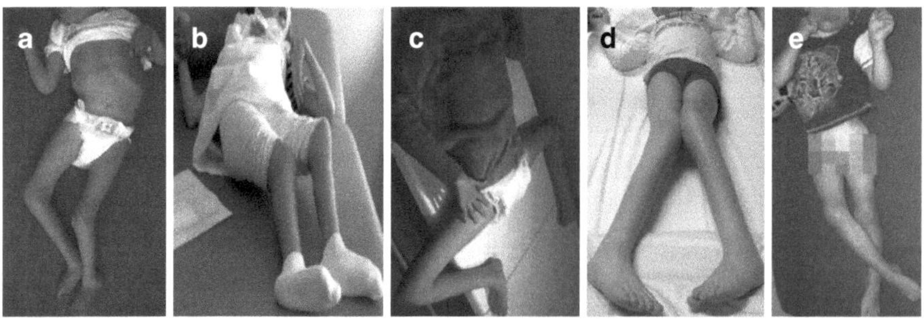

Fig. 11.1 Postures in relaxing position in frontal plane of inferior limbs in nonambulatory children. (**a**) Right windswept, (**b**) left windswept, (**c**) batracoid, (**d**) crossed-like legs, (**e**) scissor-like legs

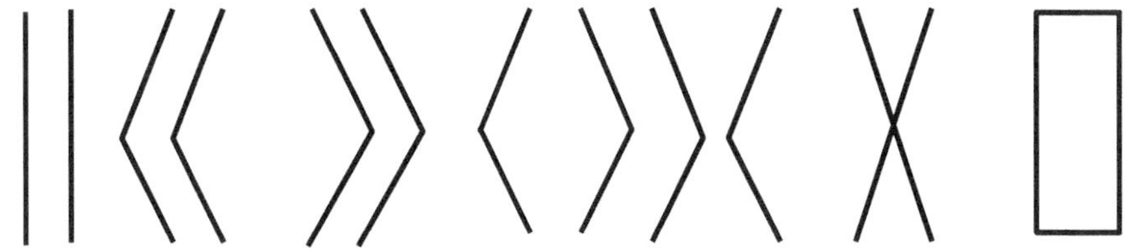

Fig. 11.2 Frontal-plane schemes of lower-limb postures in relaxing position (nonambulatory children)

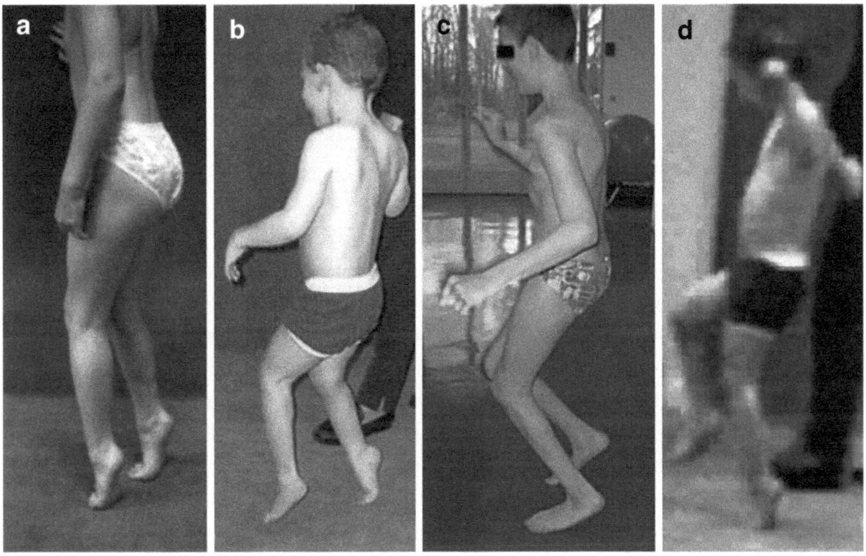

Fig. 11.3 Gait patterns of ambulatory patients with spastic diplegia. (**a**) True equinus, (**b**) apparent equinus, (**c**) crouch gait, (**d**) jump gait (taken from video)

Table 11.1 Classification of common gait patterns on the sagittal plane in ambulatory children with spastic diplegia

Gait pattern	Pelvic tilt	Hip flexion/ extension	Knee flexion/ extension	Ankle dorsiflexion/ plantar flexion
True equinus	Normal or anterior	Normal	Normal or recurvatum	Equinus
Jump gait	Normal or anterior	Normal or flexed	Flexed (on motion)	Equinus
Apparent equinus	Normal or anterior	Flexed	Flexed	Normal
Crouch gait	Anterior or normal or posterior	Flexed	Flexed	Calcaneus

In addition to the patterns defined in this table, there are asymmetric gait patterns the true equinus gait; the gastrocnemius, hamstrings and psoas for the jump gait; and hamstrings and psoas for the apparent equinus and crouch gait.

It is important to identify which muscular groups harbor a harmful spasticity that disturbs function and should be the target of the treatment and which muscular groups are weak and whose decrease in tone by surgery would be dangerous. Clinical examination should also determine whether or not there are additional irreducible muscular retractions, i.e., contractures that would require adjuvant orthopedic procedures, as they would not be reversed by neurological surgery alone.

11.2 Assessment of Range of Motion

Contractures and deformities in extremities may develop, particularly hip dislocations, knee flexion, ankle plantar flexion, rocker bottom feet. Also spinal deformity, especially scoliosis, may appear. Assessment of the range of motion detects possible permanent and fixed contractures, which are inaccessible to neurosurgical treatment. Complete assessment includes goniometric measurements in supine and prone positions [5]. The examination should have a logic order and require minimal effort from the patient. After a single turn of the child, the measurements in supine position are followed by the tests in prone position.

The measurement of the passive range of motion determines the angle of arrest upon slow stretch of the muscle group assessed, which provides insight on soft-tissue length and extensibility. Each muscle group is first evaluated by very slow but powerful stretching. One must keep in mind that the degree of range of motion is only a static evaluation after a slow and passive solicitation.

For examination of the passive motion, any displacement from the rest position should be made with the maximal possible stretch but at slow speed in order to avoid any spastic involvement by retriggering the myotatic response. Moreover, excessive manipulations could cause microhemorrhages and subsequent chronic microcalcifications that would further restrict the range of motion and increase musculotendinous retraction, as well as articular capsular calcifications and subsequent ankylosis. The angle at which soft-tissue resistance is no longer overcome by the clinician is defined as the passive range of motion against the muscle group assessed. The stretching maneuver is ceased when the clinician appreciates that muscular and articular integrity is threatened or if pain occurs during examination.

If differentiation between permanent contracture and severe spastic posture is uncertain but such distinction becomes critical for therapeutic decisions, complementary techniques may be applied. They include a motor nerve block with local anesthetic, injections of botulinum toxin, or even the assessment of the passive range of motion under general anesthesia and relaxant agents.

Moreover, the active range of motion is measured. It evaluates the net result of the recruitment of the agonist muscle group minus the combined resistance from

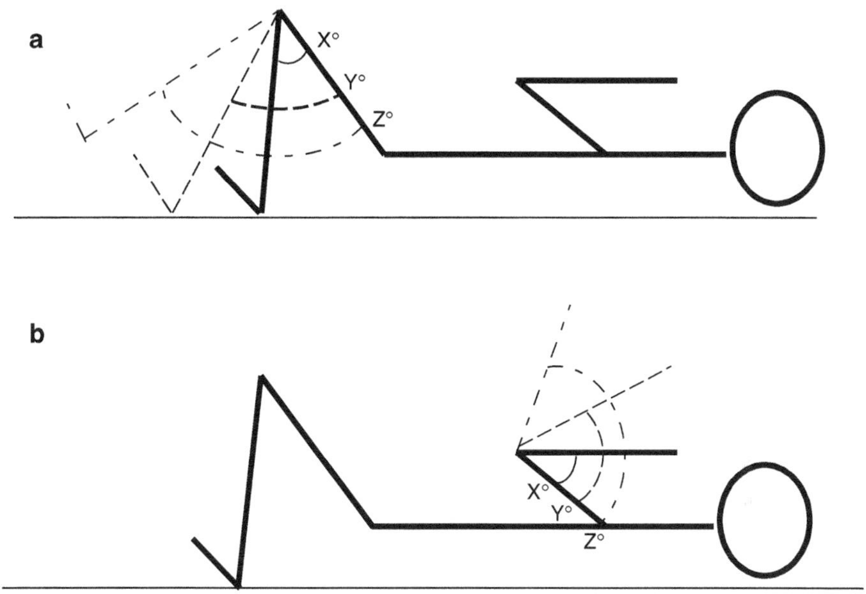

Fig. 11.4 Range of motion assessment for spastic patients in supine position. *X*° Angle of active range of motion, *Y*° angle of passive range of motion under slow stretching, *Z*° angle of range of motion after motor nerve block, botulinum toxin injection, or general anesthesia with relaxants. (**a**) Lower limb, (**b**) upper limb

passive soft-tissue stiffness and spastic abnormal posture. For each passive movement, the clinician asks the patient to perform an active movement against the muscle group evaluated, as far as possible until the active force produced by the agonist muscle group is neutralized by the combination of passive resistance and spastic formation coming from the stretched antagonist. The maximal range of active motion is thus obtained. Then the difference between the passive and active range of motion is determined, which expresses the ability for potential therapeutic benefit up to the limit of possible contractures (Fig. 11.4).

11.3 Quantification of Spasticity

Two scales are available for quantifying the spasticity in children with CP: the Ashworth scale (Table 11.2) [6, 7] and the Tardieu scale (Table 11.3) [8, 9].

With the patient lying, evaluation is performed by rapidly moving the segments of the limbs: flexion and extension of the knees, flexion and extension and abduction of the hips, dorsiflexion of the ankle with the knee in extension and in flexion.

Both scales are useful. The Tardieu scale appears appropriate for young children who walk and have no contractures. This scale was especially designed for the assessment of triceps spasticity and is very useful in this case. The Ashworth scale

Table 11.2 Ashworth scale for evaluation of spasticity in lower limbs

Criterion	Score
No increase in tone	0
Slight increase in tone giving a "catch" when limb is moved during flexion or extension	1
More marked increase in tone but limb easily flexed	2
Considerable increase in tone – passive movement difficult	3
Limb rigid during flexion or extension	4

The scale rates the exaggeration of the stretch reflex

Table 11.3 Tardieu scale for evaluation of spasticity associated with cerebral palsy

Criterion	Symbol or score
Speeds at which affected part(s) are passively moved:	
As slow as possible	V1
Intermediate speed	V2
As rapid as possible	V3
Parameters measured:	
Type of muscle reaction	X
Angle at which muscle reaction occurs	Y
Types of muscle reaction:	
No increase in muscle tone throughout the range of motion	0
Slight increase in muscle tone without any "catch" at a particular angle	1
"Catch" interrupting the movement at a particular angle, followed by muscular release	2
Exhaustible clonus (less than 10 s for a permanent stretch) appearing at a particular angle	3
Inexhaustible clonus (more than 10 s for a permanent stretch), appearing at a particular angle	4

is simpler to deal with and allows a global assessment of spasticity, whilst the Tardieu scale, which is more sophisticated, provides a finer approach for the determination of the degree of the spasticity.

11.4 Quantification of Dystonia

When dystonia predominates in generalized form, the Barry–Albright Dystonia (BAD) scale provides a reliable total score for its quantification in children with cerebral palsy or traumatic brain injury [10]. It is a reasonable method of assessing the patient for dystonia in each of the following regions: eyes, mouth, neck, trunk, each upper and lower extremity (eight body regions) (Table 11.4). Severity rating with the BAD scale is based only on dystonia as evidenced by abnormal movements or postures without involving spasticity and other disorders of muscle tone.

Table 11.4 Barry–Albright Dystonia scale for assessment of children with generalized dystonia

Region and criterion	Score
Eyes, signs of dystonia (include prolonged eyelid spasms and/or forced eye deviations)	
Absent	0
Slight: dystonia less than 10 % of the time and does not interfere with tracking	1
Mild: frequent blinking without prolonged spasms of eyelid closure, and/or eye movements <50 % of time	2
Moderate: prolonged spasms of eyelid closure and/or eye movements >50 % of the time that interfere with tracking	3
Severe: prolonged spasms of eyelid closure, with eyelids closed >30 % of the time, and/or eye movements >50 % of the time that prevent tracking	4
Unable to assess eye movements	
Mouth, signs of dystonia (include grimacing, clenched or deviated jaw, forced open mouth, and/or forceful tongue thrusting)	
Absent	0
Slight: dystonia <10 % of the time and does not interfere with speech and/or feeding	1
Mild: dystonia <50 % of the time and does not interfere with speech and/or feeding	2
Moderate: dystonia >50 % of the time and/or dystonia that interferes with speech and/or feeding	3
Severe: dystonia >50 % of the time and/or dystonia that prevents speech and/or feeding	4
Unable to assess mouth movements	
Neck, signs of dystonia (include pulling of the neck into any plane of motion: extension, flexion, lateral flexion or rotation)	
Absent	0
Slight: pulling <10 % of the time and does not interfere with lying, sitting, standing and/or walking	1
Mild: pulling <50 % of the time and does not interfere with lying, sitting, standing and/or walking	2
Moderate: pulling >50 % of the time and/or dystonia that interferes with lying, sitting, standing and/or walking	3
Severe: pulling >50 % of the time and dystonia that prevents sitting in a standard wheelchair	4
Unable to assess neck movements	
Trunk, signs of dystonia (include pulling of the trunk into any plane of motion: extension, flexion, lateral flexion or rotation)	
Absent	0
Slight: pulling <10 % of the time and does not interfere with lying, sitting, standing and/or walking	1
Mild: pulling <50 % of the time and does not interfere with lying, sitting, standing and/or walking	2
Moderate: pulling >50 % of the time and/or dystonia that interferes with lying, sitting, standing and/or walking	3
Severe: pulling >50 % of the time and dystonia that prevents sitting in a standard wheelchair, standing and/or walking	4
Unable to assess trunk movements	
Upper limb, signs of dystonia (include sustained muscle contractions causing abnormal postures; score each limb separately)	
Absent	0
Slight: dystonia <10 % of the time and does not interfere with normal positioning and/or functional activities	1

(continued)

Table 11.4 (continued)

Region and criterion	Score
Mild: dystonia <50 % of the time and does not interfere with normal positioning and/or functional activities	2
Moderate: dystonia >50 % of the time and/or dystonia that interferes with normal positioning and/or upper extremity function	3
Severe: dystonia >50 % of the time and/or dystonia that prevents normal positioning and/or upper extremity function	4
Unable to assess upper extremity movements	
Lower limb, signs of dystonia (include sustained muscle contractions causing abnormal postures; score each limb separately)	
Absent	0
Slight: dystonia <10 % of the time and does not interfere with normal positioning and/or functional activities	1
Mild: dystonia <50 % of the time and does not interfere with normal positioning and/or functional activities	2
Moderate: dystonia >50 % of the time and/or dystonia that interferes with normal positioning and/or lower extremity function	3
Severe: dystonia >50 % of the time and/or dystonia that prevents normal positioning and/or lower extremity function	4
Unable to assess lower extremity movements	

11.5 Evaluation of Functional Abilities

11.5.1 Gross Motor Function Measure

Assessment of spasticity is just one element of global function measurement. The gross motor function measure (GMFM) [11, 12] was designed to evaluate motor function capability and changes in children with CP. There are two versions of the GMFM: the original 88-item measure and the more recent 66-item GMFM.

The GMFM is a criterion-referenced measure based on normal gross motor developmental milestones. All items are achievable by a 5-year-old child without any motor disability. With the GMFM-88 it is possible to obtain scores for 5 separate dimensions: (a) lying and rolling, (b) sitting, (c) crawling and kneeling, (d) standing, (e) walking, running, and jumping. A goal total score is calculated as the mean of the individually selected GMFM dimension scores.

The GMFM-66 includes a subset of the 88 items that has been shown to be unidimensional. For the GMFM-66, the ordinal scale is converted into an interval scale. This transformation increases the accuracy of the child's ability estimate and provides a measure that is equally responsive to change across the spectrum of ability. An assessment with the GMFM scale every 6 or 12 months gives a curve of evolution and therefore provides an objective basis for therapeutic decisions. Quantifying the patient's functional abilities with the GMFM score is particularly helpful in the longitudinal evaluation of patients who are selected for neurosurgical treatment.

The gross motor function classification system (GMFCS) [12] allows defining five functional levels for children according to their categories of age: between 1 and 2 years, 2 and 4 years, 4 and 6 years, and 6 and 12 years (Fig. 11.5) (http://www.canchild.ca).

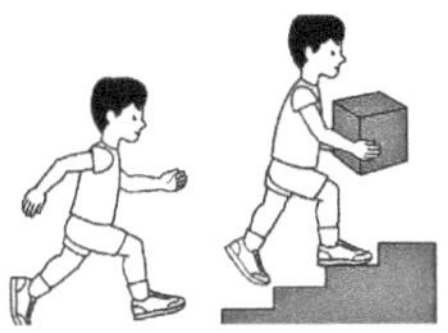	**GMFCS level I** Children walk at home, school, outdoors and in the community. They can climb stairs without the use of a railing. Children perform gross motor skills such as running and jumping, but speed, balance and coordination are limited.
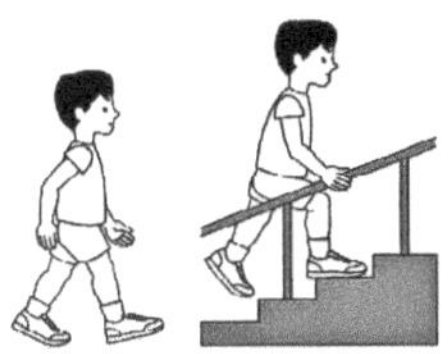	**GMFCS level II** Children walk in most settings and climb stairs holding onto a railing. They may experience difficulty walking long distances and balancing on uneven terrain, inclines, in crowded areas or confined spaces. Children may walk with physical assistance, a hand~held mobility device or used wheeled mobility over long distances. Children have only minimal ability to perform gross motor skills such as running and jumping.
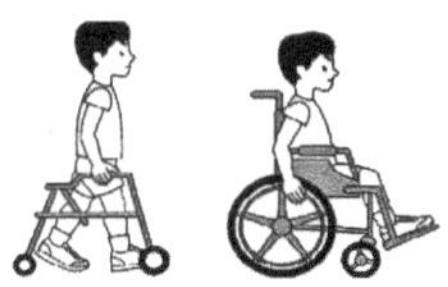	**GMFCS level III** Children walk using a hand-held mobility device in most indoor settings. They may climb stairs holding onto a railing with supervision or assistance. Children use wheeled mobility when traveling long distances and may self-propel for shorter distances.
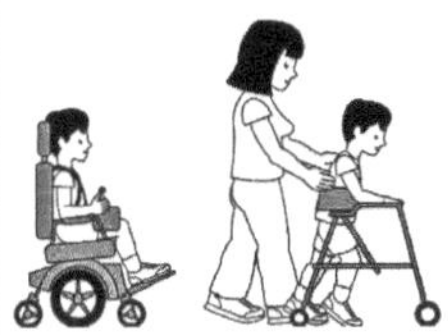	**GMFCS level IV** Children use methods of mobility that require physical assistance or powered mobility in most settings. They may walk for short distances at home with physical assistance or use powered mobility or a body support walker when positioned. At school, outdoors and in the community children are transported in a manual wheelchair or use powered mobility.
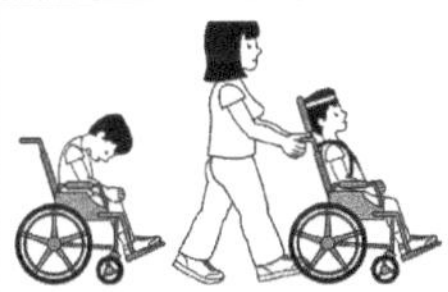	**GMFCS level V** Children are transported in a manual wheelchair in all settings. Children are limited in their ability to maintain antigravity head and trunk postures and control leg and arm movements.

Fig. 11.5 Gross motor function classification system (*GMFCS*), or levels of Palisano, for children between 6 and 12 years of age [13]

This classification is used worldwide to grade the child, make a prognosis, follow his (her) evolution, and communicate between caregivers and centers, and also to characterize and quantify functional status for publications.

11.5.2 New York University Classification System

Patients are categorized according to the severity of their functional locomotor impairment by a grading scale based on the New York University classification system conceived by Abbott et al. [14] (Table 11.5). Noteworthily, this classification was dedicated to the selection of children with CP as candidates for dorsal

Table 11.5 New York University classification system of candidates for dorsal rhizotomy

Preoperative function	Postoperative goal	Group
Walks without assistive devices	Improve appearance and efficiency of walking	I
Walks with assistive devices	Improve quality of walking and decrease amount of assistance (use of canes, crutches, walkers) required for ambulation	II
Quadruped crawler, limited ability to stand and reciprocally move legs	Improve ability to reciprocally move the legs in the standing position with assistive devices	III
Commando or belly crawler	Improve ease of care taking and facilitate function in sitting position	IV
No locomotive abilities, fully dependent	Improve ease of care taking and facilitate positioning in adaptive equipment	V

rhizotomy. For patients able to ambulate independently (group I), the goal of surgery is to improve the efficiency and appearance of gait. The quality of locomotion is anticipated to improve in patents who require assistive mobility devices (group II), thus reducing their need for assistive devices to achieve independent ambulation. The goal for group III patients (reciprocal and nonreciprocal quadruped crawlers) is to ambulate with braces or other assistive devices. Nonambulatory patients (groups IV and V) seldom obtain functional motor gains despite elimination of spasticity; therefore they are not considered good candidates for rhizotomy. These severely disabled children can be offered other treatment modalities to relieve their spasticity, such as tendon-lengthening surgery or implantation of an intrathecal baclofen pump in elder ones.

11.5.3 Pediatric Evaluation of Disability Inventory

The pediatric evaluation of disability inventory (PEDI) is a standardized instrument used by a multidisciplinary team for the evaluation of functional performance, program monitoring, documentation of functional development, and clinical decision-making [13, 15, 16]. The target group are children aged 0.5–7.5 years. It is also suitable for children older than 7.5 years if their functional ability is below that of nondisabled 7.5-year-olds. The PEDI contains 197 items in three parts; functional skills, caregiver's assistance, and used modifications and adaptive equipment. Each part has three domains: self-care, mobility, and social function (Fig. 11.6). The activity items are rated by a parent or caregiver and are judged on the basis of the following five-point rating scale: (0) unable to do; (1) with much difficulty; (2) with some difficulty; (3) with a little difficulty; (4) without any difficulty.

11.6 Video Recordings

For a comprehensive approach of pediatric patients complete methodical use of textual data, scores and scales, also series of photographs and, even more useful, of video recording should be made. Video recordings of the child's capabilities

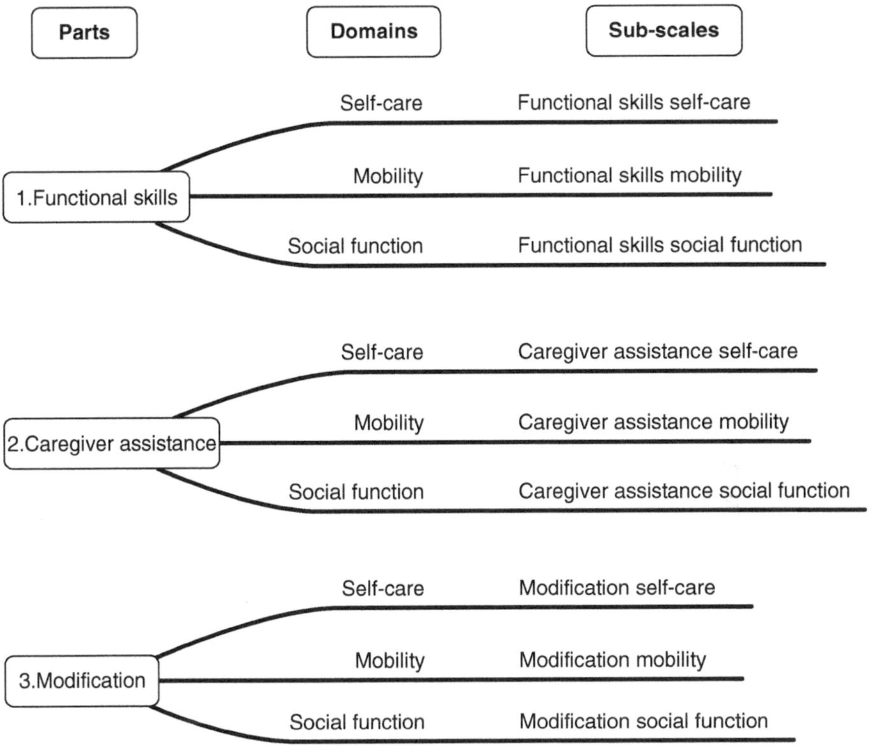

Fig. 11.6 Parts, domains, and subscales of PEDI (Pediatric Evaluation of Disability Inventory)

(gait and aspects of static lying) are of paramount value in the evaluation of clinical outcome. This utility is further enhanced by split-screen, two-dimensional recordings with a freeze-frame facility.

As a matter of fact, simple observation of the child at the outpatient unit is not sufficient for a detailed analysis of locomotor gait, walking, and motor fixation and discrimination of movement disorders. It is difficult to analyze simultaneously all of the articulations at the same moment and at different directions. Video recording permits a profound investigation without time limits, at slow-motion viewing or with an image held on screen. The reliability of comparisons between recordings necessitates a strict protocol that compiles different systematic views (static, dynamic, frontal, sagittal). The reproduction of the clinical image as a "movie" helps memorizing each case easily. Those scenes interesting from the clinical point of view can be reviewed in circles providing emphasis on particular segments. The evaluation of the objectives is made by the parallel comparison of the preinterventional goals and the postinterventional outcomes with a dynamic approach showing the differences in plasticity, speed, sequence of motion before and after. A step-by-step analysis helps to evaluate what the child won and what she (he) didn't lose after the surgical procedures. Finally, the reproduction of video recordings facilitates the complete construction of the patient's files and the further discussion in a multidisciplinary team.

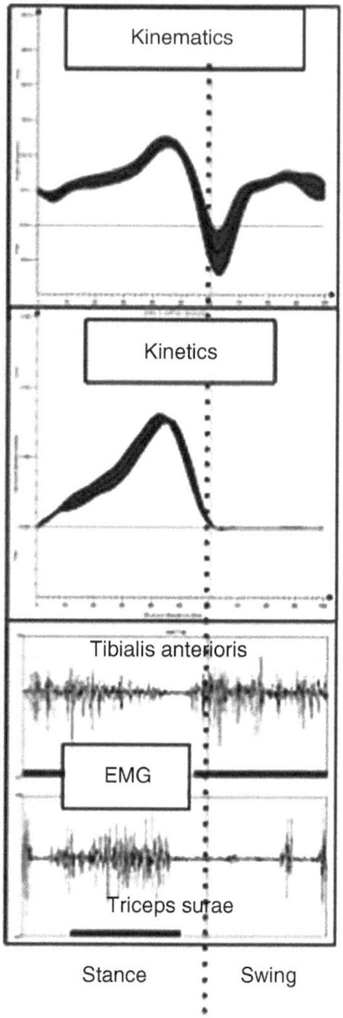

Fig. 11.7 Dynamic gait analysis at level of ankle, including kinematics, kinetics, and electric muscle activity in tibialis anterioris and triceps surae

11.7 Dynamic Gait Analysis

Dynamic gait analysis is the most productive method of motion analysis [17]. It is commonly used by the reference centers specialized in the study and management of spasticity. It provides objective and reproducible data, together with functional assessment scales, to plan treatments and evaluate outcomes of interventions (see Sect. 4.2.3). Dynamic gait analysis includes recordings of kinematics, kinetics, and electrical muscle activity during motion (Fig. 11.7).

Kinematics explores the spatial movement of the body. Displacement of the body markers is captured by an optoelectronic system with multiple cameras.

Kinetics explores the mechanisms that cause movement. Mechanic constraints are studied with a force platform that measures the ground reaction force generated by a body standing or moving on it. Kinetics helps to understand the pathogenesis of gait problems.

Polyelectromyography recordings are made with surface electrodes and depict any decrease in activity of weak muscles and hyperactivity of spastic muscles and co-contractions between agonist and antagonist muscles.

As with adult patients, dynamic gait analysis with children has substantial limitations. It can be done only with patients able to perform certain functional skills according to their age, in which motion is involved, without major equilibrium disturbances and without assistive devices. Practically, kinematics easily explores abnormalities in the sagittal plane (equinus of foot, hyperextended position of knee, flexion of hip), but does much less reliably so for abnormalities in the frontal plane.

Dynamic gait analysis is nowadays a prerequisite to evaluate the benefits or detriments of interventions and to make a postoperative quantitative appraisal of their effects. Dynamic gait analysis provides useful information to plan treatment. It helps to verify and characterize spasticity among abnormal deformities of a patient's body and to define underlying mechanisms. Dynamic gait analysis under anesthetic blocks is of prime importance to predict effects of an eventual intervention (e.g., botulinum toxin injections, peripheral neurotomies, dorsal rhizotomies, intrathecal baclofen, orthopedic surgery).

Many other techniques are accessible for assessing and quantifying the motor disorders and functional status of children affected with CP. They are listed and detailed in the very clear and well-documented handbook by C. Bérard [18].

Conclusion

Detailed and in-depth assessment of the child provides a professional and objective evaluation of the spastic and the movement disorder components, as well as eventual deformities, and an understanding of their respective mechanisms. By helping to define which component(s) is (are) harmful and to what extent and to appraise the evolution of the child, it permits an objective choice of treatments against spasticity. After a therapeutic intervention, benefits and eventual detriments can be evaluated in comparison with the preinterventional status, according to the preplanned objectives.

References

1. Bax M (1964) Terminology and classification of cerebral palsy. Dev Med Child Neurol 6:295–297
2. Surveillance of Cerebral Palsy in Europe (2000) Surveillance of cerebral palsy in Europe: a collaboration of cerebral palsy surveys and registers. Dev Med Child Neurol 42:816–824
3. Hodgkinson I, Jindrich ML, Duhaut P, Vadot JP, Metton G, Bérard C (2001) Hip pain in 234 non-ambulatory adolescents and young adults with cerebral palsy: a cross-sectional multicentre study. Dev Med Child Neurol 43:806–808

4. Rodda JM, Graham HK, Carson L, Galea MP, Wolfe R (2004) Sagittal gait patterns in spastic diplegia. J Bone Joint Surg Br 86:251–258
5. Viehweger E, Bérard C, Berruyer A, Simeoni MC, Groupe Varax (2007) Testing range of motion in cerebral palsy. Ann Readapt Med Phys 50:258–265
6. Bohannon RW, Smith MB (1987) Interrater reliability of a modified Ashworth scale of muscle spasticity. Phys Ther 67:206–207
7. Damiano D, Quinlivan J, Owen B, Payne P, Nelson K, Abel M (2002) What does the Ashworth scale really measure and are instrumented measures more valid and precise? Dev Med Child Neurol 44:112–118
8. Mackey AH, Walt SE, Lobb G, Stott NS (2004) Intraobserver reliability of the modified Tardieu scale in the upper limb of children with hemiplegia. Dev Med Child Neurol 46:267–272
9. Tardieu G (1983) Spasticity: an ill-defined condition. In: Abstracts of restorative neurology in the central and peripheral nervous system, World Federation of Neurology, Venice, 24–26 May, 1983
10. Barry MJ, Van Swearingen JM, Albright AL (1999) Reliability and responsiveness of the Barry–Albright Dystonia Scale. Dev Med Child Neurol 41:404–411
11. Russell DJ, Rosenbaum PL, Avery LM, Lane M (2002) Gross motor function measure (GMFM-66 & GMFM-88). Mac Keith, London
12. Palisano R, Rosenbaum P, Walter S, Russell D, Wood E, Galuppi B (1997) Development and reliability of a system to classify gross motor function in children with cerebral palsy. Dev Med Child Neurol 39:214–223
13. Sanger TD, Delgado MR, Gaebler-Spira D, Hallett M, Mink JW, Task Force on Childhood Motor Disorders (2003) Classification and definition of disorders causing hypertonia in childhood. Pediatrics 111:e89–e97
14. Abbott R, Johann-Murphy M, Shiminski-Maher T, Quartermain D, Forem SL, Gold JT, Epstein FJ (1993) Selective dorsal rhizotomy: outcome and complications in treating spastic cerebral palsy. Neurosurgery 33:851–857
15. Sanger TD, Chen D, Delgado MR, Gaebler-Spira D, Hallett M, Mink JW, Taskforce on Childhood Motor Disorders (2006) Definition and classification of negative motor signs in childhood. Pediatrics 118:2159–2167
16. Haley SM, Coster WJ, Ludlow L, Haltiwanger JT, Andrellos PJH (1992) Pediatric evaluation disability inventory (PEDI), version 1,0. New England Medical Center Hospitals, Boston
17. Novacheck TF, Gage JR (2007) Orthopedic management of spasticity in cerebral palsy. Childs Nerv Syst 23:1015–1031
18. Bérard C (ed) (2010) La paralysie cérebrale de l'enfant: guide de la consultation, examen neuro-orthopédique du tronc et des membres infèrieurs, 2nd edn. Sauramps Médical, Montpellier

12 Decision-Making for Treatment of Children with Disabling Spasticity

Effective treatments are available for spasticity in children with cerebral palsy: botulinum toxin [1, 2], neurotomies [3], dorsal rhizotomies [4–7], intrathecal baclofen therapy [8, 9]. Each child represents a particular situation; therefore treatment should be adapted to every given case [10]. The goal is to reduce excess of spasticity in order to avoid deformity and improve function. Expectations of both the child and the family can be quite different from what can be achieved; it may be hoped that the child be able to walk even if this capability cannot be obtained as a realistic goal. Therefore, objectives should be precisely defined and formalized in form of a written consent. If a child's disability is severe, significant functional benefits may not be obtained. However, together with complementary orthopedic surgery, reduction of contractures and deformities can be achieved [11] and thereby care can be made easier and subsequent improvement in quality of life may be expected [12].

12.1 Preoperative Considerations

12.1.1 Clinical Examination

Assessment should distinguish "useful" spasticity, e.g., the potential to stand for transfers or walking, from "harmful" spasticity. The examination should not be limited to the analytic assessment of spasticity but also consider the child's general state (e.g., hypotrophy, respiratory restrictive syndrome, swallowing difficulties), the orthopedic status, namely, the musculoskeletal contractures and deformities, the evolution of the motor function as accurately quantified by the Gross Motor Function Measure (see Sect. 11.5.1), and also the child's cognitive and psychological abilities that are crucial for participation in the reeducation program. The child's and family's lifestyle, the habits, and the educational framework must also be considered, as well as the environmental factors that could be an obstacle to the child's surgical experience [13].

M. Sindou et al., *Neurosurgery for Spasticity*,
DOI 10.1007/978-3-7091-1771-2_12, © Springer-Verlag Wien 2014

12.1.2 Therapeutic Planning

Controlling spasticity is part of a global treatment that extends over years and includes physiotherapy, orthotics, and mobility aids. If spasticity becomes refractory to noninvasive treatments, neurosurgical treatment can be considered (Fig. 12.1). If spasticity is prominent, neurosurgical intervention should precede orthopedic surgery and should be performed before contractures become irreversible and deformities appear. Contractures and deformities are related to imbalances around an articulation, caused by spasticity; they increase progressively with time [14]. Reducing excessive spasticity prior to orthopedic corrections may help improve the outcome of the orthopedic surgery. In brief, neurosurgery should be considered long before any fixed contractures and deformity appear [15].

12.2 Lower-Limb Spasticity

The motor potential of a diplegic child can be evaluated objectively by an assessment with the Gross Motor Function Measure every 6–12 months. The evolution of that score is for us the most "powerful" indicator for surgical decision. Surgery is suggested to be performed without delay once the curve plateaus or decreases (Fig. 12.2). The armamentarium varies according to whether disabling spasticity is global or focal (Fig. 12.3).

12.2.1 Global Spasticity

When spasticity affects both lower limbs, techniques with global effect are considered: dorsal rhizotomy or intrathecal baclofen therapy. Intrathecal Baclofen therapy has the advantage of being a conservative method, but imposes regular medical visits every 3–6 months to refill the pump. Thus, child and family must be motivated to comply with such obligation. Besides, the size of the pump is an obstacle in younger children. Dorsal rhizotomies, which are a lesioning procedure, have the advantage to be a definitive treatment. It is currently preferred before 6 years of age or for hypotrophic patients. The procedure is tailored in accordance with the location and the importance of the harmful components of the spasticity.

12.2.2 Focal Spasticity

When disabling spasticity is limited to a (few) muscular group(s), that is, considered focal, botulinum toxin injections are usually proposed alone or as a complement to a plaster cast or a splint. This allows neurosurgical treatment to be delayed until the child reaches the later optimal age for neurotomy, which is all the more relevant as

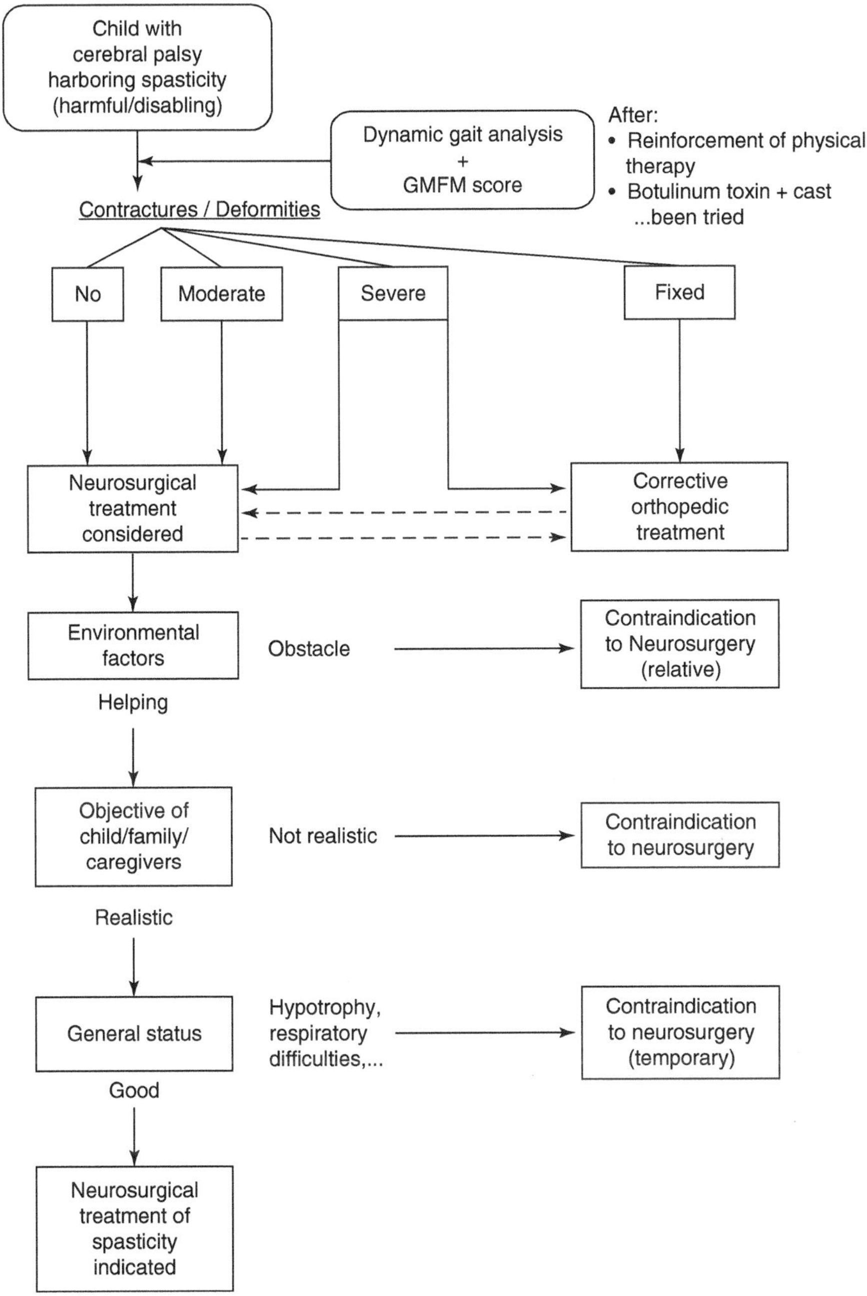

Fig. 12.1 Algorithm for neurosurgical treatment of spasticity in children (general principles)

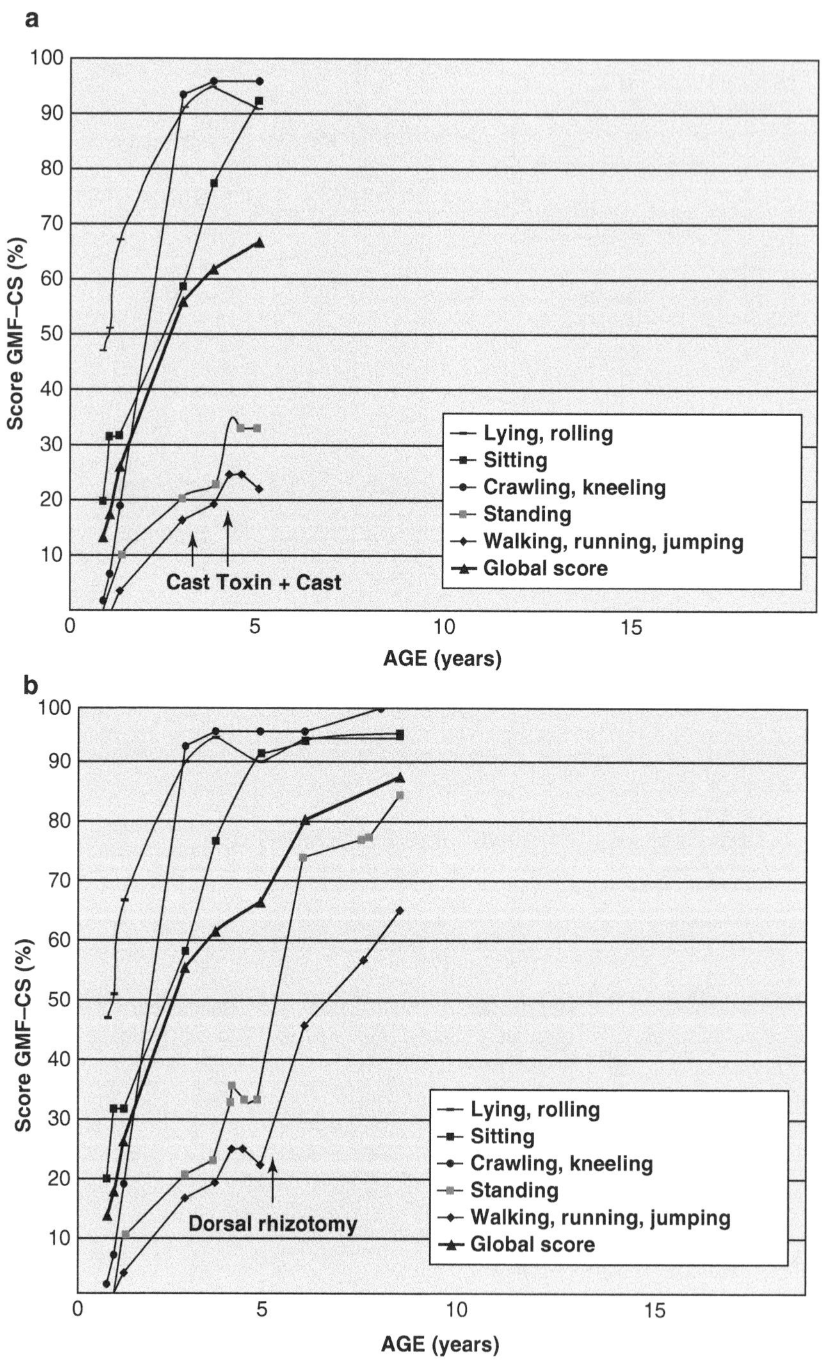

Fig. 12.2 Time course of five dimensions, together with the global score, on the Gross Motor Function Measure for a child with spastic diplegia from cerebral palsy. (**a**) Decision-making for dorsal rhizotomy, slow decrease in Gross Motor Function Measure score. Only temporary and slight amelioration after cast and combination of cast and botulinum toxin. Decision: indication for dorsal rhizotomy. (**b**) After the dorsal rhizotomy, dramatic improvement in standing and walking, running, and jumping and global score

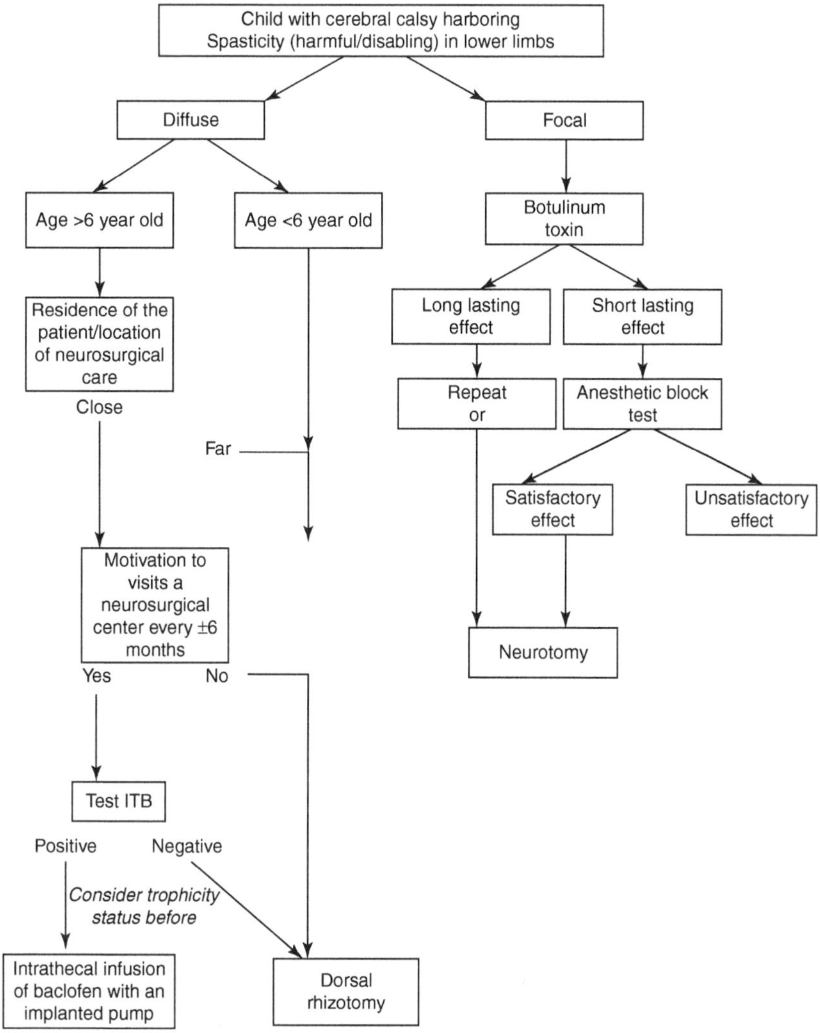

Fig. 12.3 Decision-making algorithm for neurosurgical treatment of lower-limb spasticity in children

in younger children spasticity tends to recur after neurotomy [16, 17]. Botulinum toxin injections can be tried on several muscles at one time if spasticity is not quite focal. If many muscles must be injected, general anesthesia is necessary, particularly for the iliopsoas. The dose of the toxin must not exceed a proscribed level, which limits effectiveness. Moreover, its action is rarely definitive; generally injections have to be repeated every 6–12 months. The most frequently targeted muscles are the triceps surae for equinus, tibialis posterior for varus, and flexors of toes for claw toes, and also adductors for spastic hip with adduction and internal rotation. Botulinum toxin injections may also be used as a predictive test before indicating interruptive surgery, especially peripheral neurotomies (Fig. 12.4), as it mimics their effects.

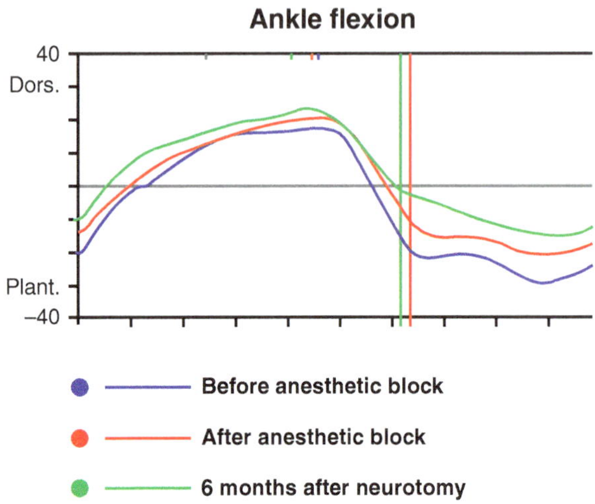

Fig. 12.4 Kinematic recordings of lower-limb motion at ankle in a hemiplegic child with equino-varus before (*blue curve*), after anesthetic block with bupivacaine of the tibial nerve to predict the effect of a tibial neurotomy (*red curve*), and 6 months after completed neurotomy (*green curve*). Note improvement under anesthetic block and even more improvement after tibial neurotomy

When an abnormal posture tends to increase and is predominant in well identifiable muscular groups, as the ankle plantar flexors or the hamstrings, consideration may be given to tendon-lengthening procedures. For thigh adductors, sectioning alone or combined with obturator neurotomy may be indicated.

Before a peripheral neurotomy is suggested, a dynamic gait analysis under anesthetic motor block provides important help for the decision of both the patient and the caregivers (Fig. 12.4).

12.3 Upper-Limb Spasticity

For spasticity in the upper limb, botulinum toxin is currently proposed as the first step of treatment [18, 19], the more so as most of the muscles of the upper limbs are considered small in most situations. The allowable dose is most often sufficient to be effective. Injections are generally to be repeated every 6–12 months. These necessary multiple visits are a constraint. Patients may also develop immunoresistance that decreases effectiveness of the treatment with time. Botulinum toxin injections have an important predictive value when they are tried before considering neurosurgical treatment, especially peripheral neurotomies. Because the effects of botulinum toxin injections mimic those of the latter, they allow the child, family, and caregivers to appreciate the benefit that could follow a neurotomy and help to establish the objectives of the treatment. These objectives may be cosmetic (e.g., to allow the child to put his or her hand in his or her pocket) or related to nursing cares (e.g., to wash the palm of the child's hand) or functional.

For children with cerebral palsy and quadriplegia, intrathecal baclofen infusion even at the thoracolumbar level, or dorsal rhizotomies onto the lumbosacral roots, may alleviate spasticity in the upper limbs through the so-called distant-effect phenomenon. Those distant effects can be explained by the inputs originating from the spastic lower limbs onto the brainstem reticular formation, as well as through the propriospinal interneuron system. They can also exert favorable influence on, e.g., swallowing and respiratory disturbances and more generally on the state of emotional "overreactivity" that is frequently observed for children with cerebral palsy.

12.4 Children with Cerebral Palsy Presenting with Mixed Spasticity and Dystonia

Although not spasticity by definition, associated dystonia may be influenced by neurosurgical procedures under certain circumstances. According to the classical definition given by Fahn et al. [20], "dystonia is a condition characterized by sustained muscle contractions, frequently causing twisting and repetitive movements, or abnormal postures". Different from spasticity, which is velocity dependent and mediated by exaggerated stretch reflexes, the continuous muscle contraction maintaining dystonic hypertonia is present without limb movements and does not depend on afferent input from the limb [21]. The motor drive behind dystonia is not a spinal reflex; but efferent mediated rather than afferent mediated [21]. Motor neuronal hyperexcitability could sustain it.

From his large experience Steinbok in his excellent synthetic review article [22] builds guidelines for indications on the following basis: Dorsal rhizotomies improve spasticity but not dystonia, whereas intrathecal baclofen can improve both spasticity and dystonia. This is well in accordance with Denny-Brown's work [23], which showed that dystonic phenomena persist after dorsal root sectioning. In children with cerebral palsy, dystonia mainly develops in those quadriparetic, especially as they become older. Therefore Steinbok [22, p.985] states: "We do not recommend dorsal rhizotomies in spastic quadriplegic children until they are at least 8 years old, by which time dystonia will generally have declared itself. If significant and disabling dystonia develops, intrathecal Baclofen clearly is the appropriate treatment."

Intraventricular baclofen may be also the first option for children with generalized dystonia. The site of baclofen activity when treating dystonia may be at the cortical level. Intraventricular infusion may result in higher baclofen concentrations over the cortex than intrathecal infusion does [24–26].

Because of its mechanisms, dystonia can be favorably influenced by procedures that modify the motor nerve of muscle activity. Botulinum toxin injections are widely used under this indication. In case of resistance to botulinum toxin injections, intensity of hypertonia and amplitude of abnormal postures, as well as parasite movements, can be reduced by lesioning procedures, especially peripheral neurotomies, which act by interrupting both the sensory IA and the motor alpha fibers.

Conclusion

Indications for neurosurgical treatment of spasticity in children must consider not only the motor function and the functional evolution of the child but also his/her general conditions and orthopedic status and the environmental factors.

This approach requires a multidisciplinary team and the comprehensive and active participation of the child, family, and caregivers. Additional orthopedic surgery(ies) is frequently indicated; therefore, a high level of cooperation between orthopedic and neurological surgeons is most desirable.

References

1. Fattal-Valevski A, Giladi N, Domanievitz D, Zuk L, Masterman R, Harel S, Wientroub S, Hayek S (2002) Parameters for predicting favorable responses to botulinum toxin in children with cerebral palsy. J Child Neurol 17:272–277
2. Ubhi T, Bhakta BB, Yves HL, Allgar V, Roussounis SH (2000) Randomised double blind placebo controlled trial of the effect of botulinum toxin on walking in cerebral palsy. Arch Dis Child 83:481–487
3. Sindou MP, Simon F, Mertens P, Decq P (2007) Selective peripheral neurotomy (SPN) for spasticity in childhood. Childs Nerv Syst 23:957–970
4. Kim DS, Choi JU, Yang KH, Park CI (2001) Selective posterior rhizotomy in children with cerebral palsy: a 10-year experience. Childs Nerv Syst 17:556–562
5. Mittal S, Farmer JP, Al-Atassi B, Gibis J, Kennedy E, Galli C, Courschesnes G, Poulin C, Cantin MA, Benaroch TE (2002) Long-term functional outcome after selective posterior rhizotomy. J Neurosurg 97:315–325
6. Lazareff JA, Garcia-Mendez MA, De Rosa R, Olmstead C (1999) Limited (L4-S1, L5-S1) selective dorsal rhizotomy for reducing spasticity in cerebral palsy. Acta Neurochir (Wien) 141:743–751
7. Sindou M, Mertens P (2000) Neurosurgery for spasticity. Stereotact Funct Neurosurg 74:217–221
8. Jacobs JM (2001) Management options for the child with spastic cerebral palsy. Orthop Nurs 20:53–59; quiz 59–61
9. von Koch CS, Park TS, Steinbok P, Smyth M, Peacock WJ (2001) Selective posterior rhizotomy and intrathecal baclofen for treatment of spasticity. Pediatr Neurosurg 35:57–65
10. Boop FA, Woo R, Maria BL (2001) Consensus statement on the surgical management of spasticity related to cerebral palsy. J Child Neurol 16:68–69
11. Gerszten P, Albright L, Johnstone G (1998) Intrathecal baclofen infusion and subsequent orthopedic surgery in patients with cerebral palsy. J Neurosurg 88:1009–1013
12. Hodgkinson I, Bérard C, Jindrich ML, Sindou M, Mertens P, Bérard J (1997) Selective dorsal rhizotomy in children with cerebral palsy: results in 18 cases at one year postoperatively. Stereotact Funct Neurosurg 69:259–267
13. Fougeyrollas P, Cloutier R, Bergeron H, Côté J, Côté M, St Michel G (1996) Révision de la proposition québécoise de classification: processus de production de handicap. Réseau International sur le Processus de Production du Handicap, Lac St-Charles
14. Morell DS, Pearson JM, Sauser DD (2002) Progressive bone and joint abnormalities of the spine and lower extremities in cerebral palsy. Radiographics 22:257–268
15. Abbott R (1991) Indications for surgery to treat children with spasticity due to cerebral palsy. In: Sindou M, Abbott R, Keravel Y (eds) Neurosurgery for spasticity: a multidisciplinary approach. Springer, Wien/New York, pp 215–217
16. Berard C, Sindou M, Berard J, Carrier H (1998) Selective neurotomy of the tibial nerve in the spastic hemiplegic child: an explanation of the recurrence. J Pediatr Orthop B 7:66–70
17. Deltombe T, Gustin T, Laloux P, De Cloedt P, De Wispelaere JF, Hanson P (2001) Selective fascicular neurotomy for spastic equinovarus foot deformity in cerebral palsy children. Acta Orthop Belg 67:1–5

18. Autti-Rämö I, Larsen A, Taimo A, von Wendt L (2001) Management of the upper limb with botulinum toxin type A in children with spastic type cerebral palsy and acquired brain injury: clinical implications. Eur J Neurol 8(Suppl 5):136–144
19. Boyd RN, Morris ME, Graham HK (2001) Management of upper limb dysfunction in children with cerebral palsy: a systematic review. Eur J Neurol 8(Suppl 5):150–166
20. Fahn S, Marsden CD, Calne DB (1987) Classification and investigation of dystonia. In: Marsden CD, Fahn S (eds) Movement disorders 2. Butterworths, London, pp 332–358
21. Sheean G (2008) Neurophysiology of spasticity. In: Barnes MP, Johnson GR (eds) Upper motor neurone syndrome and spasticity: clinical management and neurophysiology, 2nd edn. Cambridge University Press, Cambridge, pp 9–63
22. Steinbok P (2007) Selective dorsal rhizotomy for spastic cerebral palsy: a review. Childs Nerv Syst 23:981–990
23. Denny-Brown D (1966) The cerebral control of movement. Liverpool University Press, Liverpool
24. Albright AL (2007) Intrathecal baclofen for childhood hypertonia. Childs Nerv Syst 23:971–979
25. Albright AL, Ferson SS (2009) Intraventricular baclofen for dystonia: techniques and outcomes. Clinical article. J Neurosurg Pediatr 3:11–14
26. Turner M, Nguyen HS, Cohen-Gadol AA (2012) Intraventricular baclofen as an alternative to intrathecal baclofen for intractable spasticity or dystonia: outcomes and technical considerations. J Neurosurg Pediatr 10:315–319

13 Dorsal Rhizotomies for Children with Cerebral Palsy

Since the late nineteenth century, dorsal rhizotomies (DR) have been known to alleviate spasticity. But only in the last 20 years, DR became commonly used after refinements in surgical indications and selection of roots and rootlets on their topographic and/or functional responses to stimulation.

History started in 1898, when Sherrington demonstrated that division of posterior roots reduced tone in decerebrate cats [1]. On this basis, Foerster applied the technique to spasticity in humans and in 1913 published a review of posterior-root resections in 159 children with cerebral palsy [2]. His technique consisted in dividing the entire dorsal roots from L2 to S2, excluding the "antigravity root" L4. He used intraoperative electrical stimulation to identify segmental levels and to discriminate between ventral and dorsal roots. In the 1960s, Gros and co-workers in Montpellier separated the dorsal roots into rootlets and performed partial dorsal rhizotomies with nonselective sectioning of 80 % of the rootlets of each root to limit postoperative sensorial deficits. Later on with the quest of rendering DR more selective in its topographic effects [3], the Montpellier school developed the "sectorial posterior rhizotomy". The procedure aimed at limiting the sectioning to those roots only that correspond to what the authors categorized as "handicapping" spasticity, in opposition to "useful" spasticity, which is the one that maintains lower limbs in extension for antigravity. By the Montpellier method the roots were identified according to their topographic muscular responses. In 1976, Fasano and colleagues in Turin introduced a different concept of dorsal rhizotomy: the "functional posterior rhizotomy". The method is based on identification of "abnormal" muscular responses to electrical stimulation of roots and rootlets [4]. Responses were categorized as abnormal when repetitive dorsal root and rootlets stimulation with a train at a frequency of 50 Hz and a duration of 1 s provoked sustained responses in the corresponding segmental muscles, and also responses spread to other territories either ipsilateral or contralateral. In Fasano's original technique, the approach consisted in a limited laminotomy. At the beginning of the 1980s, for achieving more precise identification of the whole lumbar and sacral rootlets, Peacock and Arens extended the exposure to the entire cauda equina through an L1–S2 laminectomy [5].

M. Sindou et al., *Neurosurgery for Spasticity*,
DOI 10.1007/978-3-7091-1771-2_13, © Springer-Verlag Wien 2014

13.1 Technical Variants

13.1.1 Whole Cauda Equina Exposure by Laminotomy from L1/L2 to S1/S2

The exposure of the entire cauda equina, popularized by Peacock [5], was the most commonly used modality over the past decades [6–8].

Under general anesthesia with endotracheal intubation and after an indwelling urinary catheter has been placed, the child is positioned on the operating table in prone position, on bolsters to minimize intra-abdominal pressure. An S1–L1 laminotomy is performed with a high-speed drill or a craniotome saw. The dura and arachnoid are longitudinally opened. The S2–L2 sensory roots are separated from the motor roots at their exit to the dural sleeves.

According to the description by Farmer and McNeely [8], the selection of rootlets to be divided is guided by the muscular responses to electrical stimulation. The motor roots, especially S1 and S2, are stimulated orthodromically to confirm levels. Then the sensory roots from S2 up to L2 are stimulated sequentially. Roots and rootlets with the most abnormal responses are selected for lesioning. As a rule, no more than 75 % of the sensory rootlets are lesioned at any given level. To avoid urinary disturbances, no more than 50 % of the combined (i.e., right and left) dorsal S2 rootlets are cut. For example, if three sensory rootlets are identified at S2 on either side and two of the three rootlets on one side are cut, then only one of the three on the other side is cut. Also, no more than 50 % of the dorsal L4 rootlets are divided, in order to maintain tonal stability at the knee.

The dura is tightly closed. Laminoplasty is then secured by drilling holes through each lamina and spinous process and sutured.

Postoperative management begins with a 3-day period of bed rest and analgesic therapy. Pain may be controlled with an epidural infusion of bupivacaine, the catheter being removed on the third postoperative day. The urinary catheter is withdrawn 24 h later. The child is transferred to a rehabilitation facility at the end of the first postoperative week, for an average 6- to 8-week course of intensive physiotherapy and rehabilitation.

13.1.2 Limited Exposures

Extensive laminectomies or laminotomies from L1/L2 to S1/S2 have the advantage of allowing complete identification of the roots and rootlets of the entire cauda equina but also the disadvantage of a long and painful postoperative period, plus the risk of secondary spine kyphosis and instability. Therefore, it may be preferred to limit exposure in order to reduce invasiveness.

13.1.2.1 Limited Root Approaches at Conus Medullaris

In the 1980s and 1990s we commonly used osteoplastic laminotomy limited to the three vertebrae T11, T12, and L1 (Fig. 13.1). Through this approach, the ventral (and corresponding dorsal) L2 and L3 roots are reached just before they exit at their

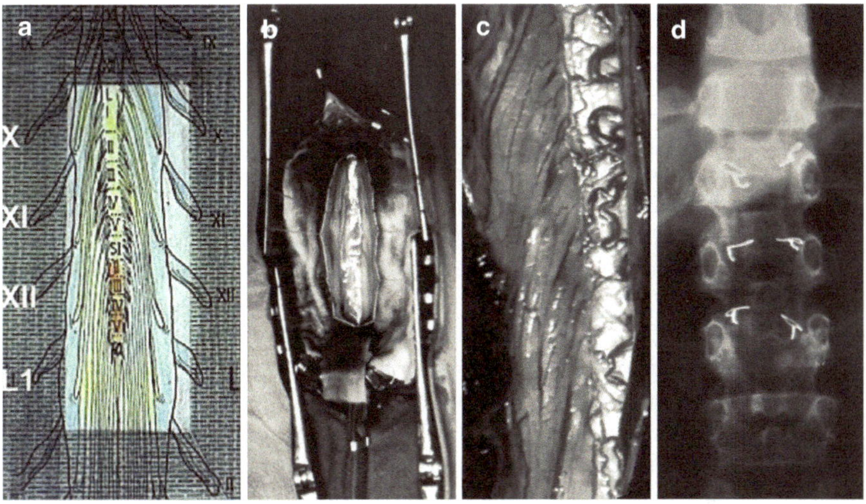

Fig. 13.1 Lumbosacral dorsal rhizotomy for children with cerebral palsy. (**a**) Classic scheme by Hovelacque of lumbosacral roots with corresponding vertebral levels. (**b**) Our former technique consisted in a limited osteoplastic laminotomy from T11 to L1 with a power saw. Operative photograph shows dura opened, arachnoid prior to opening and through it by transparence the exposed conus medullaris. (**c**) Dorsal (and ventral) L1, L2 and L3 roots can be identified intradurally at entry into their respective dural sheaths. Dorsal L4, L5 lumbar and sacral roots and rootlets can be identified at their entrance into the dorsolateral sulcus at the conus medullaris. (**d**) Laminae are then repositioned and fixed as shown on anterior-posterior X-ray

respective dural sheaths and are identified there by their muscular responses to electrical stimulation. The other (dorsal) lumbar and sacral rootlets are identified at their entry into the dorsolateral sulcus at the conus medullaris. The landmark between the S1 and the S2 medullary segments is located about 30 mm from the exit of the (tiny) coccygeal roots from the conus [9]. The medullary segments S1, L5, and L4 can be identified thanks to evoked motor responses after stimulation (in triceps surae, extensors of the toes, dorsal flexor of the ankle, and quadriceps, respectively); the roots for the bladder (S2–S3) by monitoring the vesical pressure; and those for the anal sphincter (S3–S4) by rectomanometry or simply by introducing a finger protected with a glove into the anal canal and/or by electromyography (EMG) recordings of sphincter activity. Usually on average 60 % of the total amount of the dorsal rootlets are cut, the quantity per root differs with respect to a root's level and function and its involvement in the (harmful) components of the spasticity. L4, which predominantly gives innervation to the antigravity muscle quadriceps femoris, is partly preserved.

Also Park and co-workers [10, 11] advocated a limited approach at the thoracolumbar junction. By this technique, named "single-level immediately caudal to conus medullaris approach", the T12–L1 and L1–L2 interlaminar spaces are exposed. Localization of the conus and adjacent cauda equina are confirmed by an ultrasound probe through the exposed spaces. The conus appears hypoechogenic and cylindrical, the cauda equina hyperechogenic and inhomogeneous. Once their identification is completed, a single-level laminectomy – or more if necessary – is performed. After dural and arachnoid opening, L1 and L2 roots are identified at the exit to their corresponding intervertebral foraminae. The dorsal root of L2 is separated from the ventral root and followed up to the conus. From the L2 dorsal root at dorsolateral sulcus, the subjacent dorsal rootlets – from L3 to supposedly S2 – are then progressively retracted medially, while being separated from their corresponding ventral roots. The latter are kept apart with a cottonoid placed over them. Then the S3 to S5 roots are identified at their exit from the most caudal part of the conus so that they be spared. The EMG examination is then undertaken at the individual levels of rootlets, from L2 to S2. As a first step, identification of muscular innervation of the various exposed roots is carried out by single constant square wave pulses with a duration of 0.1 ms at a frequency of 0.5 Hz, with increasing intensity until a reflex response appears. As a second step, a 50 Hz train stimulation that lasts 1 s is applied in a sequential way to each rootlet or group of rootlets individually in order to find abnormal responses and to decide on cutting or sparing.

13.1.2.2 Minimally Invasive Staged Interlaminar Approach

We recently developed a staged interlaminar (IL) approach which we designed to reduce invasiveness, depending on the roots to be targeted (Fig. 13.2) [12]. See schematic drawing of vertebral IL levels where selected roots can be targeted according to the preoperative program, at end of Section 3 in Appendix. Procedure steps are illustrated in (Figs. 13.3 and 13.4). The lumbar middle line incision is extended according to the selected IL spaces to be reached. Both the spinous processes and the interspinous ligaments are preserved. After resecting the flavum ligament at the selected IL space(s), the space is enlarged by resecting the lower half of the upper lamina and the upper half of the lower lamina. Then the dura and the arachnoid are opened on the midline for 2 cm at each of the selected interlaminar spaces. L2 and L3 roots can be reached through L1–L2 IL opening, L4 and L5 roots through L3–L4 IL opening, and S1-S2 roots through L5–S1 IL opening. At the exit from their dural sheath, the dorsal rootlets (on average 5 per root) are easily identified under the microscope; they are grouped posteriorly to the ventral root, separated from the latter by an arachnoid fold. Muscular responses to stimulation with a preferably bipolar electrode to avoid spreading of current are tested first for the ventral roots and then for the dorsal root and rootlets. The threshold for obtaining motor responses by stimulating the dorsal root is at least three times higher than that for responses to stimulation of the corresponding ventral root (0.1–1 mA for the latter). After identification of the dorsal roots to be targeted, between one third and four fifths of the constituting dorsal rootlets are divided, according to the preoperative chart. The dural incision is sutured in a watertight fashion and the dural suture line covered with fat harvested subcutaneously.

13.2 Protocol for Anesthesia

Surgery needs general anesthesia with endotracheal intubation. It is preferable to place a vesical catheter that will stay in place for a few days after the operation. Position is prone on the operating table, on bolsters to minimize pulmonary and abdominal compression.

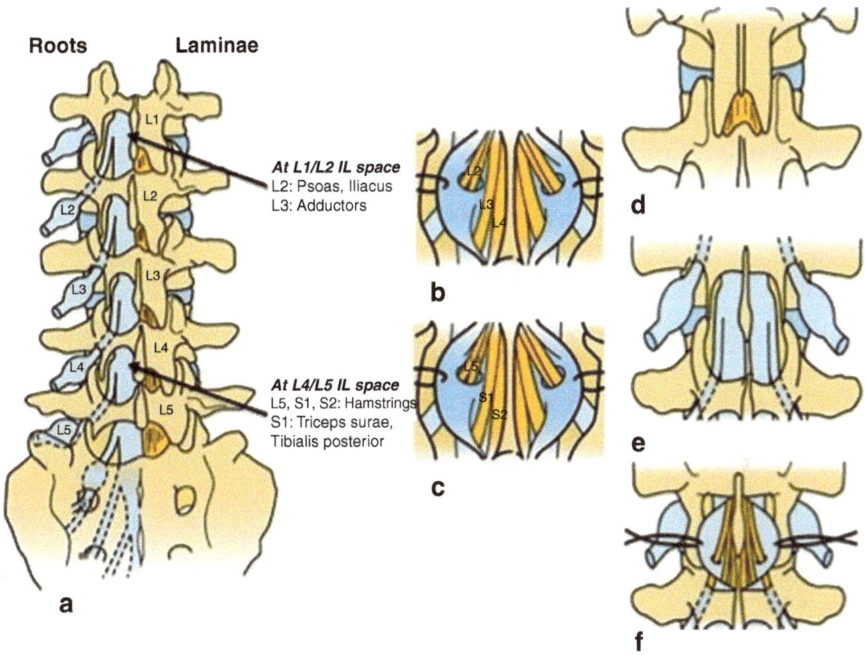

Fig. 13.2 Staged interlaminar (*IL*) approach of lumbar and sacral roots (recent personal technique). (**a**) The muscles most often attained by harmful spasticity are psoas – iliacus and adductors of the thigh, whose corresponding roots (*L2* and *L3*) can be targeted at L1-L2 interspace, and hamstrings (*L5*, *S1*, and *S2*) and triceps surae and posterior tibialis (*S1*), at L4-L5 interspace. The procedure is performed under the microscope and electrophysiological guidance. (**b**) In this example, L2, L3 roots are exposed at the L1-L2 IL space (**b**) and (**c**) L5, S1 roots exposed at the L4-L5 IL space (**c**). (**d–f**) Schematic drawings of enlarged IL midline approach. (**d**) Vertebral approach. (**e**) IL space extended by resecting the lower half of upper lamina and the upper half of lower lamina. Spinous processes and interspinous ligaments are preserved. (**f**) Dura and arachnoid are opened on midline; roots can be accessed (obliquely from contralateral side) under the operative microscope (Fig. 13.3)

Curare is administered at the induction of anesthesia and short lasting to reach only from tracheal intubation and positioning to approach. Long-lasting curarization, as well as narcotics or analgesics that could influence neural activities, should be avoided so as not to affect muscular contraction responses to stimulation. The anesthetic technique uses a combination of inhaled sevoflurane (or 50–70 % nitrous oxide) and of intravenously administered sufentanyl (or remifentanyl). For elder patients, the protocol may combine propofol with sevoflurane, although propofol may decrease activities recorded by EMG.

13.3 Topographical Mapping and Physiological Testing

Most children with cerebral palsy, especially diplegic ones, show a posture pattern called scheme of Little [13]. For children able to ambulate, the muscles contributing to the antigravity function, especially the gluteus and quadriceps, should have tone and

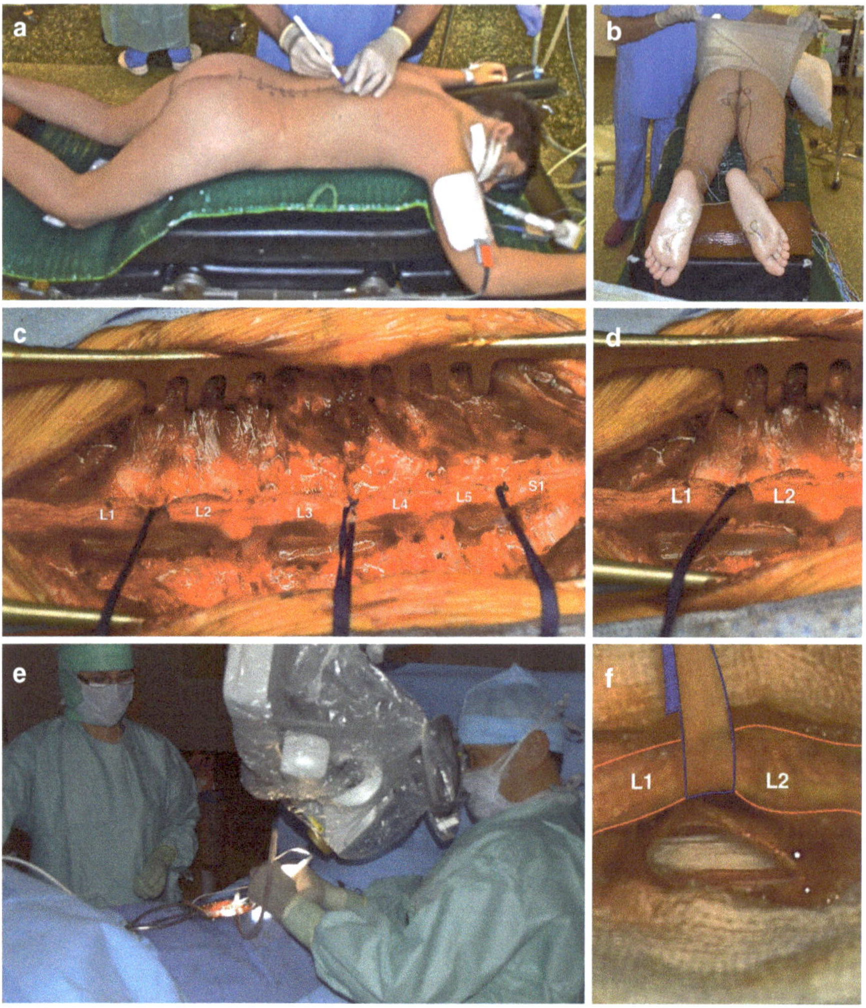

Fig. 13.3 Staged Interlaminar (IL) Microsurgical Dorsal Rhizotomy: installation and approach. (**a**) Positioning on table and landmarks for lumbosacral incision. (**b**) Needle intramuscular electrodes for EMG recordings: Adductors, Quadriceps, Tibialis anterioris, Soleus, Biceps femoris, Flexor digitorum, Anal sphincter. (**c**) Exposure of L1-S1 laminae, with L1-L2, L3-L4, L5-S1 IL openings. (**d**) Enlarged IL opening at L1-L2 level, viewed from left side of the patient. The two inferior thirds of upper lamina (L1) and the two superior thirds of lower lamina (L2) have been rongered, and flavum ligamentum removed to expose dura. Note the preservation of the spinous processes of L1 and L2 as well as of the interspinous ligament. (**e**) Surgeon operates with an oblique trajectory, at 45° angle, to target the contralateral root at entry into its corresponding dural sheath. Trajectory passes below the interspinous ligament, as shown in (**f**). (**f**) Roots of cauda equina seen after dura opened

power spared. A preoperative chart has to be established, specifying the muscular groups to be weakened in tone and to which degree and those whose tone must be preserved. Whatever the modality used, dorsal rhizotomies must be performed through electrophysiological guidance. From a conceptual point of view two methods were developed on the basis of different principles.

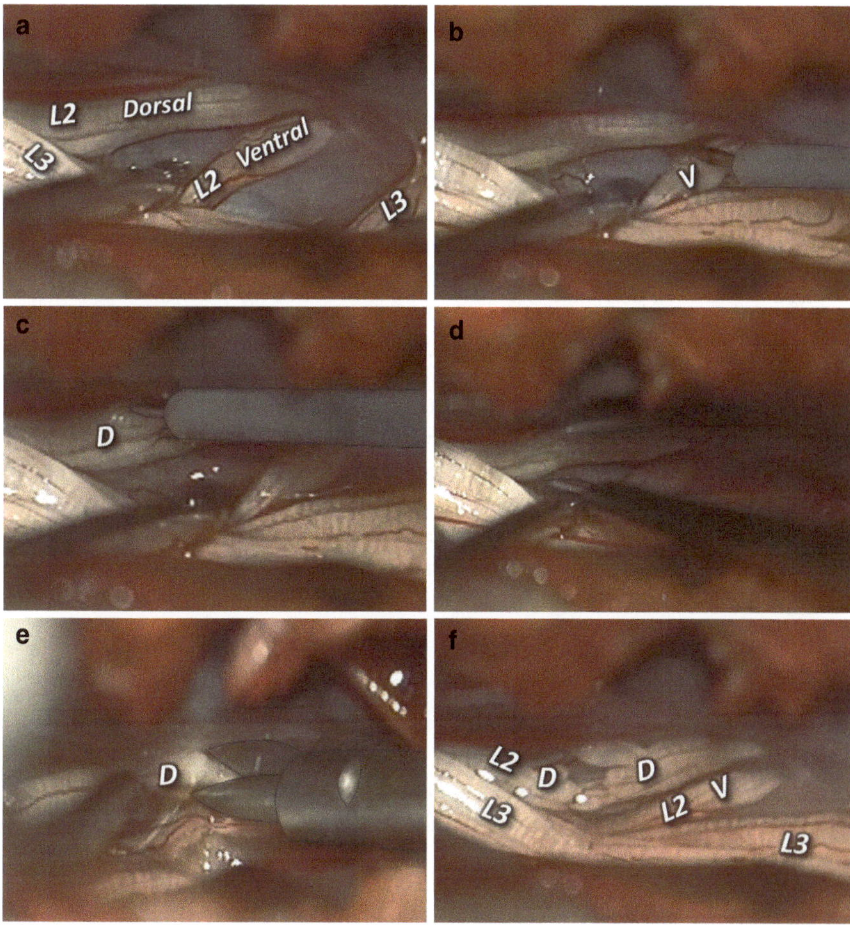

Fig. 13.4 Staged Interlaminar (IL) Microsurgical Dorsal Rhizotomy: microsurgical steps. (**a**) Exposure of the right L2 Dorsal and Ventral roots at entry into dural sheath, obliquely seen under the microscope from the contralateral side. Note L3 root pushed down with a ball-tip microsucker. (**b**) Identification of the topographical level of the root by electrical stimulation of the ventral root (V) - at 2Hz, 0.2mA - using a bipolar electrode. (**c**) Physiological testing of the dorsal root (D) - at 50Hz, 1mA - using same bipolar electrode. Coagulation with bipolar forceps (**d**) and section with microscissors (**e**) of the selected rootlets. (**f**) View of the three sectioned rootlets out of the four that constitute the dorsal root, i.e., three/fourth sectioning

The first one was based on anatomy and promoted by Gros and coworkers. It consists in identifying by electrostimulation the motor innervation of the exposed ventral and corresponding dorsal roots, in order to decide which dorsal roots and rootlets should be cut or spared [14]. Conversely, the second method, based on physiology and introduced by Fasano, consists in the identification of abnormal, i.e., excessive, muscular responses to electrical stimulation thus considered to be involved in the dysfunctional spinal circuits [4].

13.3.1 Topographical Mapping

Identification of the segmental, i.e., radicular, levels, is achieved by electrical stimulation, preferably bipolar, at an initial intensity between 0.1 and 1 mA and at a frequency of 2 Hz. For a dorsal root, the intensity required to reach the threshold of muscular responses is approximately three times higher than that for a ventral root. Briefly stimulation of L2 root produces a predominant response in iliopsoas and adductor muscles of hips; stimulation of L3 root, in adductors and quadriceps; stimulation of L4 root, in quadriceps and dorsal flexor of the ankle; stimulation of L5 root, in extensors of the toes. Stimulation of S1 root produces a motor response in the gastrocnemius-soleus group. This response can be confirmed by repeated checking of the Achilles ankle reflex before, during, and after the radicular cut. Stimulation of S2 produces motor response in flexors of the toes. Those motor responses can be felt by leg palpation of muscle groups and/or monitored by EMG recordings of activities. Stimulation of S2 to S4 roots can be assessed by recording vesical or anal response by cystomanometry and rectomanometry or EMG recordings of anal sphincter activity or simply with a gloved finger placed into the anal canal at the level of the sphincter. Table 13.1 and Fig. 13.5 summarize the pertinent features of this anatomical mapping.

13.3.2 Physiological Testing

Physiological testing estimates the level of excitability of the spinal circuitry by stimulating the dorsal roots and rootlets. Following Fasano's concept, criteria for considering dorsal roots and rootlets to be involved in dysfunctional spinal circuits include a low threshold to a single stimulus, a sustained response to a 50 Hz train stimulation at threshold, and a spread of the response outside the myotome corresponding to the stimulated root.

The present consensus for grading is to adopt the 5-grade classification of abnormal responses modified from Fasano's classification [4] by Philips and Park [16] (Table 13.2).

The protocol is as follows. First the stimulation threshold is determined with current pulses with a duration of 1 ms, beginning with an intensity of 0.1 mA, which is increased until muscular contraction appears. Once the threshold is determined, a stimulus consisting of a train at 50 Hz is delivered with an intensity two to three

Table 13.1 Predominant or specific motor response produced by stimulation of selected roots

Stimulated root	Predominantly responding muscle(s) (myotome)
L2	Iliopsoas, adductors of hips
L3	Adductors of hips, quadriceps
L4	Quadriceps, dorsal flexor of ankle (tibialis anterior)
L5	Extensors of toes, hamstrings
S1	Achilles ankle deep tendon reflex, gastrocnemius-soleus group, hamstrings, tibialis posterior
S2	Flexors of toes, hamstrings, bladder
S3	Anal sphincter, bladder
S4	Anal sphincter

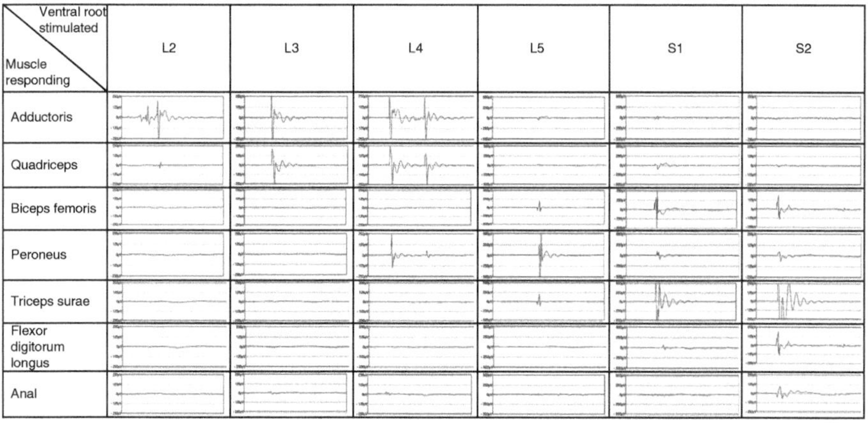

Fig. 13.5 Topographical mapping according to muscular response(s) to ventral root stimulation (at 2 Hz). Muscular responses can be observed by clinical examination and/or recorded with EMG (as shown). Stimulation of a selected root produces predominant, if not specific, motor responses in corresponding myotomes [15]

Table 13.2 Grading of muscular responses to dorsal root stimulation for decision about sectioning and its extent [4, 7, 16]

Muscular response to dorsal root stimulation with a 50 Hz stimulus train for 1 s	Grade
Unsustained motor response in muscles innervated by the segmental level of the stimulated dorsal nerve root or rootlets	0
Sustained motor response in myotome of stimulated nerve root	1
Contraction of muscles in myotomes of adjacent segmental level(s)	2
Contraction of muscles in myotomes at a distance from that of stimulated nerve root	3
Contraction of muscles in contralateral leg or upper limbs	4

times that of threshold to recruit a maximum of motor units. Then motor responses are quantified with the 5-grade system. The first trial is at the dorsal root globally; a second may be at dorsal rootlet levels after rootlet dissection.

Which grade of response would be the most reliable for determining which roots (rootlets) should be cut still is a matter of discussion [17]. It has been shown that a low threshold and sustained response of dorsal roots and rootlets to the train stimulation with a frequency of 50 Hz and a duration of 1 s may occur in nonspastic individuals. At most centers, the determination relies on the diffusion of the response much beyond the stimulated segmental level, namely, to the contralateral side or suprasegmentally onto the upper limbs [18].

13.3.3 Combined Topographical Mapping and Physiological Testing

To fulfill the surgical program as specifically tailored for each particular patient and written in the preoperative chart, our current policy is to use a combined topographical mapping and physiological testing, in two steps (Fig. 13.6).

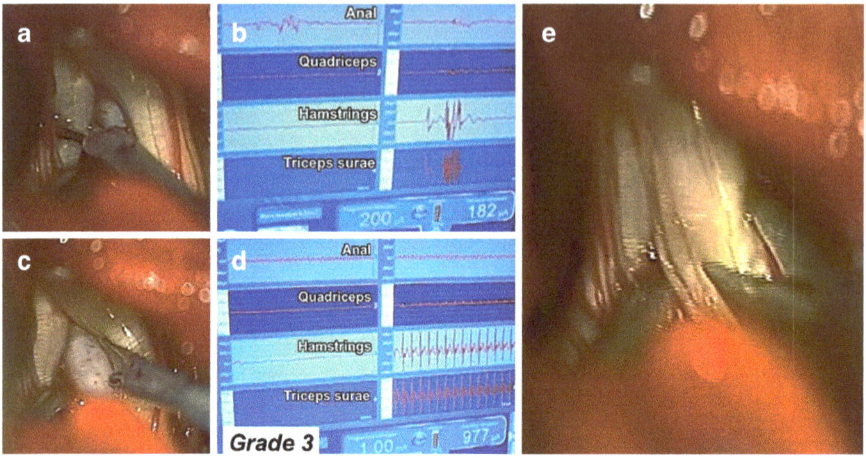

Fig. 13.6 Example of stimulation of S1 root. (**a**) Microsurgical view of stimulated ventral root. (**b**) Topographical mapping according to muscular response(s) to ventral root stimulation (2 Hz, 0.2 mA). See on screen EMG response in Hamstrings and Triceps Surae. (**c**) Microsurgical view of stimulated dorsal root. (**d**) Physiological testing by stimulation of dorsal root at 50 Hz and 1 mA. In this case, dorsal root stimulation produced a sustained response in Hamstrings and Triceps Surae, and also in adjacent and distant segmental levels, i.e. Quadriceps and Anal sphincter (Grade 3) (**e**) Microsurgical view of S1 dorsal root (75 %) sectioning

To be recalled the preoperative chart includes (a) the description of all the harmful components of the disabling spasticity, (b) the enumeration of the various muscular groups harboring excess of tone, (c) the designation of the corresponding roots supposed to convey the harmful afferents on the basis of classical anatomical knowledge, (d) the number of rootlets to be cut for each radicular target, whose estimation is proportional to the excess of tone affecting the corresponding muscular group(s), (e) the muscles whose tone should be maintained and consequently the corresponding roots and rootlets that must be maintained.

Procedure has two steps (Fig. 13.6). At the first stage, each exposed root is electrically stimulated to identify its innervation territory and thereby to confirm its anatomical level. Stimulation (at 2 Hz) is first performed on the ventral component, which is easy when the root is accessible near its foramen, and then on the dorsal component, which requires a much higher intensity. The roots corresponding topographically to the muscles harboring "harmful" spasticity are separated from the ones to be spared. Their constituting rootlets are individually dissected and isolated over a few millimeters. The number of dorsal rootlets to be cut is layed down in the preoperative chart for which the established and specified amount was set in proportion to the severity of spasticity in the corresponding muscular group(s). The amount ranges generally between 2 of 5 and 4 of 5 of the constituting rootlets of the root. Before final decision for cutting, the dorsal root/rootlets are stimulated with a 50 Hz train with a duration of 1 s for each train to evaluate the degree of their involvement in the spinal cord "excitability". Excitability is considered excessive when stimulation elicits an "exaggerated" (sustained, diffusing) response as previously described (Fig. 13.7).

As pointed out previously, the definition of an abnormal response that will justify surgical section is not quite settled yet. Some neurosurgeons admit that cutting is

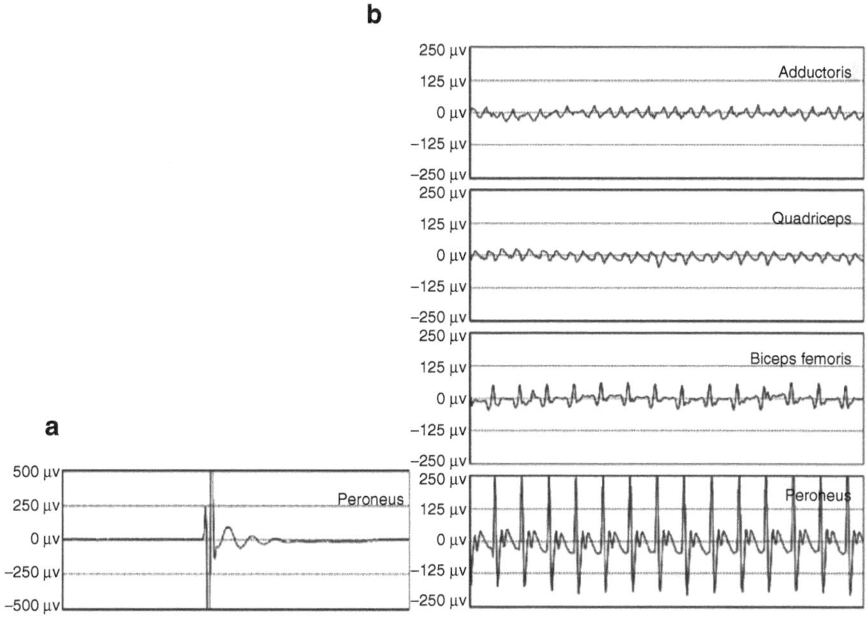

Fig. 13.7 Example of stimulation of selected L5 root. (**a**) Topographical mapping according to muscular response(s) to ventral root stimulation (2 Hz, 0.2 mA). (**b**) Physiological testing by stimulation of dorsal root at 50 Hz and 1 mA. In this case, dorsal root stimulation produced grade 3 muscular response, that is, contraction of muscles in myotomes at a distance from the stimulated root

justified if a grade 3 or 4 response is reached, others insist on grade 4 only. Because of the lack of strict physiological patterns for cutting, we favor the combination of an initial topographical mapping of roots and rootlets to be cut or spared according to the preoperative chart with a subsequent electrophysiological testing of their degree of excitability, to help quantify of rootlet cutting.

13.3.4 H-Reflex Monitoring

A few authors base their selection process on intraoperative H-reflex monitoring [19, 20]. The method consists in an intraoperative study of the H-reflex recovery curve. An increased H_2/H_1 ratio (the ratio of the second to the first H wave) indicates involvement in the spastic process. When a pair of stimuli with a varying interstimulus interval is applied to the posterior tibial nerve, as most frequently done in current practice, and the amplitude ratio of initial and subsequent H responses (H_2/H_1) is plotted against the interstimulus interval, the H-reflex recovery curve can be measured. Patients with upper motor neuron lesion, namely, patients with cerebral palsy, exhibit more rapid and complete recovery with less late inhibition than normal, due to increased excitability of the motor neuron and reduced presynaptic inhibition. According to Nishida and Storrs's [20] protocol, in intraoperative conditions stimulation can be delivered to the dorsal root proximal to the ganglion. All dorsal roots can be explored, the recording electrodes (preferably surface electrodes) being placed over the appropriate muscle group innervated by its corresponding root. Each root and rootlet was stimulated at a rate of 1, 2, 5, 10, 20, and 50 Hz, and the ratio of subsequent H (i.e., H_2) to H_1 was determined at each rate of stimulation [20]. Those roots and rootlets considered normal had a ratio of less than 50 % at all frequencies tested. Those considered abnormal had a ratio of more than 50 % or at times over 100 % at any frequency. Other criteria of abnormality which were clinically observed were sustained tonic or clonic contraction that persisted following cessation of stimulation and/or the spread of contractions to other muscle groups outside the stimulated myotome.

13.4 Quantification of Dorsal-Root Sectioning

Irrespective of the DR modality used, most surgical teams report cutting between one third and four fifths of the targeted root(s), with an average of two thirds of the constituting rootlets. Remarkably, such an amount of interrupted sensory afferents scarcely produces any noticeable hypoesthesia. In rare cases, neuropathic pain from a deafferentation mechanism may occur, its type may be electrical shooting, paroxystic, and/or allodynic. These pains are most often temporary and well controlled with anticonvulsant analgesic medications. Paresthesias may also occur, especially disabling when affecting the plantar sole after S1/S2 rootlet cutting; fortunately, they are most often transient. A personal study [21] showed that, in spite of an overall 60 % sectioning of the dorsal rootlets from L2 to S1(S2), the somatosensory evoked potentials to tibial nerve stimulation were present at the 6-month postoperative control. However, some alteration of the segmental responses was noticed, whereas reduction of cortical responses did not reach the significance level when compared with preoperative recordings. Precisely in all of the 10 patients studied, intraoperative recordings showed a reduction in the amplitude of segmental response N_{22} of 50 ± 25 % of the reference value after section of a mean 60 % of L2–S2 dorsal rootlets ($p = 0.03$), and latencies delayed ($p = 0.005$). These modifications persisted 6 months after surgery. In contrast to this, no significant changes in the cortical response P_{39} were found after surgery. This suggests that a considerable reduction of afferent inputs is compensated by a central amplification of the peripheral signal. This compensation explains that no somatosensory deficit was detectable at 6-month postoperative clinical examination.

With the combined topographical-physiological mapping as our method of choice for deciding cutting, our usual targeting was as follows. For flexion and adduction and internal rotation of hip and thigh, L2/L3 was cut by two thirds. L4, the main root for quadriceps innervation, was usually cut by no more than one third; but when the quadriceps was severely spastic with patella ascension, cutting amounted to two thirds. L5 was usually cut by one third so as not to weaken the gluteal muscles known to be responsible for hip and thigh extension and to play a role in the antigravity function and the stability of the pelvis for standing and walking. With regard to hamstring spasticity, roots to be targeted for hamstring muscles are several: L5, S1, and S2; predominant cutting depended on patients' individual patterns. S1 was usually cut by three fourths to four fifths, especially when gait was impaired by equinus or varus postures. S2 was cut by one half when there were claw toes; more cutting could impair bladder and sexual functions.

According to Abbott's report [22], when S2 was not included in the DR lesioning, there was harmful residual spasticity in the plantar flexors and hamstrings in nearly half of the children. Conversely, when S2 was included in the lesioning, the incidence of postoperative urinary disturbances amounted to 24 %. Therefore, Abbott and co-workers developed the intraoperative pudendal neuromonitoring to make surgery safer [22]. The method consists in recording the evoked potentials in the S1–S3 sensory roots and spinal cord segments after electrical stimulation of the shaft of the penis or the surface of the clitoris. Under such spinal cord monitoring, the S2 rootlets carrying "abnormal spreading muscular responses to their direct stimulation" are cut unless they contain afferent pudendal nerve activity at sensory evoked potential exploration. By doing so, postoperative urinary disturbances decreased to less than 4 % in their series.

This raises the question whether S2 dorsal roots should be targeted in patients with disabling hyperactive neurogenic bladder [23]. A hyperactive neurogenic bladder is not uncommon in children with cerebral palsy; it was estimated to occur in about 34 % of the children [24]. Noteworthily, the urodynamic exploration for such an estimation is not easy to perform and to interpret with children with cerebral palsy, as they are generally extremely anxious and tend to emotional overreactivity.

13.5 Postoperative Management

Postoperative management varies between centers and depends on the modality of dorsal rhizotomy used. In most institutions, the child stays in the intensive care unit for the following night and then returns to the ward for a 5- to 10-day hospitalization before discharge.

To decrease incidence and severity of headaches, the head is positioned downward to reduce the intracranial hypotension due to intraoperative CSF loss. Control of pain depends upon teams; arsenal includes epidural infusions of bupivacaine for a few days, intravenous infusion of morphine combined with oral or rectal acetaminophen and diazepam for the next week, morphine and clonazepam for 10 days until discharge [7]. Clonazepam may be prolonged for (rare) cases of neuropathic pain, dysesthesias, and/or disabling paresthesias. Immediately after surgery the child may have flexion spasms until operative pain disappears.

The necessity of a temporary lumbar immobilization with a corset depends on the type of the surgical approach. The staged intralaminar approach as performed in our most recently operated patients does not necessitate any prolonged immobilization and allows resuming physical therapy in the early period after surgery.

The urinary catheter is left in place for a few days until the child is able to sit down and use the toilet. After withdrawal of the catheter, a bladder scan control to rule out presence of residue is a wise precaution.

After hospitalization the child is transferred to a rehabilitation facility for on average 1 month of physical-therapy program and then to his (her) community institution or back home under an intensive physical-therapy program.

Importantly, patients and caregivers must be warned at discharge that the procedure generally produces excessive hypotonia, which may be responsible for loss of strength and make transfers difficult. The "desirable" level will be entered only after a 3- to 9-month delay, on average. This has to be mentioned in the preoperative patient's and family's consent form.

13.6 Complications and Their Prevention

Complications may occur during the surgical period and in the long term.

Children with cerebral palsy, especially if ex-premature, frequently harbor, sometimes latent, visceral dysfunctions. They have an increased incidence of bronchopulmonary dysplasia with reactive airways and risk of bronchospasm that can complicate anesthesia. Administration of a bronchodilator and also steroids prophylactically may be wise in children at such risk. In quadriplegic patients, disturbances in swallowing and ventilatory command might lead to respiratory problems that justify admission to the intensive care unit during recovery period. These children also have a high incidence of slowed gastrointestinal motility and thus risks of oesophagogastric reflux and aspirative pneumonia, which must be prevented.

A number of children with cerebral palsy have urinary dysfunction that may be latent or manifested by a history of, e.g., recurrent infections, enuresis, and incontinence. To avoid postsurgical retention, incontinence, and infections, the vesical catheter should be left in place until the child is released from bed rest; the absence of residue after withdrawal of the catheter should be checked by suprapubic echography.

CSF leakage through the wound or manifested as pseudomeningocele may happen. A light and supple lumbar corset may be worn exerting compression on the paravertebral posterior muscles in order to decrease this risk and to keep bed rest short. In addition, this has the advantage of decreasing pain when the child is encouraged to sit, stand, and walk.

Trophic ulcers and (eventual) bedsores in hypoesthetic cutaneous areas are rarely a problem, provided rhizotomy has not been performed too extensively. However, prevention should be systematic; family, nurses, caregivers, and physical therapists must be warned of the risk, especially for children depending on splints and assistive devices.

A long course after surgery, spinal deformities and instability may occur – kyphosis, hyperlordosis, or even spondylolisthesis – with severe back pain. Incidence has been evaluated to be between 4 and 14 % according to reported series and extents of laminectomies or laminotomies. Risk has been significantly diminished by limitations in the approaches. Preexisting thoracolumbar kyphoscoliosis can be aggravated after DR due to the lessening of muscular strength and, by extensive vertebral approaches, a weakening of the articular processes. In patients with spastic hip(s), especially those with subluxation, DR allows improvement or at least stabilization of the situation in most cases; decompensation of the subluxation may however happen. Generally, a subluxation does not tend to aggravate unless the preoperative Reimer index exceeds 50 %. Decompensation should be particularly feared if the hip musculature is weak and the patient is overweighted.

Table 13.3 summarizes the encountered neurological or orthopedic complications after DR. It has been established after reviewing the most pertinent publications [23, 25–54].

Table 13.3 Reported neurological and orthopedic complications after DR

Complication	Annotation
Bronchospasm	Reportedly ranges from 1 to 8.3 % according to series, mostly in children and/or ex-premature with quadriplegia; limited to 1 % by bronchodilator premedication
Urinary disturbances	Transient disturbances are frequent: from 1.25 to 24 % according to series; permanent retention or incontinence are rare, mostly in patients who had more than one third of S2 rootlets sectioned
Dysesthesia, paresthesia	Reportedly ranges from 2.5 to 40 % according to series; mostly transient, rarely permanent (0–5 %)
Hypoesthesia	Not precisely reported in literature, likely underestimated; trophic ulcers and bedsores in hypoesthetic areas and at splint pressure points are rare, though likely underestimated at splint pressure points
Hip subluxation	Aggravation of preexisting hip subluxation reportedly ranges from 5 to 20 %
Spine problems	Back pain (secondary, long-lasting, disabling) reportedly ranges from 1 to 7 % according to series; aggravation of preexisting deformities or new spine deformities – scoliosis, kyphosis or hyperlordosis, spondylisthesis – variously reported; problems more frequent with multilevel laminectomies or laminotomies than with interlaminar approaches with preservation of interspinous ligament

Prevention of all these risks is better achieved when rehabilitation team, physical therapists, and caregivers are well aware of the dangers.

13.7 Indications

Before entering the selection process, all participants in the therapeutic chain, from child's family to caregivers, must agree on the objectives of the treatment (Table 13.4). For diplegic children able to ambulate, the goals are to improve functional status, mobility, and autonomy and to prevent or stop deformities. For nonambulatory diplegic or quadriplegic children, realistic goals can only be to increase ease of care, improve comfort, and reduce any pain. According to Steinbok in his masterly writing: "Relief of hypertonia or improved range of movement – per se – are not the goals but are the means to achieve the goals" [9], p. 984].

The first step of the selection process is to question whether it is the hypertonia that hampers functional status and caregiving or other dominant problems: weakness such as dystonia, dyskinesia, or ataxia or severe contractures. If the latter are prominent, orthopedic surgery has to be considered on front row. If hypertonia is dominant, one may determine the type of appropriate and useful operation(s). If contractures of some degree are present, complementary orthopedic surgery(ies) can be useful; close relationships between orthopedic and neurological surgeons working as a team are mandatory. Children most likely to benefit from DR are those with prominent spasticity compared with dystonia, dyskinesia, or ataxia and in whom spasticity limits function. DR is the procedure of choice for children with diplegia, with little upper limb involvement, and an age of less than 10 years.

For diplegic children able to ambulate, the goal of surgery is to improve quality of locomotion, with different levels to reach according to the degree of dependence

Table 13.4 Expected outcomes of DR for patients categorized preoperatively by the New York University classification

		Goal of surgery defined by		
Group	Preoperative function	Farmer and McNeely [7]	Sindou [12]	Abbott [22]
I	Walks without assistive devices	Improve efficiency and appearance of patient's gait	Improve efficiency and appearance of patient's gait	Improve efficiency and appearance of walking
II	Walks with assistive devices	Improve quality of locomotion, reduce the need for assistive devices to achieve independent ambulation	Improve quality of locomotion, reduce the need for assistive devices to achieve independent ambulation	Improve quality of walking, decrease amount of assistance (use of canes, crutches, walkers) required for ambulation
III	Quadruped crawler with limited ability to stand and reciprocally move legs	Ambulate with braces or other assistive devices	Ambulate with braces or other assistive devices	Improve ability to reciprocally move legs in standing position with assistive devices
IV	Commando or belly crawler	Functional motor gains seldom obtained; preference for other treatment modalities (tendon-lengthening surgery, implantation of intrathecal baclofen pump)	Facilitate nursing and lying positioning, reduce pain and parasite emotional overreactivity,` prevent worsening of deformities	Improve ease of caretaking, facilitate function in sitting position
V	No locomotion ability, fully dependent		Improve neck and trunk and upper limb posturing and swallowing	Improve ease of caretaking, facilitate positioning in adaptive equipment

(Figs. 13.8, 13.9 and 13.10). For characterization of these degrees, the New York University classification is currently used [22].

- For children able to walk independently without assistive devices (group I), the goal is to improve appearance of gait, velocity, and ease.
- For children who walk with assistive devices (group II), the goal is to improve ambulation and decrease the dependence to assistive devices.
- For quadruped crawlers (group III), the goal is to enable to reciprocally move the legs in the standing position, using complementary assistive devices.
- For children unable to ambulate even with assistive equipment and person helping (groups IV and V), to gain significant improvement in motor function is generally not realistic.

However, in the very disabled groups any decrease in spasticity may be useful to ease nursing for caregivers, decrease pain, and improve comfort, and to prevent worsening of deformities, which is also important. Via the (frequently observed) distant effects, i.e., suprasegmental effects, DR at the lumbosacral level can

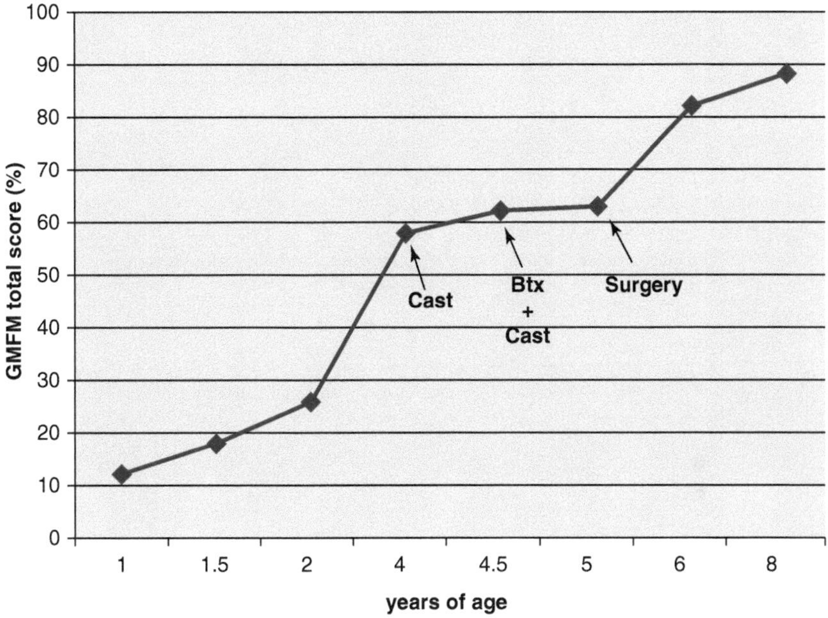

Fig. 13.8 Assessment of a diplegic child with repeated Gross Motor Function Measure score. Evolution of that score is for us the most "powerful" and reliable indicator for surgical decision. A child is proposed for surgery when the curve plateaus or decreases

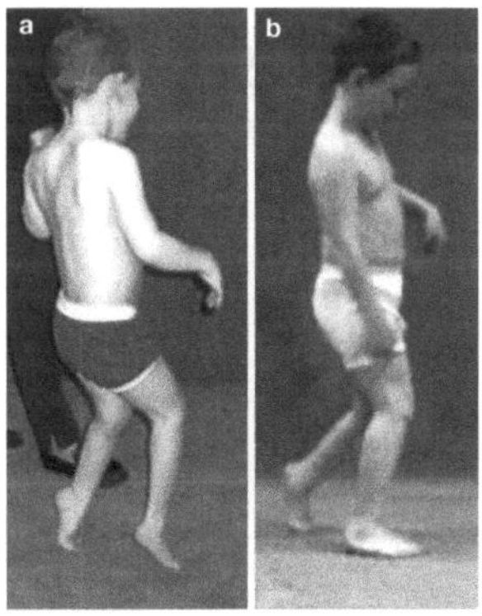

Fig. 13.9 Diplegic child (Gross Motor Function Measure score shown in Fig. 13.8) before (**a**) and 2 years after (**b**) DR (taken from video). Before surgery, the child had a jumping gait with true equinus and could ambulate autonomously only with person helping. After surgery, the child could walk autonomously and with a reestablished alternate stance and swing phase

sometimes dramatically improve neck and trunk postural maintenance, swallowing, and parasite movements of the upper limbs, as well as emotional overreactivity. For those severely affected children, complementary neuro-orthopedic surgery can be usefully indicated, especially tendon lengthening.

Absolute and relative contraindications are summarized in Table 13.5.

Techniques, patient's selection, outcome, and complications of treating spastic cerebral palsy in several series are summarized in Table 13.6.

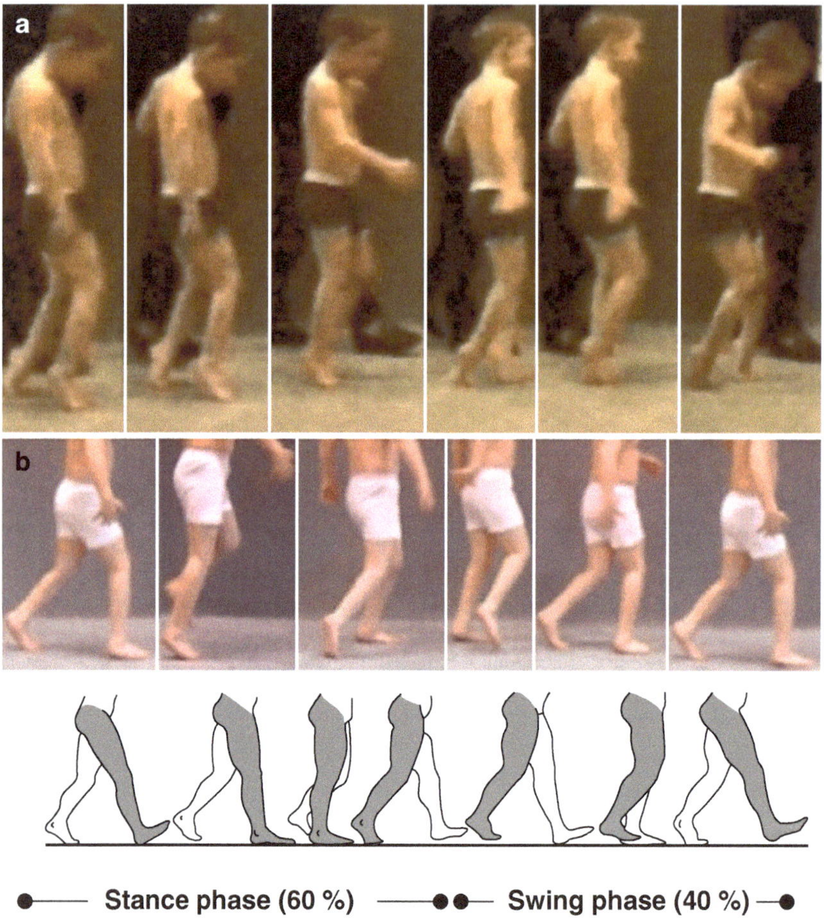

Fig. 13.10 Diplegic child before (**a**) and after (**b**) DR (taken from video). Before DR, child has jumping gait (with true equinus). After DR, alternating stance and swing phases were established. However, note that in swing phase, dorsal flexion of foot is still very weak

Table 13.5 Contraindications and relative contraindications for DR

Contraindication	Relative contraindication (poor prognostic factor)
Predominant, concomitant movement disorders (e.g., rigidity, dystonia, dyskinesia, ataxia)	Several previous orthopedic interventions
Fixed joint, severe spine deformities	Preexisting scoliosis
Severe hydrocephalus, brain atrophy, encephalomalacia	Spasticity from a progressive condition (e.g., familial spastic paraparesis)
	Epilepsy, concomitant cortical dysplasia on imaging, hydrocephalus
	Severe respiratory disturbances, bronchopulmonary dysplasia
	Severe cognitive delay, lack of motivation
	Nutritional disorders (e.g., overweight, cachexia)

Table 13.6 DR for treatment of spastic cerebral palsy (literature data)

Authors	Age (years)	NYUC	Surgical approach/roots exposed	Grade of motor response to stimulation of roots to be cut	% of root cut	Outcome (GMFM)	Complications
Abbott et al. [22, 25, 28, 29, 37]	<6	I–V	Laminotomy, L5–S2 levels/L2–S3 roots	2–4	>50	>34 % after 5 years	Immediate: bronchospasm, aspiration pneumonia, severe pain Distant: urinary tract dysfunction, spinal deformities, hip subluxation
Farmer et al. [7, 46, 49, 52]	3–7	I–III	Laminotomy, L1–S1 levels/L2–S2 roots	4	75 (S2, <50)	Functional progress	Transient: urinary retention Distant: lumbar spinal stenosis
Park et al. [10, 11, 35, 50]	3 to ≥12	I–III	Single-level laminectomy at level of conus (L1)/L2–S2 roots	3–4	65	Significant increase in GMFM score	Transient: urinary retention, dysesthesia
Sindou et al. [12, 33]	<7	I–V	Limited osteoplastic laminotomy, T11–L1/L2–S4 roots Staged interlaminar approach/L2–S2 roots	3–4	50–80 (65), antigravity L4 generally spared	Improvement of function in less affected, better comfort in more affected children	Spondylolisthesis (0.5 %), dysesthesia (1 %) None

(continued)

Table 13.6 (continued)

Authors	Age (years)	NYUC	Surgical approach/roots exposed	Grade of motor response to stimulation of roots to be cut	% of root cut	Outcome (GMFM)	Complications
Steinbok et al. [8, 26, 42, 44, 48]	3–8	I–IV	Laminoplasty, L1 or L2–L5 levels/L2–S2 roots Single-level laminectomy at level of the conus (L1)/L2–S2 roots	2–4	50–70	Significant increase in GMFM score; no significant differences between the two techniques	Bronchospasm, transient urinary retention, transient or permanent dysesthesia, back pain, hip subluxation, spinal deformities; no significant differences between the two techniques
Nordmark et al. [54]	3–7	I–V	Laminoplasty, L1–L5 levels/L2–S2 roots	Most pathological response (?)	>40	Significant functional progress after 5 years	Immediate: respiratory problems, severe pain, dysesthesia Distant: constipation

NYUC New York University classification, *GMFM* Gross Motor Function Measure

References

1. Sherrington CS (1898) Decerebrate rigidity, and reflex coordination of movements. J Physiol 22:319–332
2. Foerster O (1913) On the indications and results of the excision of posterior spinal nerve roots in men. Surg Gynecol Obstet 16:463–474
3. Privat JM, Benezech J, Frerebeau P, Gros C (1976) Sectorial posterior rhizotomy, a new technique of surgical treatment for spasticity. Acta Neurochir (Wien) 35:181–195
4. Fasano VA, Barolat-Romana G, Ivaldi A, Sguazzi A (1976) La radicotomie postérieure fonctionnelle dans le traitement de la spasticité cérébrale. Neurochirurgie 22:23–34
5. Peacock WJ, Arens LJ (1982) Selective posterior rhizotomy for the relief of spasticity in cerebral palsy. S Afr Med J 62:119–124
6. Abbott R (2009) Selective dorsal rhizotomy for the treatment of childhood spasticity. In: Sindou M (ed) Practical handbook of neurosurgery, vol 3. Springer, Wien/New York, pp 387–395
7. Farmer JP, McNeely PD (2004) Surgery in the dorsal roots for children with cerebral palsy. Oper Tech Neurosurg 7:153–156
8. Steinbok P (2007) Selective dorsal rhizotomy for cerebral palsy: a review. Childs Nerv Syst 23:981–990
9. Sindou M, Goutelle A (1983) Surgical posterior rhizotomies for the treatment of pain. In: Krayenbühl H, Brihaye J, Loew F, Mingrino S, Pertuiset B, Symon L, Troupp H, Yaşargil MG (eds) Advances and technical standards in neurosurgery, vol 10. Springer, Wien/New York, pp 147–185
10. Park TS, Gaffney PE, Kaufman BA, Molleston MC (1993) Selective lumbosacral dorsal rhizotomy immediately caudal to the conus medullaris for cerebral palsy spasticity. Neurosurgery 33:929–933
11. Park TS, Johnston JM (2008) Selective dorsal rhizotomy for spastic cerebral palsy. In: Goodrich JT (ed) Pediatric neurosurgery, 2nd edn. Thieme, New York, pp 177–183
12. Sindou M (2003) Radicotomies dorsales chez l'enfant. Neurochirurgie 49:312–323
13. Little WJ (1861) On the influence of abnormal parturition, difficult labours, premature birth and asphyxia neonatorum on the mental and physical condition of the child, especially in relation to deformities. Trans Obstet Soc Lond 3:293–344
14. Gros C, Ouaknine G, Vlahovitch B, Frèrebeau P (1967) La radicotomie sélective postérieure dans le traitment neurochirurgical de hypertonie pyramidale. Neurochirurgie 13:505–518
15. Schirmer CM, Shils JL, Arle JE, Cosgrove GR, Dempsey PK, Tarlov E, Kim S, Martin CJ, Fetz C, Moul M, Magge S (2011) Heuristic map of myotomal innervation in humans using direct intraoperative nerve root stimulation. J Neurosurg Spine 15:64–70
16. Phillips LH, Park TS (1989) Electrophysiologic studies of selective posterior rhizotomy patients. In: Park TS, Phillips LH, Peacock WJ (eds) Management of spasticity in cerebral palsy and spinal cord injury. Neurosurgery: state of the art reviews, vol 4(2). Hanley & Belfus, Philadelphia, pp 459–470
17. Mittal S, Farmer JP, Poulin C, Silver K (2001) Reliability of intraoperative electrophysiological monitoring in selective posterior rhizotomy. J Neurosurg 95:67–75
18. Cohen AR, Webster HC (1991) How selective is selective posterior rhizotomy. Surg Neurol 35:267–272
19. Storrs BB, Nishida T (1988) Use of the 'H' reflex recovery curve in selective posterior rhizotomy. Pediatr Neurosci 14:120–123
20. Nishida T, Storrs BB (1991) Electrophysiological monitoring in selective posterior rhizotomy for spasticity: principles, techniques and interpretation of responses. In: Sindou M, Abbott R, Keravel Y (eds) Neurosurgery for spasticity: a multidisciplinary approach. Springer, Wien/New York, pp 159–163
21. Parise M, Sindou M, Mertens P, Maugière F (1997) Somatosensory evoked potentials following functional posterior rhizotomy in spastic children. Stereotact Funct Neurosurg 69:268–273

22. Abbott R (1991) Indications for surgery to treat children with spasticity due to cerebral palsy. In: Sindou M, Abbott R, Keravel Y (eds) Neurosurgery for spasticity: a multidisciplinary approach. Springer, Wien/New York, pp 215–217
23. Deletis V, Vodusek DB, Abbott R, Epstein FJ, Turndorf H (1992) Intraoperative monitoring of the dorsal sacral roots: minimizing the risk of iatrogenic micturition disorders. Neurosurgery 30:72–75
24. Mertens P, Sindou M (2003) Traitement de la vessie hyperactive par drezotomie microchirurgicale sacrée. Neurochirurgie 49:399–403
25. Abbott R, Johann-Murphy M, Shiminski-Maher T, Quartermain D, Forem SL, Gold JT, Epstein FJ (1993) Selective dorsal rhizotomy: outcome and complications in treating spastic cerebral palsy. Neurosurgery 33:851–857; discussion 857
26. Steinbok P, Schrag C (1998) Complications after selective posterior rhizotomy for spasticity in children with cerebral palsy. Pediatr Neurosurg 28:300–313
27. Fasano VA, Broggi G, Barolat-Romana G, Sguazzi A (1978) Surgical treatment of spasticity in cerebral palsy. Childs Brain 4:289–305
28. Abbott R (1992) Complications with selective posterior rhizotomy. Pediatr Neurosurg 18:43–47
29. Abbott R, Forem SL, Johann M (1989) Selective posterior rhizotomy for the treatment of spasticity: a review. Childs Nerv Syst 5:337–346
30. Arens LJ, Peacock WJ, Peter J (1989) Selective posterior rhizotomy: a long-term follow-up study. Childs Nerv Syst 5:148–152
31. Fasano VA, Broggi G, Zeme S, Lo Russo G, Sguazzi A (1980) Long-term results of posterior functional rhizotomy. Acta Neurochir Suppl (Wien) 30:435–439
32. Heim RC, Park TS, Vogler GP, Kaufman BA, Noetzel MJ, Ortman MR (1995) Changes in hip migration after selective dorsal rhizotomy for spastic quadriplegia in cerebral palsy. J Neurosurg 82:567–571
33. Hodgkinson I, Bérard C, Jindrich ML, Sindou M, Mertens P, Bérard J (1997) Selective dorsal rhizotomy in children with cerebral palsy: results in 18 cases at one year postoperatively. Stereotact Funct Neurosurg 69:259–267
34. Hicdonmez T, Steinbok P, Beauchamp R, Sawatzky B (2005) Hip joint subluxation after selective dorsal rhizotomy for spastic cerebral palsy. J Neurosurg 103(1 Suppl):10–16
35. Park TS, Vogler GP, Phillips LH 2nd, Kaufman BA, Ortman MR, McClure SM, Gaffney PE (1994) Effects of selective dorsal rhizotomy for spastic diplegia on hip migration in cerebral palsy. Pediatr Neurosurg 20:43–49
36. Yasuoka S, Peterson HA, MacCarty CS (1982) Incidence of spinal column deformity after multilevel laminectomy in children and adults. J Neurosurg 57:441–445
37. Abbott R (1996) Sensory rhizotomy for the treatment of childhood spasticity. J Child Neurol 11(Suppl 1):S36–S42
38. Peter JC, Arens LJ (1993) Selective posterior lumbosacral rhizotomy for the management of cerebral palsy spasticity: a 10-year experience. S Afr Med J 83:745–747
39. Johnson MB, Goldstein L, Thomas SS, Piatt J, Aiona M, Sussman MJ (2004) Spinal deformity after selective dorsal rhizotomy in ambulatory patients with cerebral palsy. J Pediatr Orthop 24:529–536
40. Peter JC, Hoffman EB, Arens LJ (1993) Spondylolysis and spondylolisthesis after five-level lumbosacral laminectomy for selective posterior rhizotomy in cerebral palsy. Childs Nerv Syst 9:285–287; discussion 287–288
41. Spiegel DA, Loder RT, Alley KA, Rowley S, Gutknecht S, Smith-Wright DL, Dunn ME (2004) Spinal deformity following selective dorsal rhizotomy. J Pediatr Orthop 24:30–36
42. Steinbok P, Hicdonmez T, Sawatzky B, Beauchamp R, Wickenheiser D (2005) Spinal deformities after selective dorsal rhizotomy for spastic cerebral palsy. J Neurosurg 102(4 Suppl):363–373
43. Turi M, Kalen V (2000) The risk of spinal deformity after selective dorsal rhizotomy. J Pediatr Orthop 20:104–107

44. Steinbok P, Reiner A, Beauchamp RD, Cochrane DD, Keyes R (1992) Selective functional posterior rhizotomy for treatment of spastic cerebral palsy in children: review of 50 consecutive cases. Pediatr Neurosurg 18:34–42
45. Salame K, Ouaknine GE, Rochkind S, Constantini S, Razon N (2003) Surgical treatment of spasticity by selective posterior rhizotomy: 30 years experience. Isr Med Assoc J 5:543–546
46. Mittal S, Farmer JP, Al-Atassi B, Gibis J, Kennedy E, Galli C, Courchesnes G, Poulin C, Cantin MA, Benaroch TE (2002) Long-term functional outcome after selective posterior rhizotomy. J Neurosurg 97:315–325
47. Laitinen LV, Nilsson S, Fugl-Meyer AR (1983) Selective posterior rhizotomy for treatment of spasticity. J Neurosurg 58:895–899
48. Gul SM, Steinbok P, McLeod K (1999) Long-term outcome after selective posterior rhizotomy in children with spastic cerebral palsy. Pediatr Neurosurg 31:84–95
49. Farmer JP, Sabbagh AJ (2007) Selective dorsal rhizotomies in the treatment of spasticity related to cerebral palsy. Childs Nerv Syst 23:991–1002
50. Engsberg JR, Ross SA, Collins DR, Park TS (2006) Effect of selective dorsal rhizotomy in the treatment of children with cerebral palsy. J Neurosurg 105(1 Suppl):8–15
51. Taira T, Hori T (2008) Selective peripheral neurotomy and selective dorsal rhizotomy. Brain Nerve 60:1427–1436
52. Golan JD, Hall JA, O'Gorman G, Poulin C, Benaroch TE, Cantin MA, Farmer JP (2007) Spinal deformities following selective dorsal rhizotomy. J Neurosurg 106(6 Suppl):441–449
53. Nishida T, Thatcher SW, Marty GR (1995) Selective posterior rhizotomy for children with cerebral palsy: a 7-year experience. Childs Nerv Syst 11:374–380
54. Nordmark E, Lundkvist Josenby A, Lagergren J, Anderson G, Strömblad LG, Westbom L (2008) Long-term outcomes five years after selective dorsal rhizotomy. BMC Pediatr 8:54

Part IV

Complementary Treatments and Brief on Decision-Making for Neurosurgery

14 Orthopedic Surgery for Correction of Spastic Disorders

Excess of spasticity generates musculotendinous retraction that must be prevented or at least reduced before it becomes irreducible. In addition, disharmony in the intensity of muscular hypertonia creates an articular imbalance that promotes deformities and requires compensatory treatment. Therefore, it is mandatory to decrease harmful hypertonia before the appearance of irreducible locomotor disorders and beneficial to restore articular function by rebalancing the tonicity of agonist and antagonist muscles.

Neurosurgery is the first-line option when spasticity or dystonia predominates, although orthopedic surgical procedures may reduce per se spasticity through muscle relaxation resulting from tendon release or lengthening. Orthopedic surgery (OS) is indicated primarily or as an adjuvant when contractures and ankyloses are predominant or associated to spasticity, respectively.

Table 14.1 lists the different categories of OS for the treatment of spastic disorders or sequelae. Common techniques available for correcting shortness of a muscle–tendon unit are muscle slide (en bloc detachment of muscular origins, mobilized musculotendinous body remains on neurovascular bundle), tenotomy (simple tenotomy allows an extension that does not limit the correction of deformation, but the possibilities of functional muscles are lost), or lengthening tenotomy (at the musculotendinous junction, retaining a bundle of muscle fibers, preserving the functional capacity of muscle; at the tendon level by double or triple hemisection [e.g., medial, lateral, and medial] or by splitting and suturing, i.e., a Z-plasty in sagittal or frontal plane).

Tendon transfer has a different goal: It may correct articular misalignment due to muscular imbalance. It may be performed either for active function (attachment to another muscle or tendon to restore the action that muscle has lost) or for passive function (attachment to a bone or ligament for stabilization or fixation; tenodesis). Tendon transfer for the restoration of an action is useful only if the muscular strength of the transferred tendon was scored at least 4 out of 5 (0, no visible motor contraction; 5, normal motor strength). Transfer of spastic muscles must be avoided; suppression of spasticity has to be achieved first by botulinum toxin injections or by neurosurgical procedures if necessary.

M. Sindou et al., *Neurosurgery for Spasticity*,
DOI 10.1007/978-3-7091-1771-2_14,

Table 14.1 Categories of OS methods

Method	Goals and indications	Potential adverse effects and limitations
Lengthening of tendon–muscle unit (muscle slide, tenotomy, lengthening tenotomy)	Achievement of a more functional position	May reduce muscle power
Tendon transfer (shift or bifurcation for active or passive function)	Correction of articular alignment due to muscular imbalance, compensation for absent antagonist	Difficult to predict whether a spastic muscle is transferred, functional risk to transfer a tendon to its antagonist in sagittal plane, e.g., a flexor to an extensor
Osteotomy	Correction of bone deformities due to morphogenetic growth pathology, especially rotational; treatment of stiffened articulation with irreducible abnormal postures	May increase spasticity because of pain in postoperative period; by change of muscular insertion points, tension of those muscles may be increased
Articular surgery (arthrodesis, arthrolysis, arthroplasty)	Correction of osteoarticular structural deformities not correctable by osteotomy, correction of articular imbalance not correctable by tendon surgery	Arthrodesis must not be performed before the end of growth and is counterindicated for hip or knee and for shoulder or elbow, whose mobility should be preserved

Osteotomies aim at correcting bone deformities caused by pathological growth or at treating stiffened joints.

Articular surgery is indicated only when deformities cannot be corrected by osteotomy or tendon surgery alone. Arthrodesis must not be performed in children until growth is complete and should be restricted to the foot and the wrist. For arthrolysis to maintain articular stability, the main ligaments must be respected if the capsule has been retracted. For neurogenic paraosteoarthopathy, resection of heterotopic ossification may be indicated. If arthroplasty is required, it should precede any treatment of spasticity. Spasticity should be treated only if it persists after arthroplasty; as it relieves pain, arthroplasty by itself may diminish spasticity.

14.1 Spasticity in Lower Limb

Deformities in the lower limb(s) may concern hip, knee, ankle, and/or foot and present with a wide range of clinical patterns.

Examination should include standing and if possible walking, with and without shoes and orthoses, etc. Gait and kinesiologic analysis with polyelectromyography, possibly under anesthetic blocks, is of prime importance for decision-making and choice of the technique(s).

The objective of treatment may be an improvement of function in walking, standing, and transfers or at least a gain in comfort for the patient and caregiver assistance. In any case, it must be clarified with the patient, the patient's family, and caregivers.

The specific orthopedic surgical methods are indicated in Table 14.2.

Table 14.2 OS for spastic lower limb

Region and deformity	Goals and evaluation	Procedures	Limitations and risks
Hip			
Adduction, flexion and/or internal rotation (isolated or combined), internal-rotation bone deformity, hip dislocation	Reduction of abnormal postures, prevention of hip subluxation	Section of long adductor, short adductor, and gracilis to free abduction and also extension; for deformity in flexion, section of tensor fascia lata, sartorius, and rectus femoris is sufficient Derotation osteotomy Arthroplasty	Derotation osteotomy for internal-rotation bone deformity should take into account possible complications in the entire limb Treatment of spastic dislocation requires complementary bone and/or articular surgery
Knee			
Flexum	Improvement of extension	Detachment of semitendinosus (possibly with transfer to femur) and lengthening of semimembranosus and biceps If necessary, incision of (retracted) posterior popliteal aponeurosis, proximal detachment of (retracted) gastrocnemius Knee extensor (quadriceps) may be stretched with suture of patellar tendon (shortening of ligamentum patellae)	Avoid hypercorrection of extension, take care of necrosis and/or peripheral nerve (sciatic) and arterial ischemia due to stretching of vasculonervous structures
Foot			
Equinus deformity	Conservation of a 5° equinus may be necessary for standing position and ability to walk	Desinsertion of gastrocnemius if it is the sole cause or lengthening of Achilles tendon Enhancement of antagonist muscle power; if muscular force is present, by physical therapy; if muscular force is absent, by tendon transfer of tibialis posterior for varus, of flexor digitorum longus for claw toes	Avoid hypercorrection in talus

(continued)

Table 14.2 (continued)

Region and deformity	Goals and evaluation	Procedures	Limitations and risks
Varus deformity	Differentiation of types secondary either to hypertonia and retraction of posterior calf or to dystonia of anterior calf	Lenghtening of tibialis posterior, split posterior tibial tendon transfer to external aspect of calcaneus If tibialis anterior shows sufficient activity upon examination, split anterior tibial tendon to cuboid tendon; attachment of distal peroneus brevis tendon to tibialis anterior (Bardot procedure)	Risks of transfers
Valgus deformity	Deformity is awkward but usually painless and not very disabling in walking; may be due either to shortening of Achilles tendon with foot deformity characterized by eversion of calcaneus and flattened medial longitudinal arch or to hypertonia and retraction of peroneal and extensor muscles	Lengthening of Achilles tendon or lengthening of peroneal and extensor muscles	
Equino-varus deformity (irreducible deformities)	Attempt at strong mobilization to ascertain irreducibility	Triple arthrodesis (subtalar and midtarsal), Chopart arthrodesis (talonavicular or calcaneocuboid joints for stabilization of diversion or inversion), posterior tibiotarsal arthrolysis	If anterior tibialis shows inactivity in standing position, triple arthrodesis is preferable to muscle transfer; risks of 10-week immobilization
Toes			
Claw toes	Difficulty to identify which flexor muscles (intrinsic or extrinsic) are really retracted	Depending on muscles and tendons concerned, either detachment or tenotomy; possibly, arthrolysis of ankylosed joints	Trophic cutaneous lesions, infections
Hitchhiker's great toe (permanent Babinski sign)		Section or lengthening of extensor hallucis longus tendon	

14.2 Spasticity in Upper Limb

Deformities in the upper limb(s) may concern shoulder, elbow, wrist, and fingers with a range of presentations even wider than that of deformities of the lower limb.

Examination should detect and quantify the imbalance between agonists (flexors) and antagonists (extensors) in tone and also evaluate the deficiency in motor command and movement coordination. Examination should also establish whether dystonic components or synkinesis, etc., exist. It is of primary importance to differentiate contractures, fixed retractions, and ankyloses, as well as their degree, from the hypertonic components that can or even must be reduced prior to considering orthopedic correction. Short-duration anesthetic blocks and/or long-duration botulinum toxin injections can help discriminate those diverse components.

The objective of treatment has to be clarified with the patient, the patient's family, and the caregivers. It may range from an improvement in function by realigning the arm and hand in space and facilitating the capacity of extension and prehension to a matter of cosmetics or hygiene. Improvement in function requires existence of motor power and also sufficient sensory function at the hand level. All items must be checked by careful examination prior to any decision being made.

The specific orthopedic surgical methods are indicated in Table 14.3.

14.3 Main Indications

Indications of OS are particularly well described in publications by Denormandie et al. [1], Bouttens and Delecourt [2], Novacheck and Gage [3], and Bardot et al. [4].

14.3.1 Hemiplegic Adults

OS is indicated when there are evolving or fixed muscular contractures and/or irreducible articular deformities.

For wrist and fingers in flexion, release or lengthening of tendons may offer better comfort and cosmesis; in a hand with residual motor power, function can be improved. For spastic foot, OS is indicated when equinus deformity is irreducible, varus makes stance unstable, and toes are irreducibly deformed and cannot be relieved by neurosurgical treatment.

14.3.2 Paraplegic or Tetraplegic Adults

OS may be indicated for correction of deformities that may induce pressure sores and cannot be influenced by neurosurgery. Procedures are directed most frequently to hip flexors and adductors, hamstrings, and Achilles tendon.

OS for improving function in upper limbs in tetraplegic patients, especially tendon transfers, initially employed to compensate deficits after peripheral nervous

Table 14.3 OS for spastic upper limb

Region and deformity	Goals and evaluation	Procedures	Limitations and risks
Shoulder			
Adduction, internal rotation	Realignment of arm and hand, relief of pain and stiffness, improvement of hygiene in axillary region	Subscapular tenotomy, pectoralis major lengthening, transfer of latissimus dorsi and teres major, osteotomy of derotation	Anterior instability
Elbow			
Flexion	Realignment of arm and hand, relief of pain and stiffness	Brachialis tenotomy, biceps lengthening, arthrolysis (plus excision of heterotopic ossifications); to be considered, neurotomy of musculocutaneous nerve	"Dangling arm", especially if there is a brachioradialis deficit (as may result from associated extensive neurotomy)
Associated pronation		Tenotomy of pronator teres and pronator quadratus; to be considered, neurotomy of corresponding nerves	
Wrist			
Flexion (with or without ulnar or radial deviation)	Enablement of hand opening; in still functional hand, lengthening should be made with such precision that residual muscular tension maintains each finger in slightly flexed position	Detachment of flexor muscles (Scaglietti procedure), detachment of epitrochlear pronators (Page procedure), lengthening or transfer of tendon of flexor carpi radialis, flexor carpi ulnaris, flexor pollicis longus, flexor digitorum longus (for long finger flexors, the proximal end of each flexor digitorum profundis tendon can be transferred to the distal end of the flexor digitorum superficialis tendon (Keenan procedure), transfer of flexor carpi ulnaris to extensor carpi radialis brevis or longus (Green procedure)	When hand is useless due to permanent motion or sensory deficits, OS can only offer benefits of comfort and esthetics.
		Arthrodesis of first intermetacarpal space, radiocarpal joint, or phanlanges	Hypocorrection of pronation in absence of flexor-pronator lengthening, hyperextension that impedes mobility, septic pseudoarthrosis, cutaneous disunion, postoperative "swan neck" deformity; transfer of spastic muscle must be avoided (suppressed before transfer)

Table 14.3 (continued)

Region and deformity	Goals and evaluation	Procedures	Limitations and risks
Fingers			
Clenched fist, flexion–adduction of thumb (thumb in palm)	Hand opening and prehension when voluntary control exists, elevation of thumb out of palm, preservation of pincer grasp function of thumb and index finger, reestablishment of capacity of oppositon	For extrinsic type due to hypertonia of flexor pollicis longus, lengthening of this muscle and neurotomy of corresponding nerve; for intrinsic type, OS or neurotomy of intrinsic branches of ulnar nerve; flexor lengthening; to be considered, neurotomies for spasticity before OS	

system lesions, can also be applied to patients with central nervous system lesions. Muscles to be transferred should not be spastic. If necessary, reduction of their spasticity has to be achieved by neurological surgery.

The same applies to patients with severe hypertonia after brainstem or cerebral injury or pathologies.

14.3.3 Patients with Cerebral Palsy

In children, the morphology of the skeleton is conditioned by muscular tensions. These are sustained by hypertonia and contracture, the latter resulting from asynchronous longitudinal growth of muscular fibers and bones. In children with cerebral palsy, those mechanisms are aggravated by an imbalance in tone and strength between agonist and antagonist muscular groups for one given joint.

In the lower limb, imbalance is preponderant in flexors, adductors, and internal rotators of hip, flexors of knee, and plantar flexors of foot. For patients able to walk, gait analysis is an important step before any decision about surgery, either neurosurgical or orthopedic [3].

According to Bardot et al. [4, p. 205]: "The proper age for surgery is a question of common sense. Before the age of walking, orthopedic surgery is only urgently indicated for prevention of hip dislocation or for major equinus deformity of the foot. Later on, time of surgery is conditioned by the severity and speed of deterioration, and with the concern of preventing scoliosis."

Conclusion

OS occupies a major position in the treatment of the sequelae of spasticity and hypertonia. However, it must not bypass neurological surgery; both must be considered in combination or in a sequential way. OS has its proper indications, risks, and limitations. Indications should be discussed in an interdisciplinary frame of dedicated specialists; children must be followed by an experienced rehabilitation team.

References

1. Denormandie P, Kiefer C, Mailhan L, Even-Schneider A, Sorriaux G, Martin JN, Judet T (2003) Surgical treatment of orthopedic deformities due to spasticity in the lower limb. Neurochirurgie 49:339–352
2. Bouttens D, Delecourt C (2003) Orthopedic treatment of consequences of upper limb spasticity. Neurochirurgie 49:353–357
3. Novacheck TF, Gage JR (2007) Orthopedic management of spasticity in cerebral palsy. Childs Nerv Syst 23:1015–1031
4. Bardot A, Delarque A, Curvale G, Peragut JC (1991) Orthopedic surgical corrections of spastic disorders. In: Sindou M, Abbott R, Keravel Y (eds) Neurosurgery for spasticity: a multidisciplinary approach. Springer, Wien/New York, pp 201–208

15 Management of Hyperactive Bladder

Overactive bladder, with its complications on the upper urinary tract, is a frequent occurrence after damage of the central nervous system, especially at the spinal cord level.

15.1 Mechanisms

The lower urinary tract has two main functions, storage and periodic micturition, that depend on the reciprocal activity of two functional units, a reservoir – the bladder – and an outlet, which includes the bladder neck and the smooth and striated sphincters of the urethra. During storage, the bladder outlet is closed and the bladder wall quiescent. During voiding, the initial event is relaxation of the pelvic floor and striated sphincter, which is followed by a contraction of the detrusor and the opening of the bladder neck.

In normal conditions, when stimulated by filling, the bladder sends messages to the micturition center, which is located in the sacral spinal cord at the S2/S3 level and hence to the brain. At the appropriate time to void, the brain sends its release message down to the bladder through the micturition center.

After lesions of the pathways between the micturition center and the brain, the bladder is no longer under voluntary control. Voiding becomes reflexive, with the message to empty coming only from the micturition center. In addition, the threshold for the release of the detrusor reflex is lowered, resulting in detrusor hyperreflexia. When the dysfunction is chronic, the bladder wall thickens and becomes fibrotic, and thus hypertonic, which reduces the bladder capacity. This bladder dysfunction leads to vesicoureteral reflux and eventually to kidney damage.

For an assessment of bladder function in storage and voiding the following parameters are studied [1]: **bladder capacity** (the normal capacity is 350–500 ml, with the first normal desire to void elicited at 200–300 ml); **bladder residue**, which is the volume of urine remaining in the bladder immediately after completion of micturition (it can be estimated by palpation, catheterization, or ultrasonics); **cystometric capacity**, which is the volume at which the patient has an urge to void or

M. Sindou et al., *Neurosurgery for Spasticity*,
DOI 10.1007/978-3-7091-1771-2_15, © Springer-Verlag Wien 2014

urinary incontinence (total of the volume voided and any residual volume); and **uninhibited detrusor contractions** (sudden involuntary increase in detrusor pressure, usually at more than 15 cmH_2O).

Dysfunctions to be differentiated are **hyperactivity with detrusor hyperreflexia** (uninhibited contractions elicited at a low volume of urine and at a low bladder pressure), **hyperactivity with detrusor hypertonicity** (uninhibited contractions elicited at a low volume of urine and high bladder pressure), **detrusor sphincter dyssynergia** (involuntary contraction of the striated sphincter during an involuntary detrusor contraction, leading to a "conflicting" bladder), and **bladder neck obstruction** (a delay and/or a failure in bladder neck opening, synchronous with detrusor contraction, due to fibrous narrowing of the bladder neck or dyssynergia of [adrenergic] smooth muscle).

15.2 Clinical Presentation

The hyperactive bladder, because of involuntary contractions, fails to store urine adequately. The symptoms most commonly experienced by the patients are the following: **urinary frequency**, which is an increase in the number of voiding; **urinary urgency**, which is a feeling of having to empty the bladder immediately, combined with inability to retain urine once the urge to void is felt; and **urge incontinence**, which is involuntary loss of urine.

15.3 Urodynamic Exploration

The first step is study of the **spontaneous voluntary micturition** with calculation of flow in milliliter per second.

The second step is **cystometric exploration** under bladder filling (300–400 ml on average). It consists of simultaneous recordings of the intravesical and intraurethral pressure, with measurement of the abdominal pressure with a rectal catheter. Examination can be completed by electromyography of the striated urethral sphincter. Contrast medium can be used as the infusate for cystometry so that the entire process can be monitored under fluoroscopy.

Among the parameters studied by cystometry are the **volume at which the patient feels the first desire to void**; the **maximum cystometric capacity**, which is the volume at which the patient feels – sometimes painfully – not to be able to delay voiding any longer; the **detrusor pressure**, which is determined by subtracting the intra-abdominal pressure from the intravesical pressure and corresponds to the intravesical pressure due to active and passive forces in the bladder wall; and the **compliance**, which indicates the change in volume in relation to the change in bladder pressure (a bladder with low compliance is characterized by a steep filling curve indicating hypertonicity of the detrusor; a bladder with high compliance accepts a large volume of urine without significant rise in pressure).

For a **hyperactive bladder**, cystometry shows uninhibited detrusor contractions during the filling phase, a decrease in capacity, and detrusor hyperreflexia, that is, contractions triggered by suprapubic tapping.

Intravenous or intramuscular injections of anticholinergic agents or sacral anaesthetic block allow to **differentiate hyperactivity with detrusor hyperreflexia from that with detrusor hypertonicity**. By suppressing hyperactivity, bladder capacity and compliance are increased in the former situation, but not in the latter. Hypertonicity corresponds to an alteration of the bladder wall by fibrosis.

Cystography during storage and voiding reveals a small-sized bladder with bladder trabeculations, and sometimes diverticuli. The presence of vesicoureteral reflux provoked by bladder contractions has to be carefully searched as it threatens the kidneys.

15.4 Treatment

At first, factors prone to increase lower-limb or general spasticity and bladder hyperactivity should be searched for, and treated before any form of functional treatment is considered. These factors are generally of the "nociceptive" type; the most frequently encountered are urinary tract infections, bladder stones, transit bowel disturbances, pressure sores, and phlebitis. Also neuropathic pain can play an aggravating role.

Medical treatment is essentially pharmacological (Table 15.1), aiming principally at reducing the parasympathetic tone of the urinary tract. The anticholinergic agents, especially the most often used muscarinic receptor antagonists, act through a decrease of the transmission of impulses from the micturition center to the detrusor. Owing to their muscle-relaxant properties, the class of the benzodiazepines (γ-aminobutyric acid agonists) may be useful adjuvants.

15.4.1 Urologic Surgery

Indications for urologic surgery have to be discussed critically before taking a decision, as this type of surgery modifies anatomy definitively.

Surgery on the **bladder neck** aims to decrease resistance to voiding when striated sphincter becomes hypertonic and thus constitutes an obstacle to micturition. It is mainly indicated for males; because of the lack of an effective external device for urine collection in females, intermittent catheterization is currently preferred for them. Sphincterotomy of the striated sphincter has become less invasive thanks to the modern endoscopic techniques. However, urethral endoprostheses (stents) are preferable due to the reversibility of the method.

For patients with **poor bladder compliance**, enhancement of the capacity of the bladder reservoir is required to decrease incontinence and avoid irreversible damages to the upper urinary tract. Detrusor myectomy, which aims at creating bladder

Table 15.1 Methods for treatment of hyperactive bladder

Method	Goal and indication	Limits, advantages, and disadvantges
Pharmacological treatment		
Anticholinergics (muscarinic receptor agonist mostly used)	Reduction of parasympathetic tone	
Benzodiazepines	Myorelaxant effect	
Intravesical treatment		
Vanilloids (capsaicin, resiniferatoxin)	Lasting, but reversible desensitization of sensory afferent C fibers that trigger detrusor reaction	Only recommended for patients being reliant on intermittent catherization; contraindicated for urinary retention manifested in bladder residue, vesiculoureteral reflux
Botulinum toxin	Neuronal blockade by inhibition of acetylcholine release	Injections to be repeated several times per year
Urological surgery		
On bladder neck		
Sphincterotomy of striated sphincter	Reduction of striated-sphincter hypertonicity, to be done before upper urinary tract deterioration appears; indicated for bladder neck obstruction	Risk of incontinence – in that event, male patients may be equipped with an external collector, female patients may have intermittent catheterization; risk of erectile or ejaculation dysfunction; and of restenosis
Urethral stent implantation	Goal and indication as for sphincterotomy	Risks of incontinence, erectile or ejaculation dysfunction, and stent migration
On detrusor wall		
Detrusor myectomy	Indicated for refractory urge incontinence	Inconsistent effect; alternative to enterocystoplasty
Enterocystoplasty (with bowel ileum segment)	Creation of large-capacity reservoir, protection of upper urinary tract, improvement of continence	Effective in cases with poor bladder capacity, but major operation with high rate of complications
Urinary diversion		
Incontinent (ileal conduit) or continent (reservoir) cutaneous diversion with catheterizable stoma, linked to bladder or neo-bladder	Last surgical remedy for drainage	Psychologically hard to accept
Neurosurgery		
Sacral sensory denervation (S2/S3/S4) guided by intraoperative mapping		

Table 15.1 (continued)

Method	Goal and indication	Limits, advantages, and disadvantges
Open dorsal rhizotomy or microsurgical DREZotomy	Reduction of bladder or sphincter hyperreflexia in order to increase bladder capacity and decrease hyperactivity; mainly indicated for urine leakage around permanent catheter or in between intermittent catheterizations	Allows to denervate selectively the sensory fibers only and precisely at the selected sacral levels
Percutaneous lesioning techniques through sacral foramina (either chemical, e.g., with alcohol or phenol, or thermal by thermocoagulation)	Goal and indication as for open procedures	Less invasive, but entails risks: for chemical rhizotomies, that of substance diffusion to neighboring levels; for thermocoagulation, that of not sparing the ventral (motor) roots; regional anesthesia provoked in corresponding cutaneomucosal territory by any of the procedures
Electrical stimulation of sacral roots combined with S2–S5 selective dorsal rhizotomy (Brindley procedure)	Improvement of bladder continence by reduction of bladder hyperactivity through dorsal (sensory) rhizotomies, control of micturition by controlled stimulation of ventral (motor) roots	Indicated only for patients with complete spinal cord injury but intact spinal cord arc reflex at conus medullaris and bladder able to contract (i.e., not fibrotic); alternative to intermittent catheterization
Neuromodulation (stimulation of spinal cord at conus medullaris, of sacral roots at S3 level, of posterior tibial nerves, of pudental nerves)	Exertion of a favorable "neuromodulation effect" on spinal cord circuitry, as hypothesized; potential indication for urge incontinence without bladder residue or risk for upper urinary tract	Further assessment and validation required
Intrathecal infusion		
Intrathecal baclofen (γ-aminobutyric acid-B receptor agonist)	Indicated for spastic paraplegia or paresia of spinal cord origin	Useful effect on hyperactive bladder reported in several works but not all; may induce urinary retention and impair penile erection and ejaculation reflex
Intrathecal clonidine (alpha-2 agonist)	Improvement of urodynamic parameters in patients with spinal cord injuries and detrusor hyperreflexia	Reported effect is promising but mostly transient; may induce cardiovascular disturbances; bolus test required before decision on pump implantation

autoaugmentation, may be performed. However, because the effectiveness of that intervention is inconsistent, enterocystoplasty is generally preferred.

External cutaneous diversion, which is the creation of a catheterizable stoma near the umbilical level, can be a last but effective remedy.

15.4.2 Neurological surgery

The goal of neurological surgery is basically the suppression of the uninhibited bladder contractions, so as to increase bladder capacity, reduce urinary urgencies, and prevent urine leakage.

Before neurosurgery is considered, it is necessary to determine the exact functional status of the urinary tract. As a matter of fact, the neurosurgical procedures which aim at reducing detrusor hyperactivity and hyperreflexia have very limited effects once the bladder has become hypertonic, that is, affected by irreversible fibrotic degeneration. Therefore, before decision making, detailed urodynamic explorations, including anesthetic blocks if necessary, are mandatory.

For patients with complete neurological deficits, destructive procedures can be used. Decrease in bladder tone may create bladder retention that will necessitate permanent or intermittent catheterization. For patients who retain neurological functions, surgery is preferably conservative, or if destructive procedures are chosen, they must be selective.

Indication of sacral sensory denervation (S2/S3/S4) should be limited to totally paraplegic patients being reliant on catheterization, mainly to avoid urine leakage around the catheter when permanently inserted or in between catheterizations when intermittent. S2 has to be preserved at least on one side to maintain erectile capacity.

Stimulation of sacral motor roots combined with sacral dorsal rhizotomy, the Brindley procedure, is able to achieve controlled micturition [2, 3]. Strong transient electrical stimulation with an intra- or extradurally implanted electrode causes simultaneous contraction of the detrusor and striated sphincter of the urethra; but due to its smooth muscular structure, the detrusor contracts longer than the striated sphincter, which leads to urine voiding. Functional sacral ventral roots are a prerequisite for this method.

Sacral neuromodulation [4], a conservative method, may help improve control for patients with incomplete lesions affected with voiding dysfunction, especially urging incontinence, but without bladder residue.

In conclusion, whatever the technical modalities may be, surgery should be considered before fibrotic hypertonicity appears and irreversible renal damage settles.

References

1. Beneton C, Mertens P, Leriche A, Sindou M (1991) The spastic bladder and its treatment. In: Sindou M, Abbott IR, Keravel Y (eds) Neurosurgery for spasticity: a multidisciplinary approach. Springer, Wien/New York, pp 193–199
2. Brindley GS (1994) The first 50 patients with sacral root stimulation implants: general description. Paraplegia 32:795–805
3. Vignes JR, Gimbert E, Sesay M, De Seze M, Guerin J, Joseph PA (2004) Treatment of overactive bladder. Oper Tech Neurosurg 7:163–174
4. Vignes JR, De Seze M, Dobremez E, Joseph PA, Guerin J (2005) Sacral neuromodulation in lower urinary tract dysfunction. In: Pickard D, Akalan N, Di Rocco C, Dolenc V, Fahlbusch R, Lobo Antunes J, Sindou M, de Tribolet N, Tulleken CAF (eds) Advances and technical standards in neurosurgery, vol 30. Springer, Wien/New York, pp 177–224

16 Brief on Decision-Making for Neurosurgery of Adults and Children

Decision-making should follow the general principles that are based on the physiological mechanisms of spasticity and be tailored to each individual situation, including a personalized rehabilitation program. Decision-making has to obey the following steps.

16.1 Who to Operate? The Candidates Benefitting from Neurosurgery

Potential candidates are those in whom spasticity per se is harmful and refractory to medications and physical therapy. The etiology of the disease must be clearly identified and the disease estimated as not progressing or at least stabilized. All factors that likely provoke exaggeration of spasticity should have been searched for and eradicated.

Adult paraplegic (or tetraplegic) patients in whom neither rehabilitation program can progress nor physical therapies maintain efficacy are potential candidates. Neurosurgery for spasticity may also be indicated for hemiplegic patients; at lower limb, when standing and walking are impaired by excessive hypertonia; at upper limb, when abnormal postures especially in flexion turn to become irreversible and/or painful. Patients with focalized severe dystonic component may benefit.

Children affected with cerebral palsy (CP) known to develop progressive deformities frequently require recourse to surgery, orthopedic and/or neurologic, as soon as botulinum toxin injections or treatments with cast or orthosis become insufficient.

16.2 Why to Operate? The Objectives and Limits of Neurosurgery

The rationale for considering surgical treatment should be critically analyzed and, consequently, objectives clearly defined. Patients that may benefit are those patients affected with upper motor neuron syndrome for whom it has been proven that disability is mainly attributable to an excess of muscular tone and that this excess tone

M. Sindou et al., *Neurosurgery for Spasticity*,
DOI 10.1007/978-3-7091-1771-2_16, © Springer-Verlag Wien 2014

is harmful despite its beneficial effects in compensating motor weakness. Because of a frequent complexity in clinical presentations, one must be certain that hypertonia is of the spastic type or at least that the spastic component is predominant in hypertonia mixed with dystonia.

The goal is to diminish excess of tone only. As a matter of fact, a minimum of tone must be preserved, as a certain degree of hypertonia may compensate for the loss of strength especially for standing and transfers in paraplegic or tetraplegic patients or for walking in hemiplegics. By reducing spasticity, mobilization, whether passive or active, can be eased, contractures decreased, or their appearance prevented.

In patients with hyperspasticity responsible for abnormal postures, rebalancing the tone between agonist and antagonist muscular groups will increase the range of motion and facilitate mobilization. If not performed too late, contractures and deformities can be avoided. Another goal is to improve function when present or to allow its reappearance when hidden behind hypertonia.

Limitations of surgery, as well as potential risks and side effects, have to be explained to the patient, his/her family, and caregivers. Their expectations are often much above that achievable by the treatment. Objectives, limits, and risks have to be written in the signed informed consent form.

16.3 When to Operate? The Appointment of Surgery

The appropriate time to consider surgical treatment is when excess of spasticity has been recognized to be harmful per se and before contractures and articular ankyloses are a threat and irreducible deformities appear. Prior to any decision, all curable potential causes likely to increase spasticity have to be eliminated, all relaxant medications have be administered, and all forms of physical therapies performed. One must be sure that the rehabilitation program was rigorously followed.

Determination of the appropriate time for surgery is rather easy for adult patients, provided the course of disease is stabilized.

Indication and determination of the appropriate time for surgery is much more difficult for children with CP. A decision on surgery timed too early would neglect a young child's potential for developmental maturation of its central nervous system and capacities of further locomotion skills. A decision timed too late risks the appearance of contractures and deformities likely remaining irreducible. We advise that decision be based not on age itself but rather on the deterioration of the child's development, which can be objectively quantified and followed on scoring systems, especially the **Gross Motor Function Measure**.

16.4 How to Operate? The Choice of Procedure

According to literature, up to now few of the attempts to reduce spasticity by electrical stimulation or stereotactic lesioning techniques at the various potential targets at the encephalic level showed any long-term effectiveness. Neuromodulation by electrical stimulation at the spinal cord level manifested only mild, often inconstant, relaxing effects in spastic paraplegic patients; however, spinal cord stimulation may be proposed to patients affected with multiple sclerosis or degenerative spinal cord diseases.

At present, the most effective surgical way to treat spasticity is to reduce the excess of tone at the corresponding spinal cord segments by either intrathecal infusion of relaxant drugs, principally baclofen (ITB), or lesioning techniques at the selected levels in the dorsal roots or the dorsal root entry zone (DREZ). Also peripheral nerves can be targeted in order to rebalance tone between agonist and antagonist muscular groups and corresponding joints. This is indicated for patients presenting with abnormal postures in limbs. Peripheral neurotomies achieve (partial) denervation of the corresponding muscles, on both the afferent (sensory myotatic) and the efferent (motor) side.

Adults with paraplegia (or tetraplegia), if totally paralyzed, may benefit from either ITB or lumbosacral DREZotomy when spasticity is intense and diffuse to limb(s); whereas for patients not severely paralyzed, ITB is preferable. If harmful spasticity is focalized, peripheral neurotomies can be the solution when botulinum toxin injections prove insufficient.

In hemiplegic patients, the spastic leg may respond well to peripheral neurotomies, especially the one of the tibial nerve when spasticity in the foot is disabling. For a spastic upper limb, peripheral neurotomies may be a remedy when spasticity is focalized; or when it is diffuse, DREZotomy. This procedure may also be considered for patients harboring severe dystonia, provided DREZotomy would be extended deep into the spinal cord, down to the ventral horn layers. Patients with brain or brainstem insults – whatever the etiology, traumatic or vascular –, even if spasticity is mixed with dystonia, can benefit from ITB. Because of the risk of irreversible contractures, decision should be taken as soon as decortication or decerebration rigidity develops; ITB therapy may be ceased, though not abruptly, if the patient recovers.

Regarding CP children with diplegia (or tetraplegia), for the young ones dorsal rhizotomy is generally preferred; whereas for older ones ITB may be an alternative, especially if spasticity is mixed with severe (generalized) dystonia. Thanks to its so-called "distant effects", surgery for lower-limb spasticity may favorably influence any hypertonia affecting the upper limbs.

Children with spastic hemiplegia can be managed as are the adult patients.

It is important to consider and discuss at any step of the decision process what orthopedic surgery can afford as an alternative or as a complement.

Having followed the above principles, because every patient has his/her own characteristics and individual evolution, surgery should be tailored. The detailed surgical plan, as well as the objectives of surgery, together with the established rehabilitation program must be formalized in the form of a chart as it will be applied.

16.5 Where to Operate? The Necessity of a Multidisciplinary Team

There are so many factors playing a role in the disability of these handicapped patients, that analysis of the clinical presentation and of the psychological interferences requires the participation of several different medical specialties. Fields of caregivers are multiple and complementary. Caregivers have such an important role to fulfill the rehabilitation program that their participation in the decision, as well as their coordination in the conduct of the treatment, are mandatory. Operative interventions necessitate a strong and experienced team, frequently from different specialties. Therefore, working in a multidisciplinary team is indispensable.

According to our experience, dealing with spasticity in children differs from dealing with spasticity in adults. For neurosurgeons involved in both fields, there may be the necessity of collaborating with two different multidisciplinary teams, or at least one team but capable of working in an adapted "variable geometry".

Because the patient after surgery(ies) has a "new physiological or neurological status" sometimes marked by a sudden (disturbing) regression in locomotor capabilities, an intensive rehabilitation program should be organized and followed. Once more it must be stressed that this cannot be done outside the frame of a **well coordinated, multidisciplinary team**.

Appendix

In order to ease the evaluation and decision-making processes and the surgical planning, the following provides commonly used scales, schematic drawings, and forms. Important, scales are not conceived so that they can "cover" any patients' situation. A scale is not necessarily applicable to every case, even for same patient to each of his (her) evolution sequences. Therefore, before using a scoring system, it is crucial to critically check criteria relevance. Scale(s) should be chosen to appropriately evaluate the patient's particular clinical condition and to properly decide whether he (she) will be selected for one or another of the various therapeutic modalities that may be offered.

Section 1: Evaluation

- Ashworth scale
- Tardieu scale
- Tendon reflex scale
- Bohannon scale
- Hand prehension rating system
- Functional Oswestry scale
- Lyon University functional scale for paraplegic patients
- Goniometry/range of motion for spasticity in lower limbs
- Goniometry/range of motion for spasticity in upper limbs

Section 2: Surgical planning

- Patterns of spasticity and target of muscles, nerves, and roots: lower/upper limb
- Tibial neurotomy: right/left side
- Musculocutaneous neurotomy: right/left side
- Median neurotomy: right/left side
- Ulnar neurotomy at level of elbow: right/left side
- Ulnar neurotomy at level of wrist: right/left side

Section 3: Children

- Classification of gait patterns in ambulatory children with spastic diplegia
- Frontal planes schemes of Lower-limb postures in relaxing position in nonambulatory children
- New York University classification of candidates for dorsal rhizotomy
- Gross Motor Function Classification System (GMFCS)
- Operative chart for dorsal rhizotomy

M. Sindou et al., *Neurosurgery for Spasticity*,
DOI 10.1007/978-3-7091-1771-2, © Springer-Verlag Wien 2014

- Vertebral interlaminar levels for targeting selected roots
- Intraoperative checking for root identification and selection

Section 1

Ashworth scale for evaluation of spasticity in lower limbs

Family name:	
Given name:	Birth date:

Criterion	Score
No increase in tone	0
Slight increase in tone giving a "catch" when limb is moved during flexion or extension	1
More marked increase in tone but limb easily flexed	2
Considerable increase in tone –passive movement difficult	3
Limb rigid during flexion or extension	4

Tardieu scale for evaluation of spasticity associated with cerebral palsy

Family name:	
Given name:	Birth date:

Criterion	Symbol or score
Speeds at which affected part(s) are passively moved:	
As slow as possible	V1
Intermediate speed	V2
As rapid as possible	V3
Parameters measured:	
Type of muscle reaction	X
Angle at which muscle reaction occurs	Y
Types of muscle reaction:	
No increase in muscle tone throughout the range of motion	0
Slight increase in muscle tone without any "catch" at a particular angle	1
"Catch" interrupting the movement at a particular angle, followed by muscular release	2
Exhaustible clonus (less than 10 s for a permanent stretch) appearing at a particular angle	3
Inexhaustible clonus (more than 10 s for a permanent stretch), appearing at a particular angle	4

Scale for evaluation of intensity of tendon hyperreflexia

Family name:	
Given name:	Birth date:

Tendon reflex	Score
Absent	0
Present but weak	1
Normal	2
Brisk	3

Bohannon scale for quantification of spasticity in upper limbs, namely, the elbow

Family name:	
Given name:	Birth date:

Criterion	Score
No increase in muscle tone	0
No increase in muscle tone, manifested by a "catch" and release or by minimal resistance at end of range of motion when affected	1
Slight increase in muscle tone, manifested by a "catch" followed by minimal resistance throughout the remainder (less than half) of range motion	1+
More marked increase in muscle tone through most of range motion, but affected part(s) easily moved	2
Considerable increase in muscle tone, passive movement difficult	3
Affected part(s) rigid during flexion or extension	4

Scale for evaluation of prehension of hand during daily activities by patients with disturbances of muscular tone in upper limb

Family name:	
Given name:	Birth date:

Prehension	Score
Impossible	0
Possible with help and grasp	1
Present but precautious or instable	2
Functionally effective	3

Oswestry scale for quantification of functional disability

Family name:	
Given name:	Birth date:

Criterion	Score
Solely spastic No willed movement; tonic reflexes or spinal reflexes present	0
Very severe spasticity Movement very poor, total spastic synergy in one pattern only (i.e., only total extension if limb is passively flexed or only total flexion from an extended position)	1
Severe spasticity Movement poor, marked total spastic synergy but during both flexion and extension patterns (i.e., patient can flex extended limb and extend flexed limb, with or without some isolated proximal control)	2
Moderate spasticity Movement fair, spasticity synergy, but some isolated control in a small range of movement at a distal joint (ankle or wrist)	3
Mild spasticity Movement good with isolated distal control possible in good range; spastic synergy still apparent on reinforcement by resistance to the movement or by effort exerted in another part of body	4
No spasticity Movement normal; no spastic synergy	5

Global Functional Disability scale of Lyon University for paraplegic patients with spasticity in lower limbs

Family name:	
Given name:	Birth date:

Criterion	Score
Pain:	
Absent	0
Rare and mild; no disability	1
Frequent; minimal disability	2
Marked and frequent; marked disability	3
Permanent and severe	4
Spasms:	
Absent	0
Rare and mild spasms only during mobilization; no disability	1
Frequent, spontaneous but moderate spasms; some disability	2
Frequent, spontaneous and marked spasms; marked disability	3
Almost constant and severe spasms; severe disability, major problems for sitting and lying	4
Sitting position:	
Normal	0
Mild difficulty	1
Moderate difficulty	2
Severe difficulty, patient has to be tied down in position	3
Impossible	4
Body transfer:	
Normal	0
Mild difficulty	1
Moderate difficulty	2
Marked difficulty, needs one person helping	3
Severe difficulty, needs two persons helping	4
Washing and dressing:	
Normal	0
Mild difficulty	1
Moderate difficulty	2
Marked difficulty, needs one person helping	3
Severe difficulty, needs two persons helping	4
Total score	/ 20

Goniometry/range of motion for spasticity in lower limbs

Region (Motion)	"Baseline" deformity[a]	Active ROM	Passive ROM	Passive ROM under anesthetic block or general anesthesia	Remarks
Hip/thigh					
Flexion	R: / L:	R: / L:	R: / L:	R: / L:	
Extension	R: / L:	R: / L:	R: / L:	R: / L:	
Adduction	R: / L:	R: / L:	R: / L:	R: / L:	
Abduction	R: / L:	R: / L:	R: / L:	R: / L:	
Internal rotation	R: / L:	R: / L:	R: / L:	R: / L:	
External rotation	R: / L:	R: / L:	R: / L:	R: / L:	
Knee					
Flexion	R: / L:	R: / L:	R: / L:	R: / L:	
Extension	R: L:	R: / L:	R: / L:	R: / L:	
Ankle / foot					
Plantar flexion	R: / L:	R: / L:	R: / L:	R: / L:	
Dorsal flexion	R: / L:	R: / L:	R: / L:	R: / L:	
Varus	R: / L:	R: / L:	R: / L:	R: / L:	
Valgus	R: / L:	R: / L:	R: / L:	R: / L:	
Toes					
Plantar flexion	R: / L:	R: / L:	R: / L:	R: / L:	
Dorsal flexion	R: / L:	R: / L:	R: / L:	R: / L:	
Hallux extension	R: / L:	R: / L:	R: / L:	R: / L:	

[a]Spontaneous abnormal posture of the joints compared with their respective physiological position

Goniometry/range of motion for spasticity in upper limbs

Region (Motion)	"Baseline" deformity[a]	Active ROM	Passive ROM	Passive ROM under anesthetic block or general anesthesia	Remarks
Shoulder					
Adduction	R: / L:	R: / L:	R: / L:	R: / L:	
Abduction	R: / L:	R: / L:	R: / L:	R: / L:	
Int. Rotation	R: / L:	R: / L:	R: / L:	R: / L:	
Ext. Rotation	R: / L:	R: / L:	R: / L:	R: / L:	
Antepulsion	R: / L:	R: / L:	R: / L:	R: / L:	
Retropulsion	R: / L:	R: / L:	R: / L:	R: / L:	
Elbow					
Flexion	R: / L:	R: / L:	R: / L:	R: / L:	
Extension	R: / L:	R: / L:	R: / L:	R: / L:	
Forearm					
Pronation	R: / L:	R: / L:	R: / L:	R: / L:	
Supination	R: / L:	R: / L:	R: / L:	R: / L:	
Wrist					
Flexion	R: / L:	R: / L:	R: / L:	R: / L:	
Extension	R: / L:	R: / L:	R: / L:	R: / L:	
Ulnar deviation	R: / L:	R: / L:	R: / L:	R: / L:	
Radial deviation	R: / L:	R: / L:	R: / L:	R: / L:	
Fingers					
Flexion mp	R: / L:	R: / L:	R: / L:	R: / L:	
Flexion pip	R: / L:	R: / L:	R: / L:	R: / L:	
Flexion dip	R: / L:	R: / L:	R: / L:	R: / L:	
Thumb					
Flexion	R: / L:	R: / L:	R: / L:	R: / L:	
Adduction	R: / L:	R: / L:	R: / L:	R: / L:	
Opposition	R: / L:	R: / L:	R: / L:	R: / L:	

[a]Spontaneous abnormal posture of the joints compared with their respective physiological position

Section 2

Muscles involved and nerves or roots to be targeted according to clinical pattern for spasticity in lower limb

Family name:				
Given name:			Birth date:	
Clinical pattern	**Muscle(s) involved**	**Nerve**	**Roots or segments of origin**	**Sectioning quantification**
Flexed hip	Iliopsoas	Branch from lumbar plexus	L2–L3	
	Rectus femoris	Femoral	L3–L4	
Adducted thigh	Adductor group (longus, brevis, magnus), gracilis, obturator externus, pectineus	Obturator	L2–L3	
Extended knee	Quadriceps group (rectus femoris, vastus intermedius, vastus medialis, vastus lateralis)	Femoral	L3–L4	
Flexed knee	Hamstring (biceps femoris, semitendinosus, semimembranosus)	Sciatic	L5–S2	
Equinus of foot	Equinus: gastrocnemius, soleus, popliteal	Tibial	S1	
Varus of foot	Varus: tibialis posterior			
Claw toes	Flexor digitorum longus and brevis, flexor hallucis longus	Tibial	S1–S2	
Hitchhiker's great toe	Extensor hallucis longus	Peroneal	L4–L5	

Muscles involved and nerves or roots to be targeted according to clinical pattern for spasticity in upper limb

Family name:				
Given name:			Birth date:	
Clinical pattern	**Muscle(s) involved**	**Nerve(s)**	**Roots or segments of origin**	**Sectioning quantification**
Adducted and internally rotated shoulder	Pectoralis major	Lateral and medial thoracic	C5–C6 and C7–C8	
	Teres major	Inferior subscapular	C5–C8	
Flexed elbow	Coracobrachialis, biceps, brachialis	Musculocutaneous	C5–C6	
Pronated forearm	Pronator quadrates, pronator teres	Median	C6–C7	
Flexed wrist	Flexor carpi radialis, palmaris longus	Median	C6–C7	
	Flexor carpi ulnaris	Ulnar	C8–T1	
Thumb in palm	Flexor pollicis longus	Median	C7–C8	
	Adductor pollicis, opponens pollicis	Ulnar	C8–T1	
Clenched fist (fingers)	Flexor digitorum superficialis, flexor digitorum profundus	Median	C7–C8	
Swan neck (fingers)	First and second lumbrical plus interosseous	Median	C7–T1	
	Third and fourth lumbrical plus interosseous	Ulnar	C8–T1	

Section 3

Tibial neurotomy (right side)

Family name:	
Given name:	Birth date:

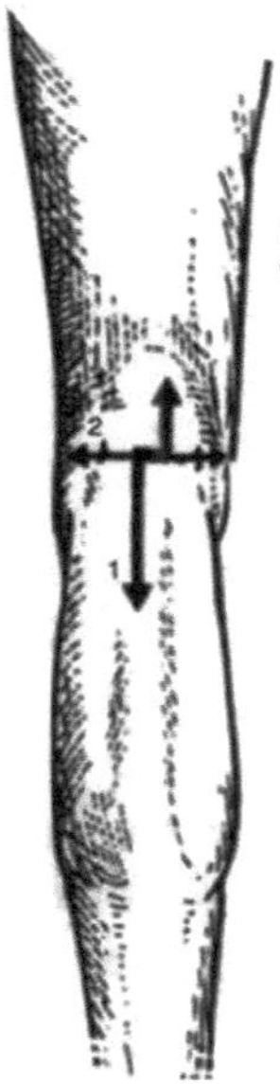

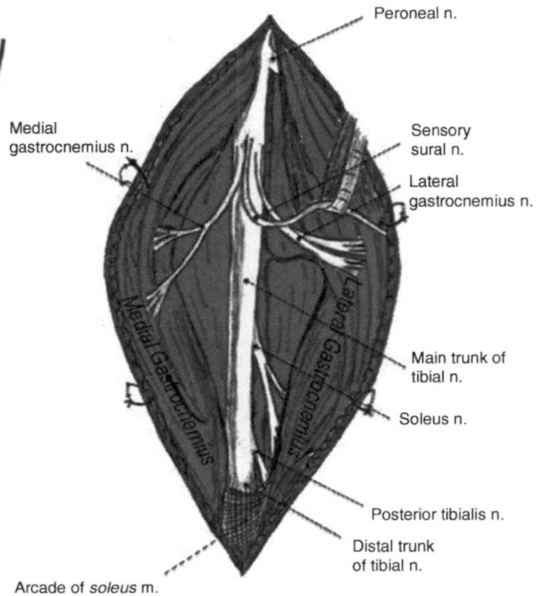

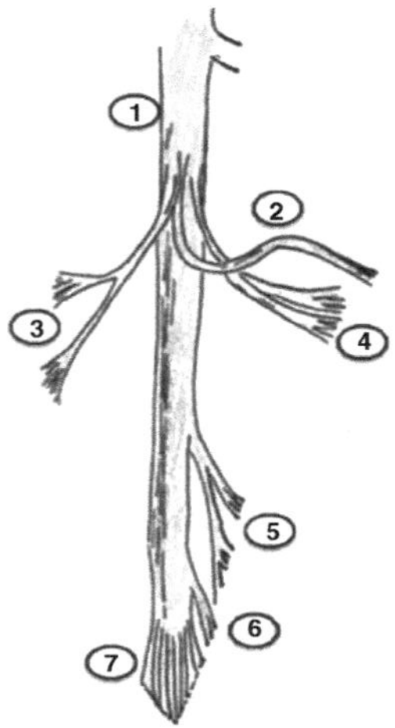

Family name:		
Given name:		Birth date:
Branch of tibial nerve	Response to stimulation	% of Section
1. Main trunk	Plantar flexion, inversion - varus, flexion of toes	Intact
2. Sural nerve	Purely sensory	Intact
3. Medial gastrocnemius	Plantar flexion	
4. Lateral gastrocnemius	Plantar flexion	
5. Soleus	Plantar flexion, equinus	
6. Tibialis posterioris	Inversion - varus	
7. Distal trunk	Flexion of toes	

Tibial neurotomy (left side)

Family name:	
Given name:	Birth date:

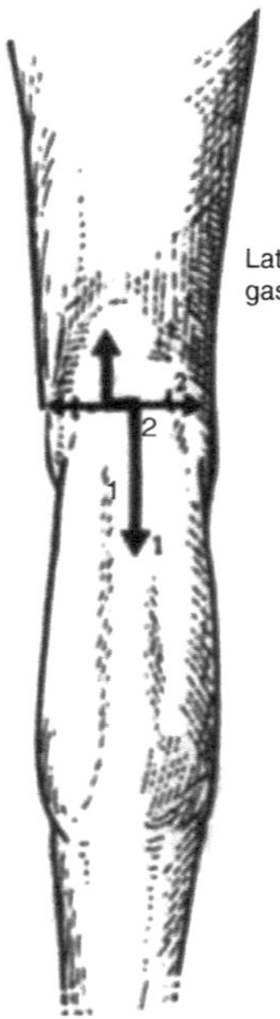

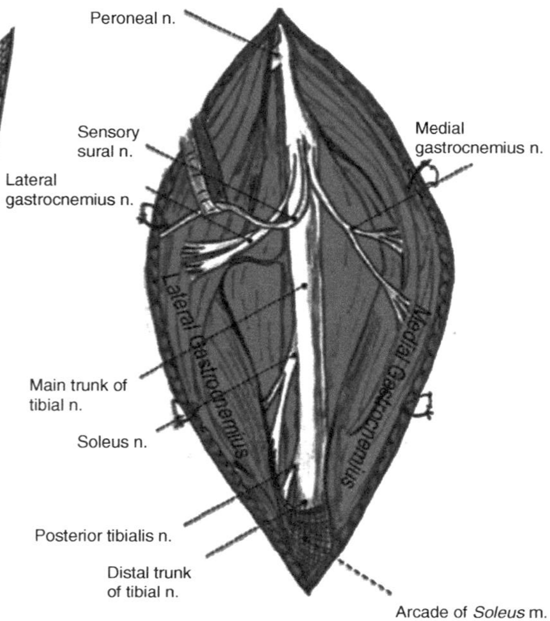

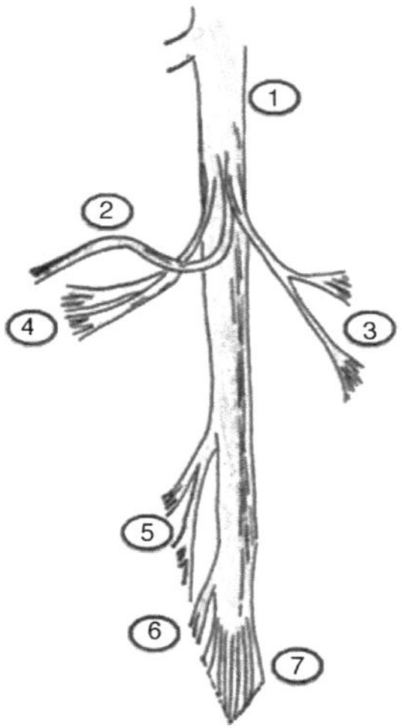

Family name:		
Given name:		Birth date:
Branch of tibial nerve	**Response to stimulation**	**% of Section**
1. Main trunk	Plantar flexion, inversion - varus, flexion of toes	Intact
2. Sural nerve	Purely sensory	Intact
3. Medial gastrocnemius	Plantar flexion	
4. Lateral gastrocnemius	Plantar flexion	
5. Soleus	Plantar flexion,	
6. Tibialis posterioris	Inversion - varus	
7. Distal trunk	Flexion of toes	

Musculocutaneous neurotomy (right side)

Family name:	
Given name:	Birth date:

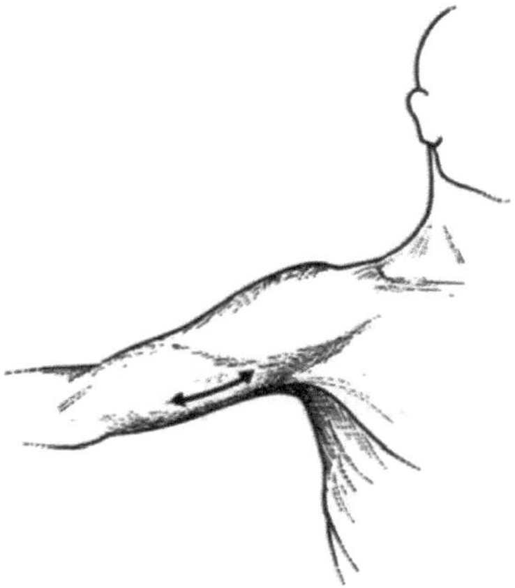

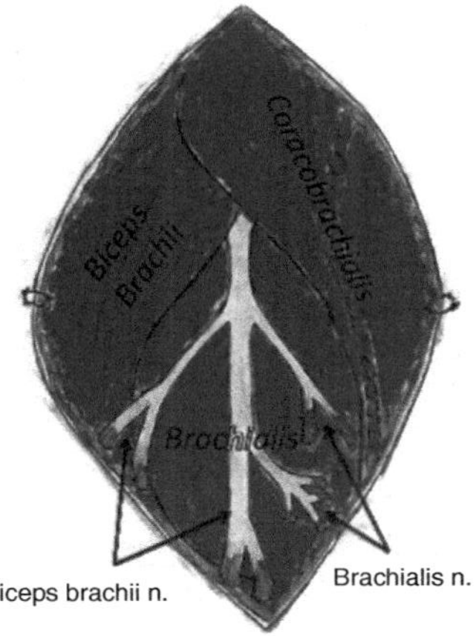

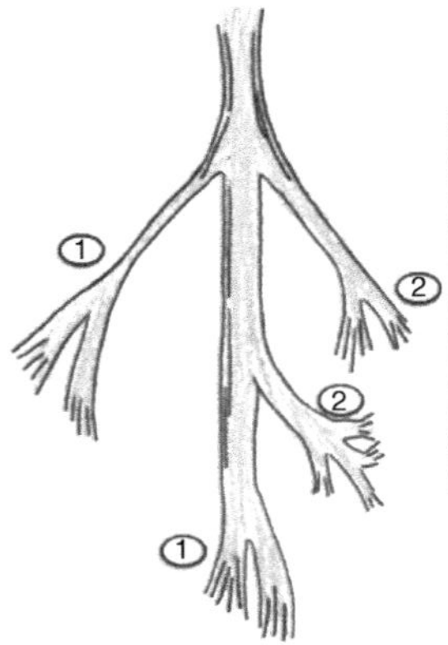

Family name:		
Given name:		Birth date:
Branch of musculocutaneous nerve	Response to stimulation	% of section
1. Biceps brachii	Flexion of elbow–supination of forearm	
2.Brachialis	Flexion of elbow	

Musculocutaneous neurotomy (left side)

Family name:	
Given name:	Birth date:

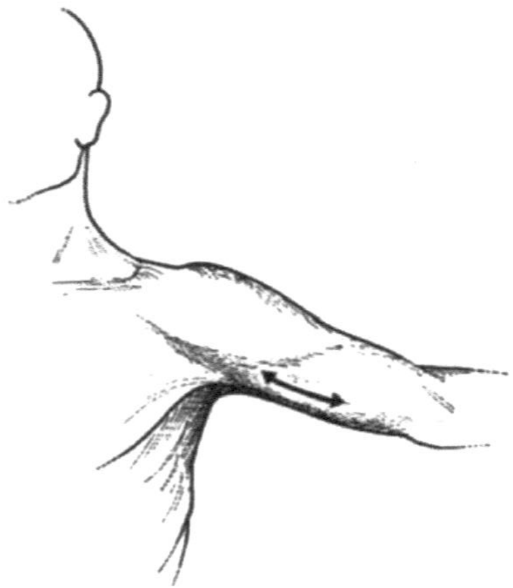

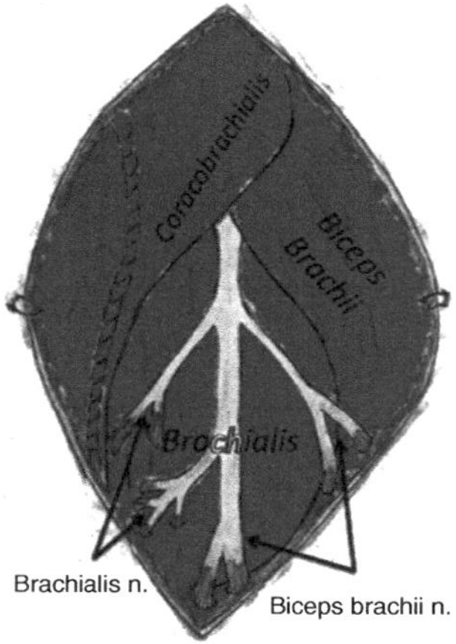

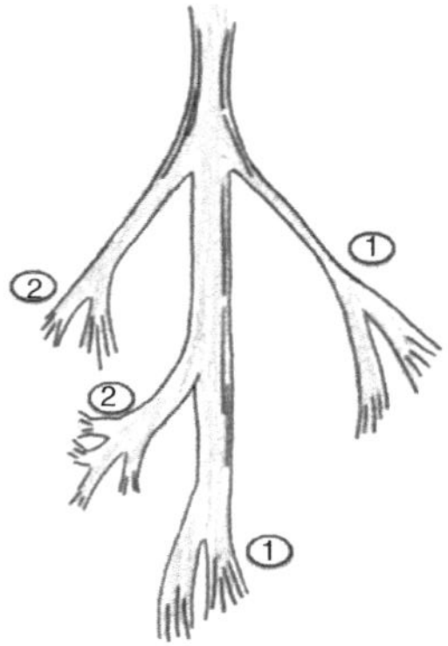

Family name:		
Given name:		Birth date:
Branch of musculocutaneous nerve	Response to stimulation	% of section
1. Biceps brachii	Flexion of elbow–supination of forearm	
2.Brachialis	Flexion of elbow	

Median neurotomy in two steps (right side)

Family name:	
Given name:	Birth date:

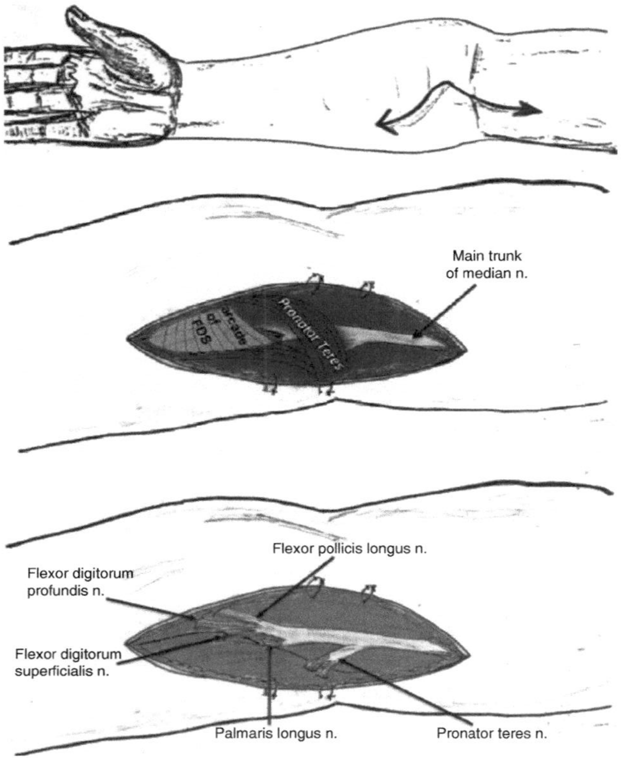

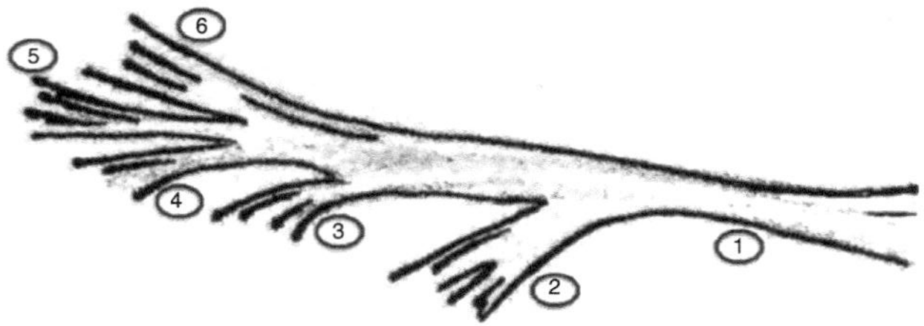

Family name:		
Given name:		Birth date:
Branch of Median nerve	Response to stimulation	% of section
1. Main trunk	Flexion of hand and wrist	Intact
2. Pronator teres	Pronation of forearm	
3. Palmaris longus	Flexion of hand and wrist–tension of palmaris aponeurosis	
4. Flexor digitorum superficialis	Flexion of medial phalanges of fingers	
5. Flexor digitorum profundus	Flexion of proximal interphalangeal joints	
6. Flexor pollicis longus	Flexion of metacarpophalangeal and interphalangeal joints	

Median neurotomy in two steps (left side)

Family name:	
Given name:	Birth date:

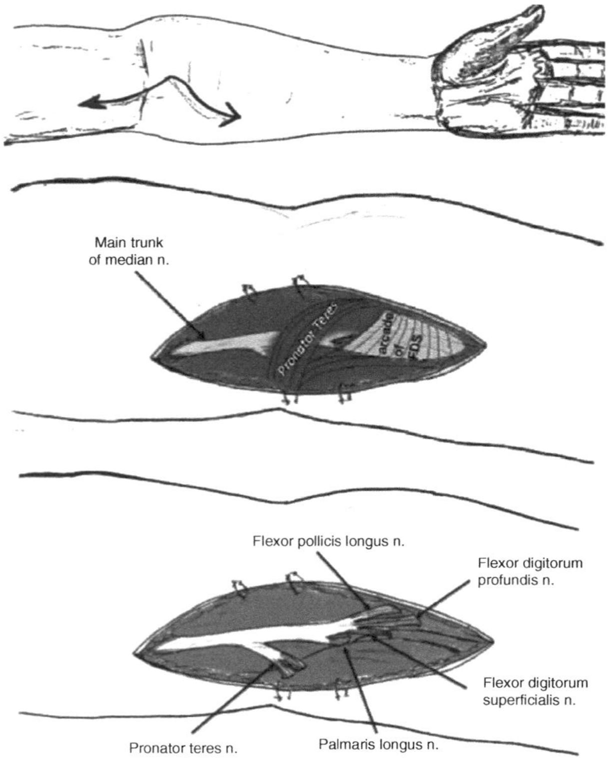

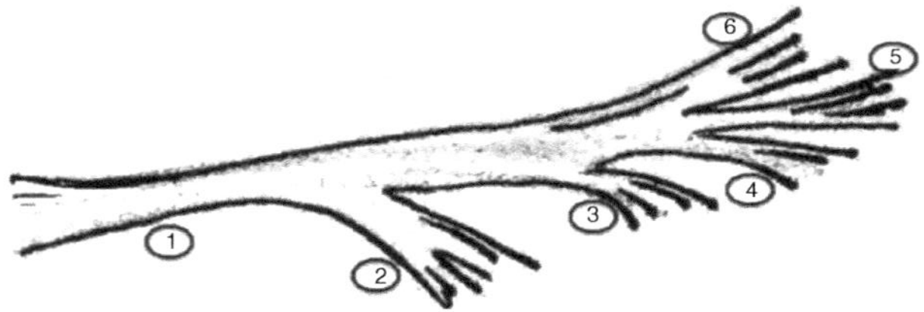

Family name:		
Given name:	Birth date:	
Branch of Median nerve	Response to stimulation	% of section
1. Main trunk	Flexion of hand and wrist	Intact
2. Pronator teres	Pronation of forearm	
3. Palmaris longus	Flexion of hand and wrist–tension of palmaris aponeurosis	
4. Flexor digitorum superficialis	Flexion of medial phalanges of fingers	
5. Flexor digitorum profundus	Flexion of proximal interphalangeal joints	
6. Flexor pollicis longus	Flexion of metacarpophalangeal and interphalangeal joints	

Ulnar neurotomy at level of elbow (right side)

Family name:	
Given name:	Birth date:

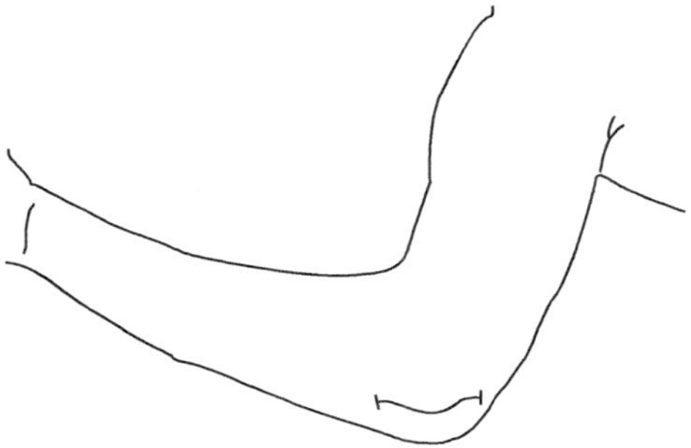

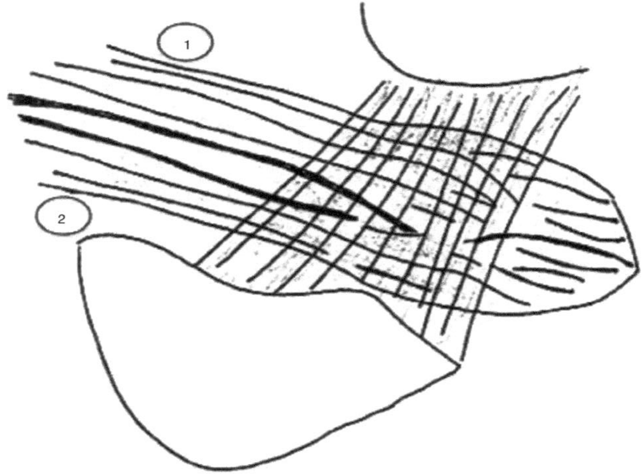

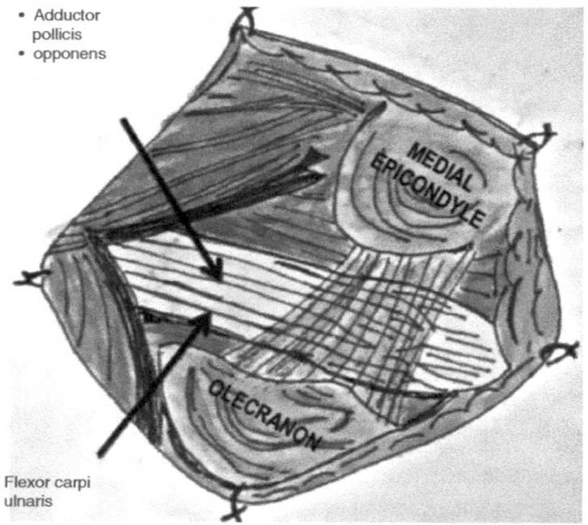

Family name:		
Given name:		Birth date:
Branch of ulnar nerve	Response to stimulation	% of section
1. Adductor pollicis/ opponens	Adduction/ opposition of thumb	
2. Flexor carpi ulnaris	Flexion of wrist with ulnar deviation	

Ulnar neurotomy at level of elbow (left side)

Family name:	
Given name:	Birth date:

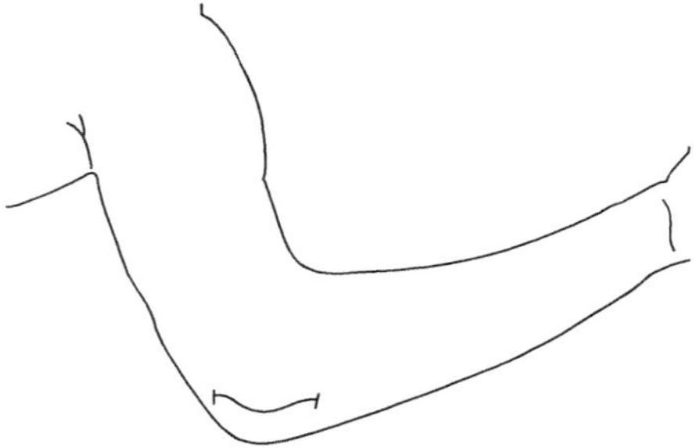

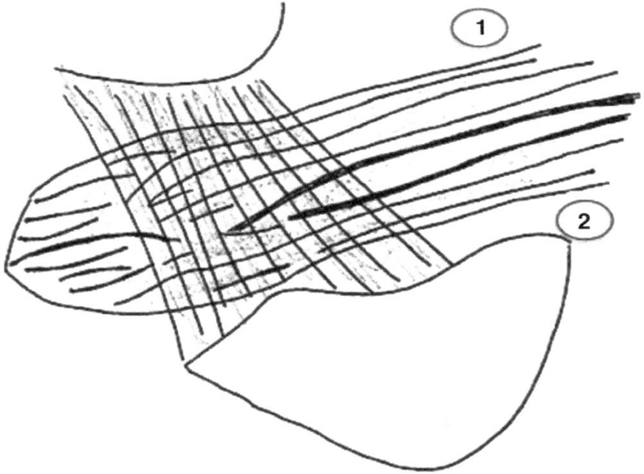

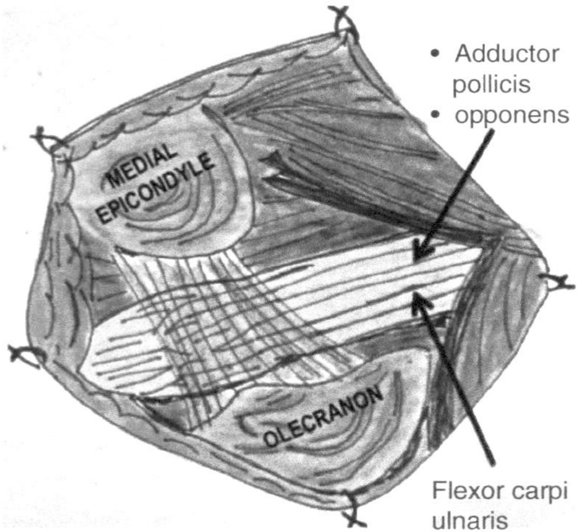

Family name:		
Given name:		Birth date:
Branch of ulnar nerve	Response to stimulation	% of section
1. Adductor pollicis/ opponens	Adduction/ opposition of thumb	
2. Flexor carpi ulnaris	Flexion of wrist with ulnar deviation	

Ulnar neurotomy at level of wrist (right side)

Family name:	
Given name:	Birth date:

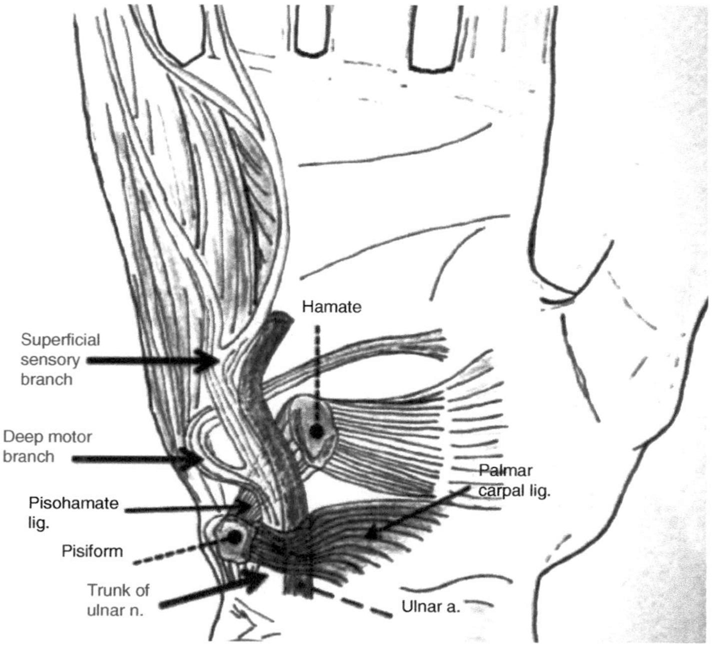

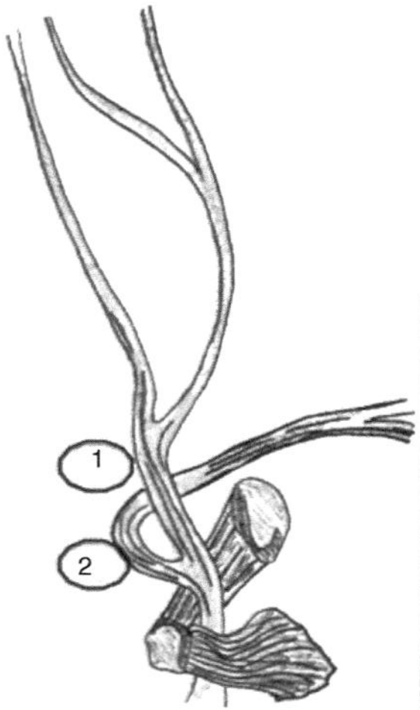

Family name:		
Given name:		Birth date:
Branch of ulnar nerve	Response to stimulation	% of section
1. Superficial sensory	Purely sensory	Intact
2. Deep motor	Hypothenar, interossei and 3rd and 4th lumbrical muscles – adduction/flexion of thumb	

Ulnar neurotomy at level of wrist (left side)

Family name:	
Given name:	Birth date:

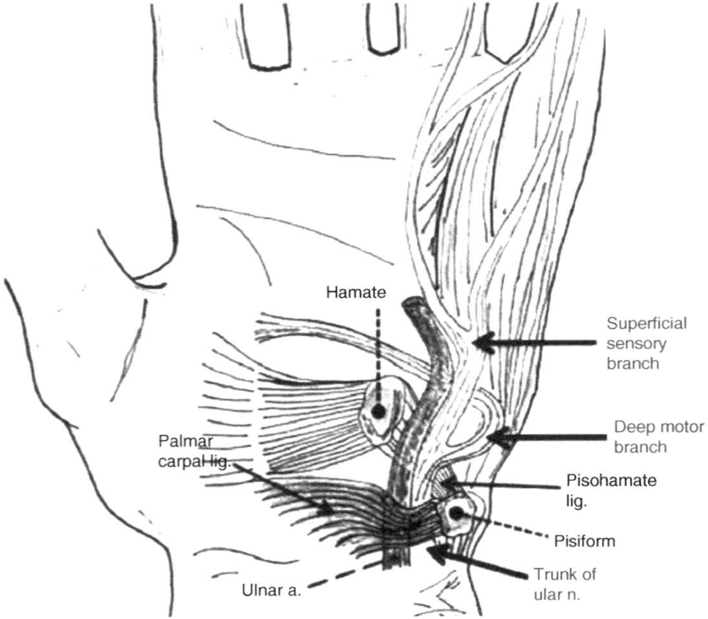

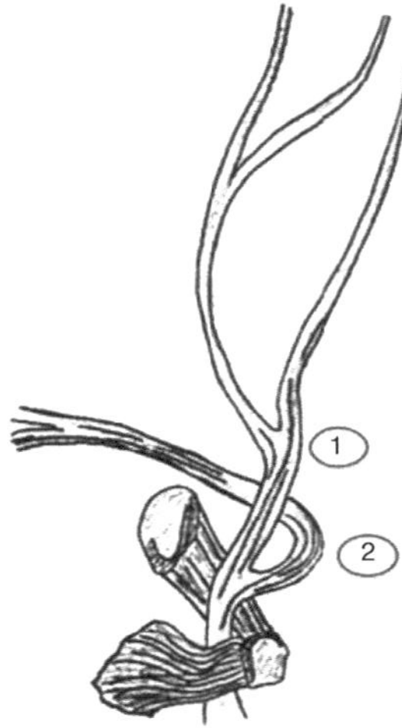

Family name:		
Given name:		Birth date:
Branch of ulnar nerve	Response to stimulation	% of section
1. Superficial sensory	Purely sensory	Intact
2. Deep motor	Hypothenar, interossei and 3rd and 4th lumbrical muscles – adduction/flexion of thumb	

Section 3

Classification of gait patterns in ambulatory children with spastic diplegia

Family name:				
Given name:			Birth date:	
Gait pattern	**Pelvic tilt**	**Hip flexion/ extension**	**Knee flexion/ extension**	**Ankle dorsiflexion/ plantar flexion**
True equinus	Normal or anterior	Normal	Normal or recurvatum	Equinus
Jump gait	Normal or anterior	Normal or flexed	Flexed (on motion)	Equinus
Apparent equinus	Normal or anterior	Flexed	Flexed	Normal
Crouch gait	Anterior or normal or posterior	Flexed	Flexed	Calcaneus
Asymmetrical gait				

Frontal-plane schemes of lower-limb postures in relaxing position (nonambulatory children)

Family name:	
Given name:	Birth date:

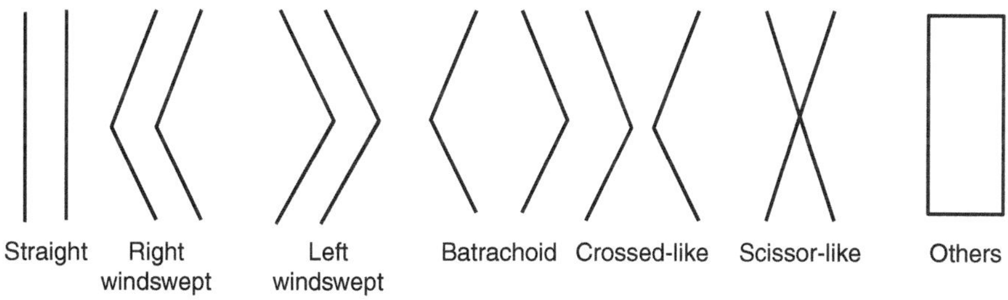

New York University classification system for candidates to dorsal rhizotomy

Family name:		
Given name:	Birth date:	
Preoperative function	**Postoperative goal**	**Group**
Walks without assistive devices	Improve appearance and efficiency of walking	I
Walks with assistive devices	Improve quality of walking and decrease amount of assistance (use of canes, crutches, walkers) required for ambulation	II
Quadruped crawler, limited ability to stand and reciprocally move legs	Improve ability to reciprocally move the legs in the standing position with assistive devices	III
Commando or belly crawler	Improve ease for caregivers and facilitate function in sitting position	IV
No locomotive abilities, fully dependent	Improve ease for caregivers and facilitate positioning in adaptive equipment	V

Gross motor function classification system (GMFCS), or levels of Palisano, for children between 6 and 12 years of age

Family name:	
Given name:	Birth date:
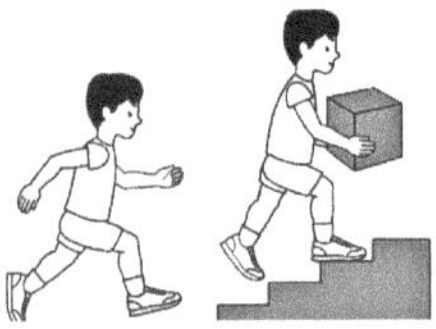	**GMFCS level I** Children walk at home, school, outdoors and in the community. They can climb stairs without the use of a railing. Children perform gross motor skills such as running and jumping, but speed, balance and coordination are limited.
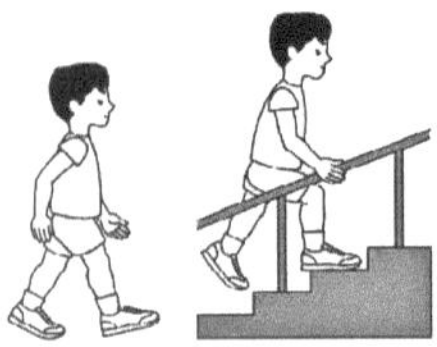	**GMFCS level II** Children walk in most settings and climb stairs holding onto a railing. They may experience difficulty walking long distances and balancing on uneven terrain, inclines, in crowded areas or confined spaces. Children may walk with physical assistance, a handheld mobility device or used wheeled mobility over long distances. Children have only minimal ability to perform gross motor skills such as running and jumping.
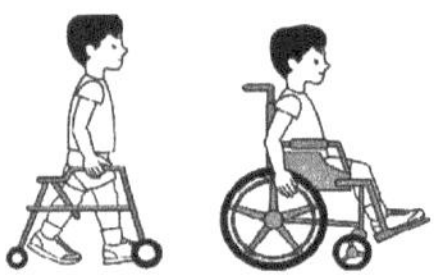	**GMFCS level III** Children walk using a hand-held mobility device in most indoor settings. They may climb stairs holding onto a railing with supervision or assistance. Children use wheeled mobility when traveling long distances and may self-propel for shorter distances.
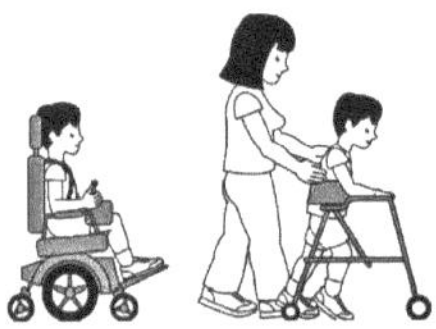	**GMFCS level IV** Children use methods of mobility that require physical assistance or powered mobility in most settings. They may walk for short distances at home with physical assistance or use powered mobility or a body support walker when positioned. At school, outdoors and in the community children are transported in a manual wheelchair or use powered mobility.
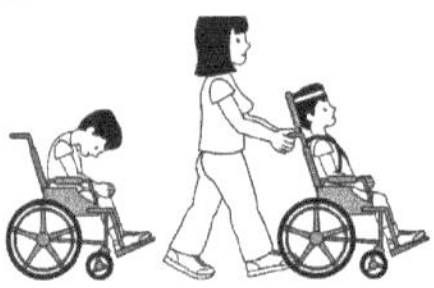	**GMFCS level V** Children are transported in a manual wheelchair in all settings. Children are limited in their ability to maintain antigravity head and trunk postures and control leg and arm movements.

Operative chart for dorsal rhizotomy: percentage of root to be sectioned according to grade of muscular response to dorsal root stimulation

Family name:			
Given name:		Birth date:	
	Criterion	Grade	
	Unsustained motor response in muscles innervated by segmental level of stimulated dorsal nerve root or rootlet	0	
	Sustained motor response in myotome of stimulated nerve root	1	
	Contraction of muscles in myotomes of adjacent segmental level(s)	2	
	Contraction of muscles in myotomes distant from that of stimulated nerve root	3	
	Contraction of muscles in the contralateral leg or upper limb(s)	4	
Stimulated root	Predominantly responding muscle(s) (myotome)	Grade of muscular response to dorsal root stimulation (1 s, 50Hz)	% of root to be sectioned
L2	Illiopsoas, adductors of hips		
L3	Adductors of hips, quadriceps		
L4	Quadriceps, dorsal flexor of ankle (tibialis anterior)		
L5	Extensors of toes, hamstrings		
S1	Achilles ankle deep tendon reflex, gastrocnemius-soleus group, hamstrings, tibialis posterior		
S2	Flexors of toes, hamstrings		
S3	Anal sphincter		
S4	Anal sphincter		

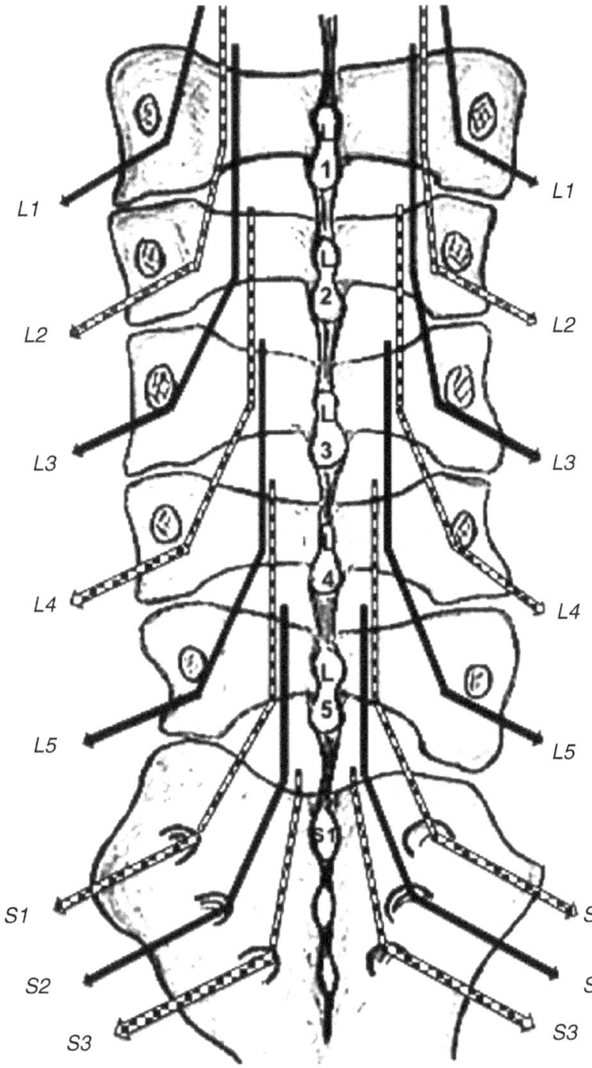

Vertebral interlaminar (IL) levels where selected roots can be targeted for DR: *L2*, *L3* at L1 – L2; *L3*, *L4* at L2 – L3; *L4*, *L5* at L3 – L4; *L5*, *S1* at L4 – L5; *S1*, *S2* at L5 – S1. IL space(s) is(are) determined according to the pre-operative program for root sectioning.

Intra-operative checking for root identification and selection

Root / Muscle	L2				L3				L4				L5				S1				S2			
	EMG		Physio-therapist		EMG		Physio-therapist		EMG		Physio-therapist		EMG		Physio-therapist		EMG		Physio-therapist		EMG		Physio-therapist	
	2Hz-200µA	50Hz -1mA	2Hz-200µA	50Hz-1mA	2Hz-200µA	50Hz-1mA	2Hz-200µA	50Hz-1mA	2Hz-200µA	50Hz-1mA	2Hz-200µA	50Hz-1mA	2Hz-200µA	50Hz -1mA	2Hz-200µA	50Hz -1mA	2Hz-200µA	50Hz -1mA	2Hz-200µA	50Hz -1mA	2Hz-200µA	50Hz -1mA	2Hz-200µA	50Hz -1mA
Adductors (L)																								
Adductors (R)																								
Quadriceps (L)																								
Quadriceps (R)																								
Tibialis ant. (L)																								
Tibialis ant. (R)																								
Hamstrings (L)																								
Hamstrings (R)																								
Soleus (L)																								
Soleus (R)																								
Flexors Digit. (L)																								+
Flexors Digit. (R)																								+
Anal																								

Assessment through clinical examination by physiotherapist and EMG recordings. Parameters of electrical stimulation used are, currently, 2Hz and 200 mA for ventral root, 50Hz and 1mA for dorsal root.

Index

M. Sindou et al., *Neurosurgery for Spasticity*,
DOI 10.1007/978-3-7091-1771-2, © Springer-Verlag Wien 2014